BIOPSY PATHOLOGY SERIES

General Editors

Professor Leonard S. Gottlieb, MD, MPH
Mallory Institute of Pathology,
Boston, USA

Professor A. Munro Neville, PhD, DSc, MD, FRC Path.
Ludwig Institute for Cancer Research,
London, UK

Professor F. Walker, MD, PhD, FRC Path.
Department of Pathology,
University of Aberdeen, UK

Other titles in the series

Biopsy Pathology of Melanocytic Disorders

Biopsy Pathology of Melanocytic Disorders

W. J. MOOI
MD
Head of Department of Pathology;
Head of Division of Tumour Biology
The Netherlands Cancer Institute
Amsterdam
The Netherlands

and

T. KRAUSZ
MD, MRCPath
Senior Lecturer and Consultant
Histopathology and Cytopathology
Royal Postgraduate Medical School
Hammersmith Hospital
London
UK

With a Foreword by

J. G. AZZOPARDI
MD, FRCPath
Emeritus Professor of Oncology
Royal Postgraduate Medical School
University of London
Honorary Consultant Pathologist
Hammersmith Hospital
London

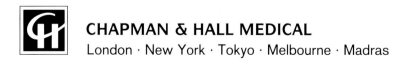

CHAPMAN & HALL MEDICAL
London · New York · Tokyo · Melbourne · Madras

Published by Chapman & Hall, 2–6 Boundary Row, London SE1 8HN

Chapman & Hall, 2–6 Boundary Row, London SE1 8HN, UK

Van Nostrand Reinhold Inc., 115 5th Avenue, New York NY10003, USA

Chapman & Hall Japan, Thomson Publishing Japan, Hirakawacho Nemoto Building, 7F, 1-7-11 Hirakawa-cho, Chiyoda-ku, Tokyo 102, Japan

Chapman & Hall Australia, Thomas Nelson Australia, 102 Dodds Street, South Melbourne, Victoria 3205, Australia

Chapman & Hall India, R. Seshadri, 32 Second Main Road, CIT East, Madras 600 035, India

First edition 1992

© 1992 W.J. Mooi and T. Krausz

Typeset in 10/12 Palatino by Best-set Typesetter Ltd, Hong Kong
Printed in Great Britain by The University Press, Cambridge

ISBN 0 412 32350 8   0 442 31592 9 (USA)

A catalogue record for this book is available from the British Library

Library of Congress Cataloging-in-Publication data available

Biopsy Pathology of
Melanocytic Disorders

BIOPSY PATHOLOGY SERIES

General Editors

Professor Leonard S. Gottlieb, MD, MPH
Mallory Institute of Pathology,
Boston, USA

Professor A. Munro Neville, PhD, DSc, MD, FRC Path.
Ludwig Institute for Cancer Research,
London, UK

Professor F. Walker, MD, PhD, FRC Path.
Department of Pathology,
University of Aberdeen, UK

Contents

Preface

The incidence of cutaneous melanoma has risen considerably over the last decades, and both the medical profession and the general public have become increasingly aware of the importance of early diagnosis of this tumour. As a consequence, pigmented lesions of the skin are submitted for pathological diagnosis more often, and melanomas are generally detected at an earlier stage of their development. Clinically important new entities such as dysplastic naevus have been identified and have added to the complexity of the differential diagnosis. Presently, several controversies continue to generate intense debate, e.g. the existence of dysplastic naevus as a distinct entity and the diagnosis of *in situ* melanoma. As a result, the diagnosis of melanocytic lesions has become more complex and difficult. Needless to say, the clinical consequences of over-diagnosis and under-diagnosis of melanoma are often far-reaching.

Reed and colleagues (1975) wrote that 'for the diagnostic histopathologist, the diagnosis of common melanocytic nevus is gestalt. He seldom, if ever, enumerates those features which clearly distinguish either a nevus or nevus cells (dermal melanocytes). When faced with an unusual melanocytic lesion, his gestalt may fail him'. In order to avoid this problem, it is important for the pathologist to follow a systematic procedure of differential diagnosis, based on concrete histological criteria. We have attempted to adhere as rigidly as possible to the use of well-defined histological features that can be used as criteria in differential diagnosis. Tables of diagnostic features are included for the large majority of entities discussed, in order to facilitate quick reference for the reader. In the text, the criteria and potential pitfalls are discussed at length, since by themselves tables are not a safe basis for pathological diagnosis. Relevant clinical data are briefly outlined, in order to enhance pathological diagnostic accuracy as well as to outline the clinical consequences of various diagnoses. Because the book is intended for surgical pathologists, we only briefly refer to aspects of molecular biology, cell biology and biochemistry of melanocytes and melanocytic lesions.

Extracutaneous melanocytic lesions are much less common, and only occasionally come to attention. However, many of them are of considerable clinical importance. Naevus cells within a lymph node may erroneously be considered to represent a micrometastasis of melanoma or carcinoma; benign naevi of the conjunctiva and iris may be misdiagnosed as melanoma; melanin–containing non-melanocytic tumours, such as pigmented schwannoma and melanotic progonoma, may baffle the pathologist insufficiently familiar with these entities. A lymph node metastasis of a histologically 'undifferentiated' malignant tumour as the first presentation of melanoma occasionally poses diagnostic problems. Cytology of metastatic melanoma is discussed in the final chapter, again emphasizing practical aspects and potential errors in diagnosis.

The diagnostic challenge posed by some melanocytic lesions is considerable and the authors dare to hope that in this respect the present book will be of some help.

The authors wish to thank the numerous fellow clinicians and pathologists who have in many ways contributed significantly to this book. We especially would like to thank Professor J. G. Azzopardi (Hammersmith Hospital, London), for his valuable advice, encouragement and detailed criticism, and for agreeing to write a foreword to this volume.

Also, we thank Professors Ph. Rümke (Netherlands Cancer Institute, Amsterdam) and N. A. Wright (Hammersmith Hospital, London) for valuable criticism. Many colleagues have contributed cases; we specifically would like to mention Dr J. Alons-van Kordelaer (Amsterdam), Dr D. De Wolff-Rouendaal (University of Leiden), Dr K. P. Dingemans (University of Amsterdam), Dr C. D. M. Fletcher (St Thomas's Hospital Medical School, London), Dr P. van Heerde and Dr J. L. Peterse (Netherlands Cancer Institute, Amsterdam), Dr R. Salm (Hammersmith Hospital, London), Dr M. B. Satti (King Fahd Hospital, Al-Khoubar, Saudi Arabia), Dr P. J. Slootweg (University of Utrecht), and Dr N. P. Smith (St John's Dermatology Centre, London).

We have been greatly helped by the expert assistance of the staff of the Library and the Department of Medical Illustration of the Netherlands Cancer Hospital and by Mr W. P. Meun, Department of Medical Illustration, University of Amsterdam.

Finally, we owe a heartfelt debt of gratitude to Suzie and Hanneke, who have put up with so much for so long during the preparation of this book.

W. J. Mooi MD
T. Krausz MD MRCPath

Reference

Reed, R. J., Ichinose, H., Clark, W. H. and Mihm, M. C. (1975) Common and uncommon melanocytic nevi and borderline melanomas. *Semin. Oncol.*, **2**, 119–47.

Foreword

Malignant melanoma, with its variants and its mimics, constitutes a major diagnostic challenge for histopathologists. The problem is an increasingly important one with the increased frequency of melanoma in many countries. The types of benign pigmented naevi proliferate remorselessly, because of increased knowledge about new clinico-pathological entities. Melanomas have acquired a certain mystique which does not apply to the same extent to lesions of, say, the gut or the thyroid. This does little to boost the confidence of the surgical pathologist approaching a difficult case. There have been many refinements of diagnosis in recent years and it clearly requires an expert to bring together the diverse strands of knowledge into an integrated whole and present the information in a way which is easily understood by a general histopathologist.

Drs Mooi and Krausz have done this admirably. The authors are primarily surgical pathologists and this has no doubt contributed to the way they tackle the subject. Histology, cytology, electron microscopy, cytochemistry and immunocytochemistry, together with some bio-chemical and embryological facets and, not least, clinical aspects are integrated in a sophisticated yet simple way. The merits and pitfalls of new methods are critically assessed. Loose undergrowth is raked away to reveal the essentials in stark relief. At the end, one is almost left wondering why one ever had difficulties, although the authors admit that the 'Spitzoid melanoma' and so-called 'malignant Spitz naevus' remain somewhat enigmatic. One could say the same of the 'deep penetrating naevus'. The reader will find topics like 'dysplastic naevus' discussed with great clarity.

I have little doubt that the Mooi–Krausz approach will meet with the approval of their peers and that this splendid monograph will come to be regarded as an essential part of the armoury of the surgical pathologist.

J. G. Azzopardi

1 Melanin and melanocytes

Melanins are a group of black, brown, red or yellow pigments, found in practically all living organisms, including bacteria, fungi and higher plants (Prota, 1980). In man, melanin is produced largely by a single cell type, the melanocyte.

In many animals melanin pigments play an important role in camouflage and mimicry, but in humans their prime function is the protection of the skin from the adverse (toxic and carcinogenic) effects of sunlight. The role of melanin in the protection of the skin is illustrated by the far more rapid development of sunburn in fair-skinned people as compared to dark-complexioned people, and by the high incidence of actinically-induced squamous carcinomas of the skin found in African negroid albinos (Okoro, 1975). Although melanin effectively absorbs light, including the ultraviolet (UV) spectrum, its efficacy as a sun-screen has remained controversial and another role, namely the removal of sunlight-induced toxic oxygen radicals, may be of greater importance (Morison, 1985; Proctor and McGinness, 1986; Nordlund *et al.*, 1989). Exposure to sunlight or other sources of UV light, such as sunbeds, leads to increased production and decreased breakdown of melanin, resulting in increased pigmentation of the skin.

The cells which synthesize the melanin, the *melanocytes*, are derived from the neural crest, whence most of its precursors (*'melanoblasts'*) travel during early embryonal life to the epidermis and hair follicles, while small numbers reach other locations such as the dermis, sebaceous glands and lactiferous ducts of the nipple (Montagna, 1970), mucous membranes of upper aerodigestive tract, genital organs and anus, orbital cavity, leptomeninges, inner ear (Savin, 1965) and, occasionally, some visceral organs (Chapter 11). The volume of the melanocyte mass in an adult human has been estimated at 1–1.5 ml (Rosdahl and Rorsman, 1983). The melanin-producing cells of the uvea are not neural crest-derived, but originate from the optic cup of the forebrain.

The numbers of epidermal melanocytes vary according to body site, age and degree of chronic exposure to sunlight. Melanocytes can be counted in sections, but an often favoured method consists of separation of the epidermis from the dermis by incubation with 2 N sodium bromide (3–4 h, room temperature), followed by the DOPA reaction (p. 23). The ratio of melanocytes to basal keratinocytes varies from about 1:4 to 1:10. Melanocytes are most numerous on the face and genitalia (more than 2000/mm^2) and least common on the upper arm (about 1100/mm^2; Fitzpatrick and Szabo, 1959). Overall, the numbers of melanocytes in sun-exposed sites are roughly double those in non-exposed sites (Quevedo et al., 1969; Gilchrest et al., 1979). During adult life the number of melanocytes decreases at a rate of about 6–8% per decade, in exposed as well as in covered sites (Gilchrest et al., 1979). Ageing also results in a decline in activity of melanin synthesis, within the epidermis as well as in hair follicles.

An increase in number of melanocytes in the vicinity of a cutaneous melanoma has been found by some workers (Wong, 1970; Cochran, 1971) and was considered a 'field change effect' induced by the tumour; however, Fallowfield and Cook (1990) recently found that the number of melanocytes in the vicinity of a melanoma is well within the range seen in sun-exposed skin, while there was no decrease in numbers with increasing distance from the melanoma, as would be expected with a 'field change'.

The marked inter-racial differences in skin pigmentation are largely the result of differences in the amount of melanin contained in keratinocytes, the numbers of melanocytes varying little between races (Szabo, 1954; Staricco and Pinkus, 1957).

Melanin is the end-product of a cascade of enzymatic reactions (the Raper–Mason pathway), starting with tyrosine as substrate (Lerner and Case, 1959). The synthesis takes place in small intracytoplasmic organelles, *melanosomes*, which travel along melanocytic dendrites during their maturation. The tips of these dendrites are eventually phagocytosed by epidermal keratinocytes (Cruickshank and Harcourt, 1964). As a result, keratinocytes often contain some melanin, especially in the basal layer of the epidermis, and they may become heavily pigmented. One melanocyte, together with the basal and suprabasal keratinocytes receiving melanin from it, are known as the so-called *'epidermal melanin unit'* (Fitzpatrick et al., 1967). In the past, keratinocytes have been thought to produce melanin themselves, which explains the misnomer 'melanocarcinoma' for melanoma encountered in the earlier literature. Within keratinocytes, melanin is usually localized in the cytoplasm bordering the 'sunny side' of the nucleus (Figure 1.1), suggesting protection of the nucleus from sunlight. In suprabasal cell layers the melanin is broken down so that the upper part of the

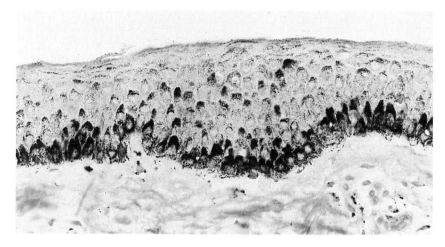

Figure 1.1 Cutaneous hyperpigmentation. Abundant melanin is present in the basal layer; in suprabasal layers it is mainly located at the 'sunny side' of the keratinocyte nuclei (Masson Fontana, × 370).

epidermis is generally not pigmented, unless there is very active synthesis and/or decreased breakdown of melanin.

In many pathological conditions affecting the epidermis, some melanin is shed into the dermis (*'pigment incontinence'*; Figure 1.2), where it is phagocytosed by tissue macrophages (*'melanophages'*; Fitzpatrick *et al.*, 1967).

1.1   Embryology

Melanocytes are derived from the neural crest, from which their non-pigmented precursors, designated *melanoblasts*, migrate during early embryonal life (Weston, 1970). The one exception to this is the uveal melanocyte, which does not derive from the neural crest but, like the uveal pigment epithelium, develops from the neuroepithelium of the embryonal optic cup.

Migration of melanocyte precursors from the neural crest has been demonstrated in a variety of vertebrates, mainly by means of ingenious embryonal tissue and organ transplantation experiments. The early experiments were reviewed by Rawles (1947, 1948) who did most of the work on the mouse model. In the human embryo, melanoblasts migrate from the neural crest to the skin in the first trimester of gestation (Gordon, 1953) and reach the epidermis by week 8–10 (Sagebiel and Odland, 1970). Akin to the development of the neural

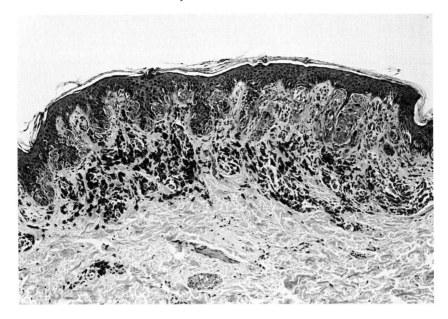

Figure 1.2 'Pigment incontinence'. Melanin produced by this naevus is shed into the upper dermis, where it is phagocytosed by macrophages (HE, × 90).

crest itself, this migration is completed in a cranio-caudal sequence, the cranial skin being the first to be colonized by these melanocyte precursors.

The large majority of melanoblasts localize in the epidermal basal layer and in the hair follicles, but some remain located within the dermis, especially in the sacral region. In races with an intermediate degree of pigmentation such as Mongolians and American Indians, the sacral area of infants often shows some bluish discolouration due to pigmentation of these dermal melanocytes ('*Mongolian spot*'; Nelson *et al.*, 1969; Warkany, 1971). Macroscopically, this pigmentation usually disappears in the first year of life, but it may persist into adulthood.

1.2   Light microscopy

Histologically, epidermal melanocytes appear as small cells located singly between the keratinocytes of the epidermal basal layer or bulging slightly downward (Figure 1.3). The melanocyte has often been designated a 'territorial' cell, to indicate that it is normally separated by several keratinocytes from the next melanocyte (Cochran, 1970). Basally, the melanocyte is attached to the epidermal basal lamina,

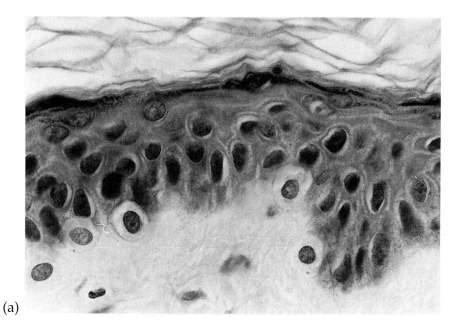

(a)

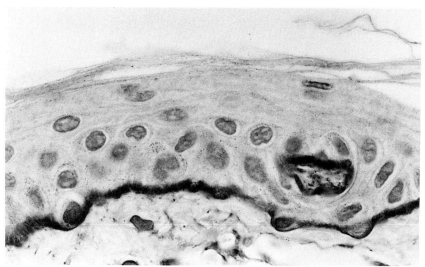

(b)

Figure 1.3 Normal skin. (a) Solitary, pale, round or oval melanocytes are situated at the dermoepidermal junction, just below the level of the basal keratinocytes. Unless they contain much melanin, melanocytic dendrites are usually invisible in HE-stained paraffin sections (HE, × 920). (b) Type IV collagen immunostain. The melanocytes are situated above the epidermal basal lamina (Immunoperoxidase, × 920).

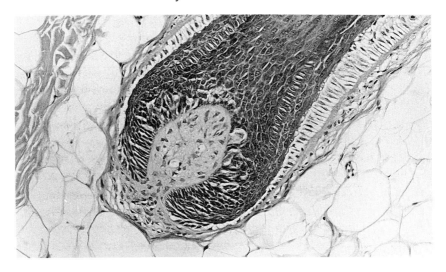

Figure 1.4   Hair follicle. Large pale melanocytes are seen within the epithelial compartment bordering the mesenchyme of the hair papilla (HE, × 370).

which is visualized by immunostaining for laminin or collagen type IV, or by electron microscopy. Melanocytes of hair follicles are also situated at the epithelial side of the basement membrane, bordering the central hair papilla (Figure 1.4).

The nucleus, which is dark and round or oval, with usually a smooth contour, is generally somewhat smaller than that of the basal keratinocyte; when it is oval in shape, it is orientated vertically, horizontally, or obliquely. There is only a small amount of pale cytoplasm (hence the old name 'Masson's clear cells'), which often shrinks and collapses against the nucleus during routine fixation, leaving an empty space between the melanocyte and the adjacent keratinocytes. Slender cytoplasmic dendrites project from the cell body and extend between keratinocytes in the vicinity. These dendrites are usually invisible on haematoxylin and eosin (HE)-stained sections, but can be visualized histochemically, or may be apparent when they are packed with melanin granules. This occurs when melanin synthesis is particularly active, or when there is a '*pigment block*', i.e. an impairment of the transfer of melanin granules to surrounding keratinocytes, so that the melanocytes become engorged with melanin.

In HE-stained sections, melanin pigment may appear absent in melanocytes. When it is seen, it is usually finely granular, but when melanin synthesis is very active, it is often dust-like, yielding a greyish tinge to the cytoplasm. Melanin within keratinocytes is always granular and the granules are often coarser, and uneven in size and shape.

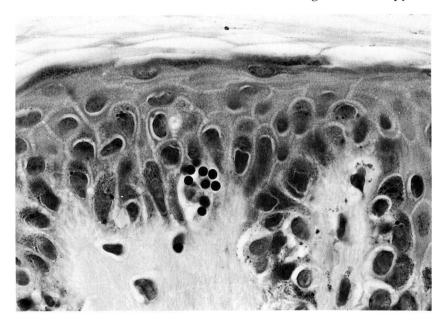

Figure 1.5   Macromelanosomes. One melanocyte contains several large round macromelanosomes, contrasting with the microgranular melanin pigment present in several other melanocytes and in keratinocytes. (HE, × 920).

Macromelanosomes (Jimbow *et al.*, 1973), also known as giant melanosomes (Konrad *et al.*, 1974), melanin macroglobules (Nakagawa *et al.*, 1984) and giant pigment granules (Morris *et al.*, 1982), are abnormally large, usually spherical melanin granules, which may reach a size of up to 6 μm (Figure 1.5). They are very rare in normal melanocytes, but occur more commonly in café-au-lait spots, especially when associated with neurofibromatosis (Szabo, 1959, Slater *et al.*, 1986), and in xeroderma pigmentosum, simple lentigo, multiple lentigines syndromes, dysplastic naevus, congenital naevus, cutaneous melanosis in disseminated melanoma, and also occasionally in common acquired naevus and Spitz naevus (Sakamoto *et al.*, 1987). Macromelanosomes are mostly located in melanocytes but they may be transferred to epidermal keratinocytes, Langerhans cells and dermal macrophages. They are usually thought to represent an abnormal form of melanosome (Jimbow *et al.*, 1973; Konrad *et al.*, 1974; Sakamoto *et al.*, 1987), although Nakagawa and colleagues (1984) demonstrated acid phosphatase activity and produced ultrastructural data (p. 14) to suggest that they may in fact be autophagosomes rather than the sites of melanin synthesis.

When melanocytes proliferate along the dermoepidermal junction, but remain arranged as individual units, one speaks of *'lentiginous melanocytic hyperplasia'* (Figure 1.6(a)). This is often accompanied by elongation of epidermal rete ridges, which retain a slender shape.

Alternatively, the melanocytes may lose their 'territorial instinct' and form small compact groups; they are then often designated *naevus cells*, a term first used by Unna (1893), and the nests are known as *'naevus cell nests'*, or *'theques'* (Figure 1.6(b)).

In the literature, the definitions of naevus cell (naevocyte) have varied; some considered all melanin-producing cells within the epidermis as melanocytes, and reserved the term naevus cell for intradermally located cells (Briggs, 1985); others abandoned the term naevus cell completely. A strict separation between melanocytic and naevocytic lesions has been attempted by some (Mishima, 1965; Pinkus and Mehregan, 1981). However, histological, histochemical, immunocytochemical and ultrastructural similarities between melanocytes and naevus cells indicate that they are the same cell type, and that the absence of the 'territorial behaviour' of the latter is not enough reason to separate them from melanocytes, and to attempt a division between melanocytic and naevocytic proliferations. Indeed, transitions from a lentiginous type of melanocytic hyperplasia to the formation of nests are very common. As Magana-Garcia and Ackerman (1990) concluded: 'If nevus cells are melanocytes, let them be called melanocytes'.

1.3   Biochemistry of melanin synthesis

Two prototypes of melanosomal melanin can be distinguished: *eumelanin*, which is brown-black, and *phaeomelanin*, which is reddish-yellow and which is the main type of melanin found in red-haired individuals (although eumelanin may also be present in the roots of red hairs; Jimbow *et al.*, 1983). There are also intermediate forms (Prota, 1980), and a single melanocyte can produce both types simultaneously (Jimbow *et al.*, 1983). Thus, there is often a mixture of eumelanin, phaeomelanin and intermediate forms; the predominant form varies between individuals.

Tyrosine is the substrate for all types of melanin and the initial two steps in their synthesis, i.e. the formation of DOPA and dopaquinone, are always the same. Dopaquinone and its subsequent metabolites are products encountered only in melanin-producing cells.

Eumelanin is a very stable polymer, composed of several different tyrosine derivatives, whereas phaeomelanin includes cystein residues and is composed largely of 5-S-cysteinyldopa and its 2-S and 6-S isomers. Importantly, phaeomelanin is far more photolabile than eumelanin, and when irradiated may give rise to toxic and potentially carcinogenic

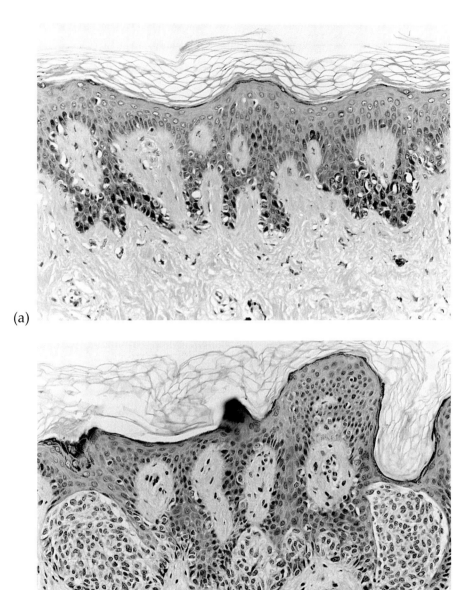

Figure 1.6 (a) Lentiginous melanocytic hyperplasia. Melanocytes are increased in number, but remain arranged as single units along the dermoepidermal junction. Note also elongation and hyperpigmentation of rete ridges (HE, × 185). (b) Melanocytic nests ('theques') in compound naevus. Melanocytes have lost their 'territorial behaviour', crowding together to form compact nests, mostly at or near the tips of rete ridges (HE, × 185).

hydroxyl radicals (Chedekel *et al.*, 1978; Tomita *et al.*, 1984), which may contribute to the sun-induced cell damage, and may thus be related to the higher incidence of melanoma in red-haired individuals.

Melanin synthesis is stimulated by a variety of hormones, including melanotropins (MSH), ACTH, prostaglandins, lipotropins, and sex steroid hormones. The latter exert their influence especially on the skin of the external genitalia and the nipples (Thody and Smith, 1977).

There are several brown pigments chemically unrelated to melanin which may cause confusion, especially because they are positive with some histochemical stains for melanin and because of the unfortunate terminology. *Neuromelanin* (Graham, 1979), which is found in the substantia nigra, locus coeruleus, trigeminal and dorsal root ganglia and occasionally in peripheral ganglion cells, is not formed *via* oxidation of tyrosine: it is a waste product of catecholamine breakdown, and is related to lipofuscin (Erlandson, 1987); it is therefore totally unrelated to 'melanosomal melanin' (Moses *et al.*, 1966). The pigment of *pseudomelanosis coli*, a brown discolouration of the colonic mucosa due to accumulation of pigment-laden macrophages within the lamina propria, and related to constipation and ingestion of certain laxatives, is also unrelated to melanosomal melanin; it is a lysosomal breakdown product related to lipofuscins. The same pigment may occasionally be encountered in mesenteric lymph nodes (Hall and Eusebi, 1978).

1.4   Electron microscopy

The melanocyte shows the general features of metabolically active exocrine cells, i.e. a prominent Golgi complex, extensive rough endoplasmic reticulum and large numbers of mitochondria (Figure 1.7). Tonofilaments and desmosomes are absent. Intermediate (vimentin) filaments are seen, and small hemi-junctions lacking the characteristic morphology of hemi-desmosomes are present where the melanocyte borders the epidermal basal lamina. Nuclei of quiescent melanocytes have a smooth outline, but active melanocytes often show lobation of the nucleus (Szabo and Flynn, 1987).

The melanocyte possesses a unique organelle, the *melanosome* (Seiji *et al.*, 1961), derived from the Golgi complex, and the site of production and packaging of melanin. Melanosomes are present in the cell body as well as in the long, slender dendrites, where they pass through various stages of development (I–IV, Figure 1.8). Melanosomes vary in size from 0.3 to about 1.0 μm; those present in highly active melanocytes, as in dark-skinned persons or due to solar radiation, are larger than those in less active melanocytes.

During their development, melanosomes travel through the mel-

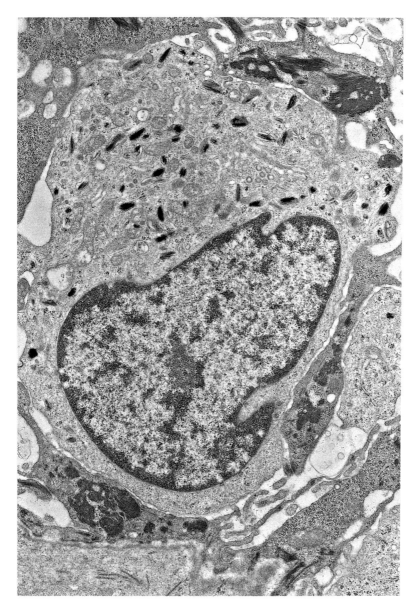

Figure 1.7   Epidermal melanocyte. A large number of small, dark melanosomes is present within the cytoplasm. *Bottom left*: Epidermal basal lamina, with a few subjacent collagen fibres (Electron micrograph, × 8250).

anocytic dendrites, and finally, the tip of the dendrite, containing the mature melanosomes, is snipped off ('apocopated'), and is phago-cytosed by the adjacent keratinocyte. Here the melanosomes fuse with lysosomes, yielding electron-dense, membrane-bound masses, de-signated 'secondary melanosomes' (a term not to be confused with stage II melanosomes). However, ultrastructural studies of a variety of pigmented epithelial tumours indicate that stage II melanosomes may also be transferred from melanocytes to keratinocytes, so that the presence of stage II melanosomes may not provide conclusive evidence that cells synthesize melanin themselves (Szpak et al., 1988). The mel-anin accumulated in dermal melanophages is also packaged in the form of secondary melanosomes. Abnormal spherical forms of mel-anosomes, with peripheral condensation of melanin, are common in dysplastic naevi and melanomas (p. 207, 292).

The ultrastructural morphology of the melanosome partly depends on the type of melanin it contains (Jimbow and Takeuchi, 1979; Jimbow et al., 1983): those containing eumelanin ('eumelanosomes'), are ellipsoid, except for the first stage of their development, and contain parallel filaments and lamellae with a distinct regular cross-striation, which later becomes obscured by melanin deposition, whereas 'phaeomelanosomes', containing phaeomelanin, are round and show a granular content.

Four stages of maturation of *eumelanosomes* (Figure 1.8) can be dis-cerned (Rhodes et al., 1988). The first stage (stage I melanosome) consists of a spherical small vesicle, about $0.3\,\mu m$ in size, which has budded off from the Golgi complex. Its morphology may not be suf-ficiently distinctive to allow recognition, unless tyrosinase activity is demonstrated histochemically, or some filaments with distinct periodicity are discernible. Subsequently, these vesicles become larger and oval in shape, and contain a larger number of filaments and membranes, which exhibit a striking cross-striation with a periodicity of about $9\,nm$ (stage II melanosome, 'premelanosome'). Melanin, which appears as an amorphous electron-dense material, is then deposited, resulting in thickening of these membranes, partially ob-scuring the internal structure (stage III melanosome). Finally, melanin almost totally fills the melanosome so that the internal structure is no longer visible (stage IV melanosome, 'melanin granule'). There often remains a peripheral electron-lucent rim. Stage II–IV melanosomes are about $0.4–1.0\,\mu m$ in length.

The development of *phaeomelanosomes* has also been divided into four stages, all of which are spherical rather than oval: stage I consists of a vacuole, which may contain a few small microvesicles. These microvesicles are more numerous in stage II; deposititation of melanin in

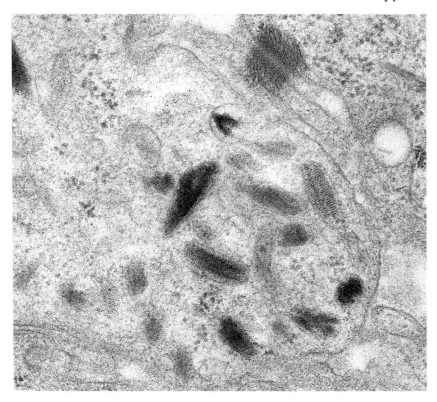

Figure 1.8 Eumelanosomes. Stage I, round vesicles; stage II, oval structures with fine cross striations; stage III and IV, increasing deposition of amorphous electron-dense melanin (Electron micrograph, × 62 500).

a spotty and granular fashion on the microvesicles as well as in the proteinaceous matrix characterizes stage III, and in stage IV the matrix is completely filled with melanin.

In whites, melanosomes are few in number, generally about 0.3–0.5 µm in size, mainly stage I and II and are found largely within melanocytes. In keratinocytes, groups of two or three melanosomes are packaged and later degraded in secondary lysosomes ('*melanosome complexes*'). Melanosome complexes can also be found in melanocytes, Langerhans cells and dermal macrophages. Sun-induced increase in pigmentation corresponds to an increase in stage III and IV melanosomes in keratinocytes. In blacks, most melanosomes are stage IV, both in melanocytes and keratinocytes. They are about 0.5–0.8 µm in length, and lie singly rather than packaged together in melanosome complexes, and are degraded more slowly (Szabo *et al.*, 1968; 1969).

Macromelanosomes (p. 7) exhibit a heavily melanized central core, which is often surrounded by one or more concentric rims of closely aggregated small electron-lucent bodies of about 30–50 nm in diameter, which, toward the centre of the macromelanosome, are buried in increasing masses of melanin. Tubular structures and filaments may also be found in the periphery. Melanosomes have been discerned in the centre of the macromelanosome by Nakagawa and colleagues (1984), who also found acid phosphatase activity. These authors therefore concluded that macromelanosomes probably represent auto-phagosomes rather than an abnormal form of melanosome. Others however reported DOPA positivity in macromelanosomes (Jimbow *et al.*, 1973; Sakamoto *et al.*, 1987) suggesting that they are the sites of melanin synthesis. Macromelanosomes and conventional melanosomes may occur together in the same melanocyte.

References

Briggs, J. C. (1985) Melanoma precursor lesions and borderline melanomas. *Histopathology*, **9**, 1251–62.

Chedekel, M. R., Smith, S. K., Post, P. W., Pokora, A. and Vessell, D. L. (1978) Photodestruction of pheomelanin: role of oxygen. *Proc. Natl. Acad. Sci.*, **75**, 5395–9.

Cochran, A. J. (1970) The incidence of melanocytes in normal skin. *J. Invest. Dermatol*, **55**, 65–70.

Cochran, A. J. (1971) Studies of the melanocytes of the epidermis adjacent to tumours. *J. Invest. Dermatol.*, **57**, 38–43.

Cruickshank, C. N. D. and Harcourt, S. A. (1964) Pigment donation *in vitro*. *J. Invest. Dermatol.*, **42**, 183–4.

Erlandson, R. A. (1987) Ultrastructural diagnosis of amelanotic malignant melanoma: aberrant melanosomes, myelin figures or lysosomes? *Ultrastruct. Pathol.*, **11**, 191–208.

Fallowfield, M. E. and Cook, M. G. (1990) Epidermal melanocytes adjacent to melanoma and the field change effect. *Histopathology*, **17**, 397–400.

Fitzpatrick, T. B. and Szabo, G. (1959) The melanocyte: cytology and cyto-chemistry. *J. Invest. Dermatol.*, **32**, 197–209.

Fitzpatrick, T. B., Miyamoto, M. and Ishikawa, K. (1967) The evolution of concepts of melanin biology. *Arch. Dermatol.*, **96**, 305–23.

Gilchrest, B. A., Blog, F. B. and Szabo, G. (1979) Effects of aging and chronic sun exposure on melanocytes in human skin. *J. Invest. Dermatol.*, **73**, 141–3.

Gordon, M. (1953) Preface. In *Pigment Cell Growth, Proceedings of the 3rd Conference on the Biology of Normal and Atypical Pigment Cell Growth* (ed. M. Gordon), New York: Academic Press.

Hu, F. (1979) Aging of melanocytes. *J. Invest. Dermatol.*, **73**, 70.

Graham, D. G. (1979) On the origin and significance of neuromelanin. *Arch. Pathol. Lab. Med.*, **103**, 359–62.

Hall, M. and Eusebi, V. (1978) Yellow-brown spindle bodies in mesenteric lymph nodes: a possible relationship with melanosis coli. *Histopathology*, **2**, 47–52.

Jimbow, K. and Takeuchi, T. (1979) Ultrastructural comparison of pheo- and eumelanogenesis in animals. *Pigment Cell*, **4**, 308–17.

Jimbow, K., Szabo, G. and Fitzpatrick, T. B. (1973) Ultrastructure of giant pigment granules (macromelanosomes) in the cutaneous pigmented macules of neurofibromatosis. *J. Invest. Dermatol.*, **61**, 300–9.

Jimbow, K., Ishida, O., Ito, S., Hori, Y., Witkop, C. J. and King, R. A. (1983) Combined chemical and electron microscopic studies of pheomelanosomes in human red hair. *J. Invest. Dermatol.*, **81**, 506–11.

Konrad, K., Wolff, K. and Hönigsmann, H. (1974) The giant melanosome: a model of deranged melanosome-morphogenesis. *J. Ultrastruct. Res.*, **48**, 102–23.

Lerner, A. B. and Case, J. D. (1959) Pigment cell regulatory factors. *J. Invest. Dermatol.*, **32**, 211–21.

Magana-Garcia, M. and Ackerman, A. B. (1990) What are nevus cells? *Am. J. Dermatopathol.*, **12**, 93–102.

Mishima, Y. (1965) Macromolecular changes in pigmentary disorders. III. Cellular nevi: subcellular and cytochemical characteristics with reference to their origin. *Arch. Dermatol.*, **91**, 536–57.

Montagna, W. (1970) Histology and cytochemistry of human skin. XXXV. The nipple and areola. *Br. J. Dermatol.*, **83**, 2–13.

Morison, W. L. (1985) What is the function of melanin? *Arch. Dermatol.*, **121**, 1160–3.

Morris, T. J., Johnson, W. M. G. and Silvers, D. N. (1982) Giant pigment granules in biopsy specimens from café au lait spots in neurofibromatosis. *Arch. Dermatol.*, **118**, 385–8.

Moses, H. L., Ganote, C. E., Beaver, D. L. and Schuffman, S. S. (1966) Light and electron microscopic studies of pigment in human and rhesus monkey substantia nigra and locus coeruleus. *Anat. Rec.*, **155**, 167–83.

Nakagawa, H., Hori, Y., Sato, S., Fitzpatrick, T. B. and Martuza, R. L. (1984) The nature and origin of the melanin macroglobule. *J. Invest. Dermatol.*, **83**, 134–9.

Nelson, W. E., Vaughan, V. C. and McKay, R. J. (1969) *Textbook of Pediatrics* (9th edn), Philadelphia: W. B. Saunders.

Nordlund, J. J., Abdel-Malek, Z. A., Boissy, R. E. and Rheins, C. A. (1989) Pigment cell biology: an historical review. *J. Invest. Dermatol.*, **92**, 53S–60S.

Okoro, A. N. (1975) Albinism in Nigeria — a clinical and social study. *Br. J. Dermatol.*, **92**, 485–92.

Pinkus, H. and Mehregan, A. H. (1981) *A Guide to Dermatohistopathology* (3rd edn), New York: Appleton-Century-Crofts, pp. 351–81.

Proctor, P. H. and McGinness, J. E. (1986) The function of melanin. *Arch. Dermatol.*, **122**, 507–8.

Prota, G. (1980) Recent advances in the chemistry of melanogenesis in mammals. *J. Invest. Dermatol.*, **75**, 122–7.

Quevedo, W. C., Szabo, G. and Virks, J. (1969) Influence of age and UV on the population of dopa-positive melanocytes in human skin. *J. Invest. Dermatol.*, **52**, 287–90.

Rawles, M. E. (1947) Origin of pigment cells from the neural crest in the mouse embryo. *Physiol. Zoöl.*, **20**, 248–66.

Rawles, M. E. (1948) Origin of melanophores and their role in development of color patterns in vertebrates. *Physiol. Rev.*, **28**, 383–408.

Rhodes, A. R., Seki, Y., Fitzpatrick, T. B. and Stern, R. S. (1988) Melanosomal alterations in dysplastic melanocytic nevi. A quantitative, ultrastructural investigation. *Cancer*, **61**, 358–69.

Rosdahl, I. and Rorsman, H. (1983) An estimate of the melanocyte mass in humans. *J. Invest. Dermatol.*, **81**, 278–81.

Sagebiel, R. W. and Odland, G. F. (1970) Ultrastructural identification of melanocytes in early human embryos. *J. Invest. Dermatol.*, **54**, 96.

Sakamoto, F., Ito, M. and Sato, Y. (1987) Ultrastructural study of macromelanosomes in a unique case of spindle and epithelioid cell nevus. *J. Cutan. Pathol.*, **14**, 59–64.

Savin, C. (1965) The blood vessels and pigmentary cells of the inner ear. *Ann. Otol. Rhinol. Laryngol.*, **74**, 611–22.

Seiji, M., Fitzpatrick, T. B. and Birbeck, M. S. C. (1961) The melanosome: a distinctive subcellular particle of mammalian melanocytes and the site of melanogenesis. *J. Invest. Dermatol.*, **36**, 243–52.

Slater, C., Hayes, M., Temple-Camp, C. and Beighton, P. (1986) Macromelanosomes in the early diagnosis of neurofibromatosis. *Am. J. Dermatopathol.*, **8**, 284–9.

Staricco, P. J. and Pinkus, H. (1957) Quantitative and qualitative data on the pigment cells of the adult human epidermis. *J. Invest. Dermatol.*, **28**, 33–45.

Szabo, G. (1954) The number of melanocytes in human epidermis. *Br. Med. J.*, **1**, 1016–7.

Szabo, G. and Flynn, E. (1987) Morphological aspects of normal human melanocytes. In *Cutaneous Melanoma: Status of Knowledge and Future Perspective* (eds U. Veronesi, N. Cascinelli and M. Santinami), London: Academic Press, pp. 127–38.

Szabo, G., Gerald, A. B., Pathak, M. A. and Fitzpatrick, T. B. (1968) Racial differences in human pigmentation at the ultrastructural level. *J. Cell. Biol.*, **39**, 132–3.

Szabo, G., Gerald, A. B., Pathak, M. A. and Fitzpatrick, T. B. (1969) Racial differences in the fate of melanosomes in human epidermis. *Nature*, **222**, 1081–2.

Szpak, C. A., Shelburne, J., Linder, J. and Klintworth, G. K. (1988) The presence of stage II melanosomes (premelanosomes) in neoplasms other than melanomas. *Modern Pathol.*, **1**, 35–43.

Thody, A. J. and Smith, A. G. (1977) Hormones and skin pigmentation in the mammal. *Int. J. Dermatol.*, **16**, 657–64.

Tomita, Y., Hariu, A., Kato, C. and Seiji, M. (1984) Radical production during tyrosinase reaction, dopa-melanin formation, and photo-irradiation of dopa-melanin. *J. Invest. Dermatol.*, **82**, 573–6.

Unna, P. G. (1893) Naevi und Naevocarcinoma. *Klin. Wochenschr. (Berlin)*, **30**, 14–6.

Warkany, J. (1971) *Congenital Malformations: Notes and Comments*, Chicago: Year Book Medical Publishers.

Weston, J. A. (1970) The migration and differentiation of neural crest cells. In *Advances in Morphogenesis* (eds M. Abercrombie, J. Brachet and T. King), New York: Academic Press, pp. 41–114.

Wong, J. A. (1970) A study of melanocytes in the normal skin surrounding malignant melanoma. *Dermatologica*, **141**, 215–25.

2 Biopsy, tissue processing and histological investigation

Although the general principles of macroscopical investigation, dissection, processing and histological investigation which apply in histopathology are no different with regard to melanocytic disorders, there are some specific points that merit attention.

First, adequate clinical information is of particular importance. It is strongly advisable not to report on pigmented lesions in the absence of basic information regarding the patient's age and site of the lesion (McGovern *et al.*, 1986). Previous trauma, such as incomplete previous removal, should always be mentioned. Other clinical data, such as a history of recent change *vs* that of a long-standing and unchanging lesion, removal for cosmetic reasons *vs* clinical suspicion, and a personal or family history of melanoma, are important, and clinicians should be urged to provide such information as well.

A macroscopical description of the lesion by the clinician is useful but not absolutely necessary; the pathologist should also assess the macrosopical features, even though the clinician is at an obvious advantage, since fine differences in pigmentation, reactive hyperaemia, palpatory features, intactness of skin lines and so on are far better evaluated before the lesion is excised.

The dissection of the specimen should always be documented in detail. Questions concerning size, form, colour, consistency, and localization of abnormalities, their relation to resection margins, and localization of lymph nodes often cannot be answered after the dissection; therefore, a faulty or incomplete macroscopical investigation and description is a serious error.

2.1 Skin biopsy of a pigmented lesion: clinical considerations

An elliptical, or sometimes hexagonal, *excisional biopsy* with narrow margins (1–2 mm from the macroscopically visible margins of the lesion) generally constitutes the proper biopsy of pigmented cutaneous lesions. The biopsy should preferably include some subcutaneous fat.

In general, *punch biopsy* and *incisional biopsy* are to be discouraged. It has been suggested that an incisional biopsy could increase the chance of local recurrence or dissemination of melanoma, but this has not been substantiated by follow-up data, and punch biopsies of melanomas do not lead to decreased survival rates (Urist *et al.*, 1985). However, there are compelling arguments in favour of an excisional biopsy. First, it allows the evaluation of the symmetry and the mode of spread at the lateral margins, which are very important in diagnostically difficult cases (Rampen and Van der Esch, 1985; Urist *et al.*, 1985). Also, excisional biopsy constitutes definitive treatment if the lesion is benign, whereas incomplete removal of a benign naevus may result in a recurrence which may have a clinically and histologically atypical appearance (p. 98), leading to diagnostic difficulties which would have been avoided had the lesion been removed in its entirety in the first instance. When the lesion is malignant, the maximal thickness and level of invasion of the entire tumour can be assessed. There is no reason to believe that the short delay in definitive treatment, caused by a diagnostic excision preceding the definitive excision, has a deleterious effect on prognosis (Epstein, 1971; Eldh, 1979; Landthaler *et al.*, 1989).

The biopsy should not be too large: when the lesion is benign, the extra margins of normal skin will have been unnecessary and, when it is malignant, the margins may still not be adequate and re-excision will remain necessary, sometimes even a larger one than one would wish, because the whole previous biopsy wound, including the deep margins, should be surrounded by a rim of normal tissue in the re-excision specimen.

The excisional biopsy should be oriented in such a way that a re-excision, when necessary, can be performed with a minimum of skin loss (Urist *et al.*, 1985); in most instances it is best taken with the long axis in the direction of the cutaneous lymphatics, which is often different from that of the skin lines (Harris and Gumport, 1975). Sometimes, a different orientation is preferred to allow better primary closure of the wound. The area is anaesthetized by field block anaesthesia, i.e. by injecting the anaesthetic just outside the area of skin to be excised; the anaesthesia fluid should never be injected into or in the immediate vicinity of the lesion, since this results in disturbing histological artefacts (Mehregan and Pinkus, 1966; Sagebiel, 1972).

A punch biopsy or incisional biopsy is occasionally justified, e.g. when the pigmented lesion is very small (so that a 6 mm punch biopsy includes a rim of surrounding normal skin), or very large (e.g. giant congenital naevus containing a suspicious area, or lentigo maligna with or without a suspected invasive focus), or when the localization is awkward, as is the case with subungual lesions. Obviously, once the diagnosis of melanoma has been made, excision of the whole lesion becomes necessary, with margins appropriate for the tumour thickness.

2.2   Macroscopical description and dissection of skin biopsy specimens

2.2.1   Punch biopsy

As indicated above, punch biopsy of a cutaneous pigmented lesion is only infrequently justified.

The macroscopical description should include the diameter of the fixed specimen (which due to tissue shrinkage during fixation is less than the diameter of the punch with which it is taken), the depth of the punch, and the presence of subcutaneous fat. The surface should be briefly described. Punch biopsies of 6 mm can be bisected with a sharp razor blade; smaller ones are best processed whole and cut at various levels; it is advisable to retain unstained sections at various levels to allow for additional stains. Special care should be taken to avoid disruption of the epidermis, which can occur when there is an extensive junctional melanocytic proliferation.

2.2.2   Excisional biopsy

The specimen is fixed whole and subsequently dissected. When there is suspicion of malignancy the surgical margins are marked with India ink or an alternative such as alcian blue (Birch et al., 1990) or Tipp-Ex fluid (Harris, 1990). In general, unless the excision specimen is large, it is unnecessary to distinguish between the two lateral sides, since these are apposed at closure of the surgical wound.

A macroscopical description of the lesion itself should be provided, although, as discussed previously, the pathologist is at a disadvantage compared to the clinician. The pathologist should form an opinion of the most likely diagnosis on the basis of his own macroscopical findings.

Assessment of the completeness of the resection is always part of the investigation. The minimal distance to the resection margin after fixation should be noted; in the initial diagnostic excision biopsy specimen, it will usually be 1 or 2 mm. When a lesion is elongated or irregular in shape, the longest axis is not necessarily parallel to the long axis of the excision specimen, since the latter depends also on other considerations, such as the direction of the cutaneous lymphatics (Roses *et al.*, 1983) and sometimes the vicinity of other structures (see above). Small excisional biopsies may be bisected and the two halves processed separately if the clinician has marked one of the ends. Larger ones should be transected at right angles to the long axis, or, when the size of cross-sections exceeds that of a paraffin block and the margin of macrosopically uninvolved skin is at least 3 mm, the resection margins can be removed first and processed separately, after drawing or photographing the specimen and the position of the blocks taken. When a lesion closely approaches a resection margin, blocks should always be taken at right angles to it, since such sections allow a far better microscopical assessment of the relation of the tumour to the resection margin.

When a lesion is too large to be embedded totally, the blocks taken should include the site of maximal thickness, areas of ulceration or crusting, and the site where the surgical margin is narrowest.

2.2.3   *Re-excision specimens*

These should be fixed whole and then transected at every 2 mm. When no suspicious lesions are seen macroscopically, and the margins of the initial diagnostic biopsy were tumour-free, we take three blocks from the scar; if the lesion was not removed totally at initial biopsy, the scar is embedded totally. In addition any suspicious lesion and any skin pigmentation present in the re-excision specimen is embedded.

2.3   Dissection of lymphadenectomy specimens

The dissection and processing of lymphadenectomy specimens of the neck, axilla and groin follows the general rules pertaining to those specimens (Rosai, 1989): all identified lymph nodes should be processed and grouped into different regions; the most proximal nodes are identified separately. As a guideline, minimal numbers of lymph nodes to be identified are: axillary lymph node dissection, 20; inguinal lymph node dissection, 12; radical neck dissection, 40. Occasionally, it may prove impossible to find this number of lymph nodes, despite a meticulous search.

One single section through the middle of each lymph node suffices, since serial sectioning of the nodes only very rarely reveals additional metastases (Reichert *et al.*, 1981). There is some debate about the usefulness of S-100 immunostaining to detect small numbers of tumour cells: this will be dealt with in Chapter 10 (p. 321).

2.4   Dissection of other specimens containing metastases

Depending on the size of the metastasis, it is wholly embedded or blocks are taken at different sites, preferably from areas with different macroscopical appearances. Blocks are taken where surgical margins are narrowest, after marking resection margins with ink.

2.5   Tissue processing and staining methods

2.5.1   Frozen section

As a rule, it is not advisable to perform frozen section diagnosis of primary cutaneous melanocytic lesions, because the morphology is inferior, multiple levels cannot be studied, a relatively large amount of tissue is lost in the cutting of sections, and the measurements of tumour thickness are not comparable to those of fixed specimens. On the basis of this, prognostic subgroups have been identified and optimal therapy can be chosen (p. 309). Obviously these considerations do not apply to frozen section diagnosis of metastatic lesions.

2.5.2   Tissue for research purposes

When one is dealing with a primary lesion over 8 mm in greatest diameter, it is acceptable to reserve for research purposes a thin slice of the lesion, excluding its thickest part and the site where the lesion most closely approximates the resection margin. This slice is snap-frozen in liquid nitrogen or another suitable fluid for immediate tissue freezing, for the purpose of immunostaining of antigens which do not withstand formalin fixation, or molecular biological investigations. At present, such work mainly serves research purposes, since the immunomarkers directly relevant to routine differential diagnosis are applicable to paraffin sections.

2.5.3   Fixation

Most lesions, certainly those smaller than 8 mm, are fixed *in toto* by immersion in neutral buffered formalin. Larger specimens, and certainly lymph node dissection specimens, should be incised, to allow adequate penetration of the fixative: a few straight, parallel incisions with a long, very sharp knife suffice, and do not jeopardize the topography of the specimen. The specimen is rinsed before fixation, because adherent blood impairs fixation, and the macrosopical investigation is hindered by it. A brief rinse with tap water does not influence tissue morphology to any appreciable extent. However, imprints for cytological investigation should be taken before rinsing the specimen.

Paraffin sections are satisfactory for practically all diagnostic purposes. Several antisera and monoclonal antibodies are available which help in the distinction between melanocytic and non-melanocytic tumours and which are applicable to paraffin sections of formalin-fixed tissue. Some antibodies which are of potential interest for refining prognosis only work on frozen sections (p. 320), but these are not of immediate concern here, since they are not included in a routine diagnostic setting.

2.5.4　Histochemical procedures; melanin stains

The identification of melanin can be achieved by a variety of staining techniques, the most widely used being reducing methods, such as the sensitive Schmorl's and Masson-Fontana's stains, which yield a blue and black staining of melanin, respectively, and the even more sensitive Warthin-Starry silver stain (Warkel *et al.*, 1980). Importantly, some lipofuscins (Senba, 1986) and endocrine cells may also give a positive reaction. Furthermore, it is always wise to perform an iron stain, such as Perls' stain, in parallel with a melanin stain.

The dark brown pigment found in *pseudomelanosis coli* (p. 10) is usually PAS-positive, while true melanin is negative, and the two can also be distinguished by alkaline diazo staining (Stevens, 1977).

Formalin pigment is a brown pigment, derived from haemoglobin when the pH drops below 6, and therefore does not form when the formalin is buffered to a neutral pH. It can be located both intracellularly and extracellularly, and can occasionally be mistaken for melanin; when present in dermal macrophages, it may lead to a diagnosis of blue naevus (p. 113). It is easily distinguished from melanin since it is birefringent and does not stain with the silver stains for melanin (Ackerman and Penneys, 1970). Formalin pigment can be rapidly dissolved by incubation of the slide in a picric acid solution.

Melanin can be *bleached* by incubation in 0.5% potassium permanganate solution, or a variety of other chemicals. After bleaching with potassium permanganate, the slides remain suitable for immunohistochemistry (McGovern and Crocker, 1987).

After formalin fixation, melanin exhibits *autofluorescence* (Fellner *et al.*, 1979). In addition, an intense autofluorescence of melanoma cells and weak fluorescence of some naevus cells in unstained paraffin sections of formalin-fixed specimens can be found (Inoshita and Youngberg, 1982); this is not due to the presence of melanin pigment.

Tyrosinase activity can be demonstrated by the *DOPA-reaction* (incubation with 0.1% 3,4-dihydroxyphenylalanine in phosphate buffer at pH 7.4, for 6 h at room temperature), which can be performed on epidermal preparations, frozen sections, or paraffin sections of suitably fixed tissue (Laidlaw and Blackberg, 1932; Rodriguez and McGavran, 1969).

2.5.5 Immunomarkers

The most important practical application of immunostaining with regard to melanocytic lesions concerns the differential diagnosis of amelanotic melanoma *vs* various other malignant tumours. *It is essential to use a panel of markers*, including markers positive for tumours which enter into the differential diagnosis (Gatter *et al.*, 1985). For the diagnosis of melanocytic *vs* non-melanocytic tumours, we use a panel of antibodies to S-100 protein, vimentin, low- and high-molecular weight keratins, leukocyte common antigen, and HMB-45 (Figure 2.1), often in conjunction with stains for melanin, mucins and reticulin. It is of importance to appreciate that some melanomas are negative for HMB-45 and occasionally for S-100 also, and that a variety of epithelial markers including keratins are by no means specific for epithelial cells and may be positive in melanoma (p. 291). This issue is discussed further in a section on the immunodiagnosis of metastatic melanoma included in Chapter 9 (p. 289).

For the distinction of benign and malignant melanocytic lesions, immunohistochemistry is of no immediate practical diagnostic use, in view of the very high specificity required to reach an acceptable predictive value (p. 28). Interesting differences have been documented in expression of a variety of antigens, including expression of *HLA class I and II* antigens (Ruiter *et al.*, 1982, 1984, 1985), which may be induced by gamma interferon produced by T-cells in the inflammatory infiltrate that is often associated with a melanoma (Van Vreeswijk *et al.*, 1988). However, the differences are not of direct help in the diagnosis of histologically difficult cases (West *et al.*, 1989). The pattern of basement membrane deposition differs between naevi and melanomas, and can be visualized using antibodies to collagen type IV and laminin but, again, this is of no immediate practical diagnostic value (Havenith *et al.*, 1989). Ki-67 immunostaining reveals differences in density of positive cells in naevi *vs* melanoma (Smolle *et al.*, 1989).

Monoclonal antibody HMB-45 recognizes a melanosomal glycoprotein which is expressed in epidermal melanocytes of fetuses and

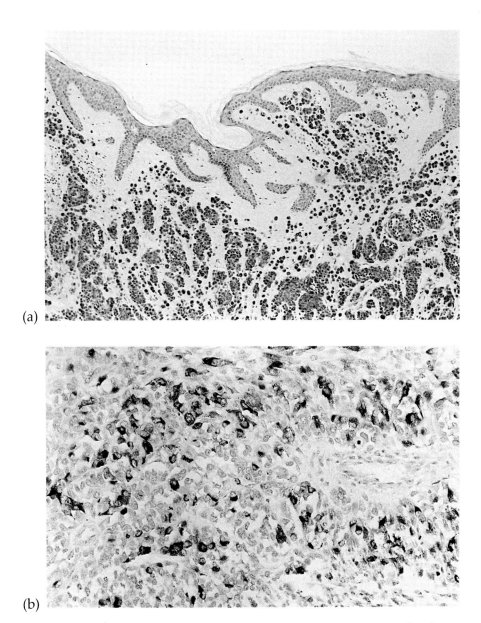

(a)

(b)

Figure 2.1 (a) Intradermal naevus, stained with an anti-S-100 monoclonal antibody. Naevus cells stand out against a negative background (Immunoperoxidase, × 90). (b) Melanoma cells, stained with monoclonal antibody HMB-45. Although this melanoma metastasis is poorly pigmented, many tumour cells are strongly positive (Immunoperoxidase, × 185).

neonates but not adults, in melanocytes in the vicinity of a hae-mangioma, a basal cell carcinoma or a scar (Smoller *et al.*, 1989a), in junctional melanocytes of junctional and compound naevi, in some melanocytes within the papillary dermis of dysplastic naevi (Smoller *et al.*, 1989b), congenital naevi, some Spitz naevi (Palazzo and Duray, 1989), deep penetrating naevi, blue naevi, melanomas (Ordónez *et al.*, 1988) and in a variety of rare non-melanocytic melanin-producing tumours (Colombari *et al.*, 1988; Sun *et al.*, 1990). Again, differences in staining patterns of various melanocytic lesions do not appear to be of direct practical diagnostic value in the differential diagnosis between different melanocytic lesions (Palazzo and Duray, 1989).

A large number of antibodies have been raised against melanoma and show differences in reactivity between naevi and melanoma (Natali *et al.*, 1983; Lehmann *et al.*, 1987; Maeda and Jimbow, 1987; Nakanishi and Hashimoto, 1987; Maeda *et al.*, 1988; Elder *et al.*, 1989). These antibodies can, therefore, be said to be associated with tumour pro-gression; however, none has yet been proven to be of direct diagnostic value and, interesting though they may be, it is too early to advocate their application in a routine diagnostic setting.

2.5.6 *Nucleolar organizer regions*

Nucleolar organizer regions are segments of DNA encoding ribosomal RNA and are present on five chromosome pairs. Their spatial distri-bution can be visualized by means of a one-step silver precipitation technique: they are then known as *AgNORs*. The numbers of AgNORs in various types of naevus and in melanoma have been investigated in order to assess their potential usefulness as an adjunct in the differen-tial diagnosis.

Most melanocytes of common naevi and many dysplastic naevi possess only one large AgNOR, whereas melanoma cells generally show several, scattered throughout the nucleus (Crocker and Skilbeck, 1987; Fallowfield *et al.*, 1988; Leong and Gilham, 1989; Howat *et al.*, 1990). However, reported average numbers of AgNORs in melanoma cells have varied markedly, from 2.1 (Howat *et al.*, 1990) to 9.2 (Leong and Gilham, 1989); these differences are probably caused by subtle differences in the silver precipitation technique used. Moreover, in many cases of Spitz naevus, and also in pigmented spindle cell naevus and some dysplastic naevi, multiple AgNORs are present, so that the diagnosis in these types of naevus, where the distinction from mel-anoma is more difficult, is not facilitated by the use of this technique (Fallowfield and Cook, 1989).

2.6   Electron microscopy

For electron microscopy, a very thin slice of tissue is fixed in a suitable fixative: Karnovsky's fixative is admirable (Karnovsky, 1965), but several others, which also contain a mixture of paraformaldehyde and glutaraldehyde, are equally satisfactory. A small slice of tissue up to about 1 mm in thickness can be fixed well in Karnovsky's fixative. A fixative containing only glutaraldehyde penetrates the tissue far more slowly, and therefore necessitates cutting tissue blocks of very small size, which is inconvenient and may damage the tissue.

After fixation, small blocks are cut, postfixed in osmium tetroxide, embedded in a suitable resin and semithin sections are cut to select areas for electron microscopy. After the blocks have been trimmed, ultrathin sections are cut and stained with uranyl acetate and lead citrate.

When only formalin-fixed tissue is available, electron microscopy can usually still yield satisfactory results, although the quality is less than optimal and more variable. The quality of paraffin-retrieved material is usually rather poor, but melanosomes may still be recognizable. However, the differential diagnostic questions can usually be solved more easily by immunohistochemistry (Jundt *et al.*, 1986), so that at present, electron microscopy is only rarely needed in the diagnosis of melanoma.

A modification of the Warthin-Starry method for the demonstration of melanin in semithin and ultrathin sections was described by Van Duinen and co-workers (1983). A combination of the DOPA reaction and the Warthin-Starry method, suitable to identify aberrant melanosomes in amelanotic melanoma (see below) has also been described (Rennison *et al.*, 1987).

2.6.1   *Ultrastructural abnormalities of melanosomes*

Electron microscopy has been used not only to distinguish between melanoma and other malignant neoplasms, but also for the distinction between common naevi, dysplastic naevi and melanoma. Part of the melanosomes in dysplastic naevi and melanoma have an abnormal ultrastructural morphology (Takahashi *et al.*, 1987; Rhodes *et al.*, 1988). In addition to melanosomes with normal morphological features, dysplastic naevi and melanomas contain abnormal melanosomes, with a spherical form and an irregular, often granular content. Such melanosomes are very rare in common acquired naevi and normal melanocytes (Rhodes *et al.*, 1988).

2.7   Other techniques in the diagnosis of malignancy

The histological distinction between benignity and malignancy in melanocytic lesions of the skin remains very much a matter for HE-stained sections. A reticulin stain may reveal some differences between naevus and melanoma: an intact subepidermal basal lamina is usually indicative of a benign naevus and reticulin surrounding most individual cells is also an indication of benignity; however, the patterns show considerable variation and, when morphology becomes difficult to interpret, this often applies also to the reticulin pattern (Briggs, 1980).

The epidermal basal lamina may be visualized by antibodies to type IV and type VII collagen, and laminin; in some melanomas, expansion of the epidermal compartment may thus be visualized (Kirkham *et al.*, 1989) so that the invasive part of the tumour is less than originally thought in HE-stained sections.

Morphometry has been applied in the distinction between benign and malignant melanocytic tumours; parameters based on nuclear size at the base of the tumour, or the ratio of nuclear size between superficial and deep parts of the tumour, appear to be promising in this respect (Lindholm and Hofer, 1986; Leitinger *et al.*, 1990).

2.8   Histological investigation and description

The histology of melanocytic lesions should be investigated systematically, assessing architectural and cytological features in a fixed order, in order to avoid overlooking inconspicuous features. Such a systematic investigation of cases, including trivial ones, will provide the critical personal experience which becomes important in difficult cases. A diagnosis should not reflect vague feelings based on past experience which although extensive, can be based on misconceptions. Instead, it should be the result of a systematic and critical evaluation of well-defined and corroborated diagnostic criteria.

When there is a proliferation of melanocytes, the localization, architecture and reactive changes in the epidermis and dermis are noted first. Subsequently, the lesion is investigated in greater detail and the nuclear and cytoplasmic features of the individual melanocytes and the presence of mitoses are assessed in different areas of the lesion. Cytological features can yield vital and conclusive diagnostic evidence in difficult cases in which the architecture does not allow a confident diagnosis.

When only the clinically relevant features are to be reported, the pathology report can usually be quite short, unless there is some doubt about the diagnosis. In the case of a melanoma, the report should include the diagnosis and those features which are of immediate prognostic importance. Other details, relevant as they are for arriving at the correct diagnosis, can usually be dispensed with in a report to the clinician. It is recommended that a statement as to the completeness of excision of the lesion should always be included, not only in melanomas but also in naevi, in view of the irregularly shaped and sometimes atypical recurrences occasionally encountered after incomplete removal of a naevus (p. 98).

While describing the morphology of the lesion, *one should refrain from using interpretative terms*, such as 'primitive', 'immature', 'active', 'irritated', and so on. The description of histological features should be based on a purely morphological terminology, describing the architectural and cytological features of the lesion and changes of the surrounding tissues. The subsequent interpretation of these morphological findings, of course, necessitates the use of interpretative terms.

2.9   Criteria for diagnosis: usefulness and limitations

Assuming well-defined morphological features have been used in describing a particular lesion, one has to appreciate the value and limitations of these features as criteria in the differential diagnosis. The application of diagnostic criteria is not always straightforward and needs some elaboration; there are some caveats which must be borne in mind in order to apply the diagnostic criteria correctly and as logically as possible. In addition, certain faults in reasoning need to be avoided as, judging from the literature, they have frequently fuelled controversy in areas which are already inherently difficult.

2.9.1   *Impact of relative prevalence of diseases on the predictive value of a given criterion*

The value of a diagnostic criterion depends, apart from its preciseness and therefore assessability, on its predictive value, i.e. the chance that, in a given differential diagnosis, the presence of a particular feature coincides with one specific diagnosis. The predictive value obviously depends on the prevalence of that feature in a certain entity, compared with its prevalence in the entities which must be distinguished from it. It is far less obvious that the predictive value depends just as much on the relative prevalence of the very entities requiring differentiation (Vecchio, 1966).

Let us suppose that a particular feature is found in 100% of melanomas and in only 5% of naevi; comparison of 100 cases of each entity in a study reported in the literature will reveal 100 cases of melanoma with this feature, but only five benign lesions, giving the erroneous impression perhaps that a lesion showing this particular feature is 20 times more likely to be malignant as benign. This, however, is clearly incorrect, since the number of excised naevi greatly exceeds that of melanomas. Supposing this ratio is 20 to 1 in favour of benign lesions, then the feature in question will actually be found in equal numbers of excised benign and malignant lesions. If the specificity of the feature is higher, so that it is found in all melanomas and only 1% of benign naevi, then a lesion with this feature will be five times more likely to be malignant than benign in diagnostic practice, a modest degree of predictability, but still nowhere near the factor of 100 that comparison of equal numbers of cases might have suggested.

Thus, the relative prevalence of lesions in the population, and more immediately in excised specimens, greatly influences the predictive value of diagnostic features. Thus, when a relatively rare entity (melanoma) has to be distinguished from a common entity (common acquired naevus), the specificity of the distinguishing diagnostic criterion needs to approach 100%, in order to achieve an acceptable predictive value. In practice, such criteria are usually not available, and this is the reason why the differential diagnosis of melanoma *vs* naevus requires the assessment of a combination of criteria rather than one only.

2.9.2   Limited usefulness of negative findings

If a diagnostic criterion is virtually 100% specific for an entity, the problem of the relative prevalence of diseases discussed under section 2.9.1 does not apply. Thus, pagetoid spread is virtually diagnostic of malignancy; indeed, this is so in almost any context, hence its supreme importance. However, for this very reason, histopathologists can be lulled into a false sense of security by the absence of pagetoid spread. The absence of pagetoid spread in Spitz naevi helps to distinguish them from superficial spreading melanomas, a point rightly stressed by many authors. However, pagetoid spread is also absent in some 'Spitzoid' spindle cell melanomas which need to be distinguished from Spitz naevus. Many signs of malignancy 'work only one way': if they are present, the lesion is definitely a melanoma, but in their absence the lesion may still be a melanoma. We believe that insufficient attention to this point accounts for a significant number of misdiagnoses of melanomas as naevi.

The absence of a highly specific diagnostic feature for malignancy (like pagetoid spread) does not equate with a benign lesion. It would only do so if the sensitivity of the feature would be 100%, which is never the case.

2.9.3   *The behaviour of resected lesions and its bearing on the nature of the lesions. Incomplete and short follow-up*

Criteria of benignity are more difficult to establish than those of malignancy; large series of incompletely removed pigmented cutaneous lesions are not available. It is usually assumed that every lesion in a given series has been diagnosed correctly, when a very small percentage of diagnoses may actually have been incorrect. This source of potential error is especially important when the significance of certain features which are both infrequent and worrisome are being assessed. For instance, atypical mitoses have been reported in a small percentage of benign lesions. However, there remains an element of doubt that a few such cases might represent underdiagnosed malignancies included in a benign series. The evidence that the lesions are benign consists in part of the fact that, after resection as for benign naevi, they do not recur after long follow-up. This evidence by itself is unsatisfactory, because it is known that small invasive melanomas have a very high cure rate with limited excisions. It is, therefore, possible that a very small percentage of lesions diagnosed as benign naevi are in fact unrecognized cured melanomas. The follow-up indicating a cure will apparently 'confirm' an incorrect diagnosis. While follow-up study can obviously demonstrate malignant behaviour, it cannot be used to demonstrate that an individual lesion is benign if that lesion has been removed. Needless to say, this problem is accentuated when follow-up data are incomplete and cover a time span of only a few years.

2.9.4   *Circular reasoning*

When a specific feature has been used to help establish a diagnosis and, thereby, for the identification of a series of cases, that feature will be represented over-frequently in that series. Thus, if Kamino bodies are used as a major means of identification of Spitz naevus, the prevalence of these bodies in that series of cases may be, say, as high as 90%. But if the diagnosis of Spitz naevus is made largely or entirely on other criteria, the prevalence of bodies may fall to a lower percentage. Thus, two series may give very different 'prevalences' of Kamino bodies. In fact, the lower figure would represent a more realistic prevalence, because the diagnosis was established on other grounds; in the first series the presence of bodies was a major factor in making the diagnosis, so that a conclusion as to the 'prevalence' of the bodies is meaningless.

Indeed, when a diagnostic feature is used as an obligatory criterion, it will of course be present in all cases. In this situation, it remains unclear whether other cases exist which are similar clinically and histologically, except for the absence of that one particular feature. There are many examples in the literature of this phenomenon manifesting itself, for instance in the diagnosis of Spitz naevus and dysplastic naevus, and in the reported frequency of an intraepidermal component in desmoplastic melanoma.

The necessity of using defined criteria to establish a series of similar cases is not in question, but these examples do illustrate how the prevalence of certain features can vary markedly between series. Reported prevalences do not necessarily reflect the real frequency of a feature in a particular tumour; they to some extent reflect the frequency with which the pathologist has identified a particular tumour, partly by virtue of the presence of this particular feature. The importance or otherwise of that feature depends on preconceived ideas of the definition of the entity, and these ideas may or may not be correct.

2.9.5 Referral bias

Cases submitted for a second opinion to a colleague, who takes a special interest in that field of pathology, are usually cases which have posed problems and therefore tend to be cases with less than classical features. This leads to over-frequency of the latter. Almost certainly, this phenomenon accounts for some of the divergent patient characteristics attributed to some entities, e.g. the age distribution of Spitz naevi. Thus, series of cases of the latter from specialist centres tend to have a greater proportion of adult patients compared with young children. The same applies to the histopathological findings. Thus, the Spitz naevi seen in a referral centre are likely to include a higher proportion without obvious telangiectasia, oedema and epithelioid giant cells in the superficial part of the lesion and, conversely, a higher proportion with transepidermal elimination of cell packets and single tumour cells, with moderately heavy pigmentation, with many mitoses, with neural involvement and so on.

'Bias' is meant to indicate that the frequency of particular features can become markedly distorted because of selection. It is not meant to indicate that referral findings *per se* are a bad thing. When an entity is first recognized, obviously only the more classical features are defined. As large numbers of cases are subsequently collected and these include many less 'typical' examples, many new cases of the entity become recognizable and thus, the limits of a lesion gradually tend to become broader, as is well exemplified by the much broader current definition of Spitz naevus.

References

Ackerman, A. B. and Penneys, N. S. (1970) Formalin pigment in skin. *Arch. Dermatol.*, **102**, 318–21.

Birch, P. J., Jeffrey, M. J. and Andrews, M. I. J. (1990) Alcian blue: reliable rapid method for marking resection margins. *J. Clin. Pathol.*, **43**, 608–9.

Briggs, J. C. (1980) Reticulin impregnation in the diagnosis of malignant melanoma. *Histopathology*, **4**, 507–16.

Colombari, R., Bonetti, F., Zamboni, G. *et al.* (1988) Distribution of melanoma specific antibody (HMB-45) in benign and malignant melanocytic tumors. An immunohistochemical study on paraffin sections. *Virchows Arch. A. (Pathol. Anat.)*, **413**, 17–24.

Crocker, J. and Skilbeck, N. (1987) Nucleolar organizer region associated proteins in cutaneous melanotic lesions: a quantitative study. *J. Clin. Pathol.*, **40**, 885–9.

Elder, D. E., Rodeck, U., Thurin, J. *et al.* (1989) Antigentic profile of tumor progression stages in human melanocytic nevi and melanomas. *Cancer Res.*, **49**, 5091–6.

Eldh, J. (1979) Excisional biopsy and delayed wide excision versus primary wide excision of malignant melanoma. *Scand. J. Plast. Reconstr. Surg.*, **13**, 341–5.

Epstein, E. (1971) Effect of biopsy on the prognosis of melanoma. *J. Surg. Oncol.*, **3**, 251.

Fallowfield, M. E. and Cook, M. G. (1989) The value of nucleolar organizer region staining in the differential diagnosis of borderline melanocytic lesions. *Histopathology*, **14**, 299–304.

Fallowfield, M. E., Dodson, A. R. and Cook, M. G. (1988) Nucleolar organizer regions in melanocytic dysplasia and melanoma. *Histopathology*, **13**, 95–9.

Fellner, M. J., Chen, A. S., Mont, M., McCabe, J. and Baden, M. (1979) Patterns and intensity of autofluorescence and its relation to melanin in human epidermis and hair. *Int. J. Dermatol.*, **18**, 722–30.

Gatter, K. C., Ralfkiaer, E., Skinner, J. *et al.* (1985) An immunocytochemical study of malignant melanoma and its differential diagnosis from other malignant tumours. *J. Clin. Pathol.*, **38**, 1353–7.

Harris, M. D. (1990) Tipp-ex fluid: convenient marker for surgical resection margins. *J. Clin. Pathol.*, **43**, 346–7.

Harris, M. N. and Gumport, S. L. (1975) Biopsy technique for malignant melanoma. *J. Dermatol. Surg.*, **1**, 24–27.

Havenith, M. G., Van Zandvoort, E. H. M., Cleutjens, J. P. M. and Bosman, F. T. (1989) Basement membrane deposition in benign and malignant naevo-melanocytic lesions: an immunohistochemical study with antibodies to type IV collagen and laminin. *Histopathology*, **15**, 137–46.

Howat, A. J., Wright, A. L., Cotton, D. W. K., Reeve, S. and Bleehen, S. S. (1990) AgNORs in benign, dysplastic and malignant melanocytic skin lesions. *Am. J. Dermatopathol.*, **12**, 156–61.

Inoshita, T. and Youngberg, G. A. (1982) Fluorescence of melanoma cells. A useful diagnostic tool. *Am. J. Clin. Pathol.*, **78**, 311–5.

Jundt, G., Schultz, A., Paul, E., Cochran, A. J. and Herschman, H. R. (1986) S-100 protein in amelanotic melanoma. A convenient immunocytochemical approach compared to electron microscopy. *Pathol. Res. Pract.*, **181**, 37–44.

Karnovsky, M. J. (1965) A formaldehyde-glutaraldehyde fixative of high osmolality for use in electron microscopy. *J. Cell Biol.*, **27**, 137A–8A.

Kirkham, N., Price, M. L., Gibson, B., Leigh, I. M., Coburn, P. and Darley, C. R. (1989) Type VII collagen antibody LH7.2 identifies basement membrane characteristics of thin malignant melanomas. *J. Pathol.*, **157**, 243–7.

Laidlaw, G. F. and Blackberg, S. N. (1932) Melanoma studies; DOPA reaction in normal histology. *Am. J. Pathol.*, **8**, 491–8.

Landthaler, M., Braun-Falco, O., Leitl, A., Konz, B. and Hölzel, D. (1989) Excisional biopsy as the first therapeutic procedure versus primary wide excision of malignant melanoma. *Cancer*, **64**, 1612–6.

Lehmann, J. M., Holzmann, B., Breitbart, E. W., Schmiegelow, P., Riethmüller, G. and Johnsen, J. P. (1987) Discrimination between benign and malignant cells of melanocytic lineage by two novel antigens, a glycoprotein with a molecular weight of 113,000 and a protein with a molecular weight of 76,000. *Cancer Res.*, **47**, 841–5.

Leitinger, G., Cerroni, L., Soyer, H. P., Smolle, J. and Kerl, H. (1990) Morphometric diagnosis of melanocytic skin tumors. *Am. J. Dermatopathol*, **12**, 441–5.

Leong, A. S. and Gilham, P. (1989) Silver staining of nucleolar organizer regions in malignant melanoma and melanocytic nevi. *Hum. Pathol.*, **20**, 257–62.

Lindholm, C. and Hofer, P.-A. (1986) Caryometry of benign compound acquired naevi, Spitz epithelioid naevi and malignant melanomas. *Acta Pathol. Microbiol. Immunol. Scand. Sect. A.*, **94**, 371–4.

Maeda, K. and Jimbow, K. (1987) Development of MoAb HMSA-2 for melanosomes of human melanoma and its application to immunohistopathologic diagnosis of neoplastic melanocytes. *Cancer*, **59**, 415–23.

Maeda, K., Maeda, K. and Jimbow, K. (1988) Specification and use of a mouse monoclonal antibody raised against melanosomes for the histopathologic diagnosis of amelanotic malignant melanoma. *Cancer*, **62**, 926–34.

McGovern, J. and Crocker, J. (1987) The effect of melanin pigment removal on the peroxidase-antiperoxidase immunoperoxidase technic. *Am J. Clin. Pathol.*, **88**, 480–3.

McGovern, V. J., Cochran, A. J., Van der Esch, E. P., Little, J. H. and MacLennan, R. (1986) The classification of malignant melanoma, its histological reporting and registration: a revision of the 1972 Sydney classification. *Pathology*, **18**, 12–21.

Mehregan, A. H. and Pinkus, H. (1966) Artifacts in dermal histopathology. *Arch. Dermatol.*, **94**, 218–25.

Nakanishi, T. and Hashimoto, K. (1987) The differential reactivity of benign and malignant nevomelanocytic lesions with mouse monoclonal antibody TNKH1. *Cancer*, **59**, 1340–4.

Natali, P. G., Aguzzi, A., Veglia, F. *et al.* (1983) The impact of monoclonal antibodies on the study of human malignant melanoma. *J. Cutan. Pathol.*, **10**, 514–28.

Ordónez, N. G., Xiaolong, J. and Hichey, R. C. (1988) Comparison of HMB-45 monoclonal antibody and S-100 protein in the immunohistochemical diagnosis of melanoma. *Am. J. Clin. Pathol.*, **90**, 385–90.

Palazzo, J. and Duray, P. H. (1989) Typical dysplastic, congenital, and Spitz nevi: a comparative immunohistochemical study. *Hum. Pathol.*, **20**, 341–6.

Rampen, F. H. J. and Van der Esch, E. P. (1985) Biopsy and survival of malignant melanoma. *J. Am. Acad. Dermatol.*, **12**, 385–8.

Reichert, C. M., Rosenberg, S. A., Weber, B. L. and Costa, J. (1981) Malignant melanoma: a search for occult lymph node metastases. *Hum. Pathol.*, **12**, 449–51.

Rennison, A., Duff, C. and McPhie, J. L. (1987) Electron microscopic identification of aberrant melanosomes using a combined DOPA/Warthin-Starry technique. *J. Pathol.*, **152**, 333–6.

Rhodes, A. R., Seki, Y., Fitzpatrick, T. B. and Stern, R. S. (1988) Melanosomal alterations in dysplastic melanocytic nevi. A quantitative, ultrastructural investigation. *Cancer*, **61**, 358–69.

Rodriguez, H. A. and McGavran, M. H. (1969) A modified DOPA reaction for the diagnosis and investigation of pigment cells. *Am. J. Clin. Pathol.*, **52**, 219–27.

Rosai, J. (1989) *Ackerman's Surgical Pathology*. St. Louis: C. V. Mosby, pp. 1871,1913–6.

Roses, D. F., Harris, M. N. and Ackerman, A. B. (1983) *Diagnosis and Management of Cutaneous Malignant Melanoma*. Philadelphia: W. B. Saunders.

Ruiter, D. J., Bhan, A. K., Harrist, T. J., Sober, A. J. and Mihm, M. C. (1982) Major histocompatibility antigens and mononuclear inflammatory infiltrate in benign nevomelanocytic proliferations and malignant melanoma. *J. Immunol.*, **129**, 2808–15.

Ruiter, D. J., Bergman, W., Welvaart, K., Scheffer, E., Van Vloten, W., Russo, C. and Ferrone, S. (1984) Immunohistochemical analysis of malignant melanomas and nevocellular nevi with monoclonal antibodies to distinct monomorphic determinants of HLA antigens. *Cancer Res.*, **44**, 3930–5.

Ruiter, D. J., Dingjan, G. M., Steijlen, P. M., Van Beveren-Hooijer, M. T., De Graaff-Reitsma, C. B., Bergman, W., Van Muijen, G. N. P. and Warnaar, S. O. (1985) Monoclonal antibodies selected to discriminate between malignant melanomas and nevocellular nevi. *J. Invest. Dermatol.*, **85**, 4–8.

Sagebiel, R. W. (1972) Histologic artifacts of benign pigmented nevi. *Arch. Dermatol.*, **106**, 691–3.

Senba, M. (1986) Staining properties of melanin and lipofuscin pigments. *Am. J. Clin. Pathol.*, **86**, 556.

Smolle, J., Soyer, H.-P. and Kerl, H. (1989) Proliferative activity of cutaneous melanocytic tumors defined by Ki-67 monoclonal antibody. A quantitative immunohistochemical study. *Am. J. Dermatopathol.*, **11**, 301–7.

Smoller, B. R., McNutt, N. S. and Hsu, A. (1989a) HMB-45 recognizes stimulated melanocytes. *J. Cutan. Pathol.*, **16**, 49–53.

Smoller, B. R., McNutt, N. S. and Hsu, A. (1989b) HMB-45 staining of dysplastic nevi. Support for a spectrum of progression toward melanoma. *Am. J. Surg. Pathol.*, **13**, 680–4.

Stevens, A. (1977) Pigments and minerals. In *Theory and Practice of Histological Techniques* (eds J. D. Bancroft and A. Stevens), Edinburgh: Churchill Livingstone, pp. 186–208.

Sun, J., Morton, T. H. and Gown, A. M. (1990) Antibody HMB-45 identifies the cells of blue naevi. An immunohistochemical study on paraffin sections. *Am. J. Surg. Pathol.*, **14**, 748–51.

Takahashi, H., Yamana, K., Maeda, K., Akutsu, Y., Horikoshi, T. and Jimbow, K. (1987) Dysplastic melanocytic nevus. Electron-microscopic observation as a diagnostic tool. *Am. J. Dermatopathol.*, **9**, 189–97.

Urist, M. M., Balch, C. M. and Milton, G. W. (1985) Surgical management of the primary melanoma. In *Cutaneous Melanoma. Clinical Management and Treatment Results Worldwide* (eds C. M. Balch and G. W. Milton) Philadelphia: J. B. Lippincott Co., pp. 71–92.

Van Duinen, S. G., Ruiter, D. J. and Scheffer, E. (1983) A staining procedure for melanin in semithin and ultrathin epoxy sections. *Histopathology*, **7**, 35–47.

Van Vreeswijk, H., Ruiter, D. J., Bröcker, E. B., Welvaart, K. and Ferrone, S. (1988) Differential expression of HLA-DR, DQ and DP antigens in primary and metastatic melanoma. *J. Invest. Dermatol.*, **90**, 755–60.

Vecchio, T. J. (1966) Predictive value of a single diagnostic test in unselected populations. *New Engl. J. Med.*, **274**, 1171–3.

Warkel, R. L., Luna, L. G. and Helwig, E. B. (1980) A modified Warthin-Starry procedure at low pH for melanin. *Am. J. Clin. Pathol.*, **73**, 812–5.

West, K. P., Priyakumar, P., Jagjivan, R. and Colloby, P. S. (1989) Can HLA-DR expression help in the routine diagnosis of malignant melanomas? *Br. J. Dermatol.*, **121**, 175–8.

3 Cutaneous Pigmented lesions not related to melanocytic naevi

Before discussing the spectrum of cutaneous melanocytic naevi and melanomas, it is useful to discuss briefly the large variety of cutaneous pigmented lesions unrelated to these entities. We shall restrict ourselves largely to lesions in which increased melanin production is an essential and sometimes striking feature; the large variety of cutaneous lesions which may show only slight increase in pigmentation of the epidermal basal layer, or which may be pigmented macroscopically for other reasons, will not be discussed. Other lesions, which appear pigmented clinically largely because of epidermal hyperkeratosis, often associated with papillomatosis, such as linear epidermal naevus, acanthosis nigricans and hypertrophic solar keratosis, will be referred to briefly.

3.1 Generalized and regional hyperpigmentation

A large number of physiological and pathological stimuli, exogenous or endogenous, systemic or localized to the skin, lead to a generalized or regional increase or decrease in cutaneous pigmentation, mainly by way of alterations in melanin production by the epidermal melanocytes. Most of these are a matter of clinical rather than histological diagnosis and are the subject of several recent reviews in the dermatological literature (Fulk, 1984; Bolognia and Pawelek, 1988). Some of the causes of epidermal hyperpigmentation are listed in Table 3.1, but the reader is referred to the reviews mentioned and to dermatological textbooks for a detailed discussion of these entities.

Exposure to light, especially *ultraviolet light*, leads to increased melanin production and transfer ('tanning'). Histologically, a slightly increased pigmentation of basal epidermal keratinocytes is seen. In the short term, the melanocytes do not increase in numbers appreciably, but, over the course of years, chronic exposure to sunlight does lead to a slight increase in number of epidermal melanocytes (p. 2).

During *pregnancy* or *oestrogen treatment*, and rarely in patients

Table 3.1 Some causes of increased general or regional skin pigmentation

Exogenous factors
  Sunlight
  Other UV sources; PUVA treatment
  Ionizing radiation
  Heat
  Chronic mechanical trauma
  Drugs (e.g. minocycline, adriamycin, busulfan, methotrexate)

'Postinflammatory hyperpigmentation'
  Many forms of cutaneous inflammatory disease
  Lichen planus
  Psoriasis
  Systemic and discoid lupus erythematosus
  Chronic solar dermatosis

Endocrine influences
  Chloasma (melasma) of pregnancy
  Oestrogen treatment
  Addison's disease
  Hyperthyroidism
  Acromegaly
  Cushing's syndrome
  ACTH and MSH-producing tumours

Dietary deficiencies
  Kwashiorkor
  Avitaminosis A
  Scurvy
  Pellagra
  Sprue

Genetically determined diseases
  Neurofibromatosis
  Albright's syndrome
  Xeroderma pigmentosum

Metabolic disorders
  Gaucher's disease
  Niemann-Pick's disease
  Wilson's disease (hepatolenticular disease)
  Haemochromatosis

Neoplasms
  Disseminated melanoma
  Cutaneous mastocytoma

with ovarian neoplasms or in the absence of a known cause, there is a varying degree of activation of cutaneous melanocytes, which is clinically apparent as darkening and sometimes growth of naevi, and as a generalized increase in cutaneous pigmentation, which is most apparent in those parts of the face most exposed to sunlight: this is known as *chloasma* or *melasma* (Sanchez *et al.*, 1981).

Increased melanin production is similarly produced by *ionizing radiation*, *heat*, and *chronic mechanical trauma*, such as friction. In these instances, there is usually in addition some degree of dermal fibrosis with increased vascularity, and pigment incontinence.

The differential diagnosis of these forms of cutaneous hyperpigmentation generally does not require biopsies; the histology of the increased pigmentation is non-specific, consisting of increased pigmentation of epidermal keratinocytes with or without enlargement of melanocytes, and some perivascular melanophages.

3.2   Ephelis (freckle)

Freckles are small lightly pigmented macules, often with an irregular border but with a sharp demarcation, usually under 3 mm in diameter, often occurring together in groups, in which case they may become confluent to form larger, irregularly bordered macules. They arise on sun-exposed skin of susceptible individuals, especially fair-skinned persons with blonde or red hair and blue eyes. They are often absent or barely visible in winter, but appear and darken during the summer months. Usually they develop in childhood and they often fade during adult life.

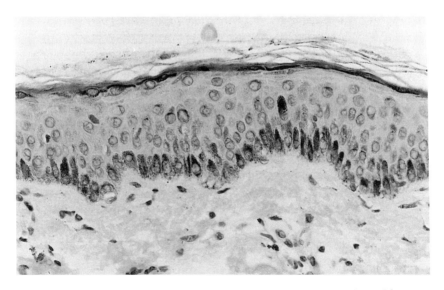

Figure 3.1   Ephelis (freckle). There is epidermal hyperpigmentation without an increase in number of melanocytes (HE, × 370).

Histologically, freckles consist of an area of hyperpigmentation of the epidermal basal cell layer, sometimes accompanied by the presence of a few melanophages near the superficial dermal vessels (Figure 3.1). Epidermal melanocytes are strongly DOPA-positive and may be enlarged, but they are not increased in number; indeed, their number is often slightly decreased (Breathnach, 1957). There is no epidermal proliferation as in lentigo simplex (p. 57). The skin appendages are not involved (Table 3.2).

Naevus spilus is a term used by some to designate a well-defined patch of uniformly light to dark brown pigmentation, with the histological features of ephelis, the only distinguishing feature being its larger size (Stewart *et al.*, 1978); in addition, some of these lesions show slight epidermal acanthosis and papillomatosis. Others, however, have used the term naevus spilus as a synonym of speckled lentiginous naevus (p. 153).

A pigmented lesion similar to a freckle occurs on the vermilion border of the lip, usually the lower lip of a female patient. It has been described as *solitary labial lentigo* (Shapiro and Zegarelli, 1971). This name is unfortunate in that there is no apparent increase in number of melanocytes in this lesion.

Table 3.2 Ephelis

Clinical features
  Small light-brown macules, usually multiple
  Occur in sun-exposed areas of the skin and arise or become more
    pronounced after increased exposure to sunlight (summer)
  Occur mainly in light-skinned people with blonde or reddish hair

Histological features
  Mild hyperpigmentation of basal epidermal keratinocytes
  Slight prominence but no increased number of melanocytes
  Normal epidermal architecture, no elongation of rete ridges
  Occasional melanophages in upper dermis.

3.3   Solar lentigo (senile lentigo; 'liver spot')

Solar lentigo is a small, darkly pigmented macule, occurring on chronically sun-exposed skin, usually in elderly persons. Despite some superficial histological resemblances to simple lentigo (p. 61), it is an altogether different lesion, related to seborrhoeic keratosis rather than to melanocytic naevi.

Histologically, most cases show elongation of rete ridges, which are slender but show an irregular, often branching contour. In some cases, rete ridges are short and club-shaped. There is increased pigmentation

Table 3.3 Solar lentigo

Clinical features
    Small pigmented macule, not palpable, occurring on sun-exposed skin

Histological features
    Irregular, club-shaped or thin, elongated rete ridges
    Increased pigmentation of epidermis
    Melanocytes normal or slightly increased in numbers
    Slight perivascular round cell infiltrate and melanophages in upper dermis
        often present
    Subepidermal fibrosis often present

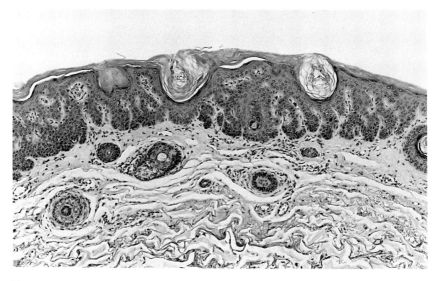

Figure 3.2   Solar lentigo. Slightly irregular elongation of epidermal rete ridges associated with mild hyperpigmentation (HE, × 90).

of the basal and suprabasal layers; however, melanocytes are normal in number (Table 3.3; Figure 3.2). When the epidermal proliferation is very pronounced, there is a gradual transition to the reticulated type of seborrhoeic keratosis.

3.4   Café-au-lait spot

Café-au-lait spots are uniformly pigmented pale brown macules, either congenital or acquired, which may reach a size of more than 1 cm, and most commonly occur on the trunk and lower limbs (Kopf *et al.*, 1985).

They are present in only about 10% of the general population, but in 90% of neurofibromatosis patients. They also show an association with spina bifida, various neurocutaneous syndromes, tuberous sclerosis, fibrous dysplasia of bone, Albright's syndrome and a variety of other rare syndromes (Fulk, 1984).

Histologically, the café-au-lait spots exhibit basal hyperpigmentation of the epidermis, some increase in number of melanocytes, hyperactive melanin synthesis as indicated by strong positivity in the DOPA reaction and, most often when associated with neurofibromatosis, macromelanosomes (p. 7).

3.5   Becker's naevus (pigmented hairy epidermal naevus)

Becker's naevus (Becker, 1949; Copeman & Wilson-Jones, 1965; Table 3.4) initially presents as an irregularly shaped area of uniformly increased pigmentation, up to 20 cm or more in diameter. The shoulder, chest and lower back are preferred sites. It usually develops in children, adolescents or young adults, most commonly in males. There may be a history of sunburn. In males, hypertrichosis often develops after several years; in this phase, the clinical appearance may suggest a congenital hairy naevus (p. 138), but the patient's history will clarify that the lesion is acquired rather than congenital. However, a very similar but congenital lesion has occasionally been reported (Karo and Gange, 1981; Slipman *et al.*, 1985). Androgen stimulation may be of importance in its pathogenesis (Person and Longcope, 1984).

Histologically there is increased epidermal pigmentation, but only a mild increase in epidermal melanocytes (Tate *et al.*, 1980). In contrast to congenital naevus, junctional nests and intradermal naevus cells are absent. The epidermis often shows mild acanthosis. Some dermal mel-

Table 3.4 Becker's naevus (pigmented hairy epidermal naevus)

Clinical features
   Irregularly shaped, evenly pigmented area of skin
   Appears mostly in childhood, adolescence, or early adulthood
   Males more commonly affected
   Hypertrichosis may develop
   Shoulder, chest and lower back preferred sites
   Association with previous sunburn in some cases

Histological features
   Mild acanthosis and increased epidermal pigmentation
   Mild increase in number of epidermal melanocytes
   Hypertrichosis and hyperplasia of arrector pili muscles in some cases

anophages are often seen. There is often hypertrichosis; terminal hairs may show follicular plugging and comedo formation.

In some cases, the hair arrector muscles are abnormally prominent. However, smooth muscle hamartomas may also occur in the absence of epidermal hyperpigmentation (Slipman *et al.*, 1985). Because of the occurrence of such partly overlapping and partly dissimilar lesions, there is some argument about the proper use of the term Becker's naevus.

In contrast to giant congenital naevus, Becker's naevus is not primarily a melanocytic tumour; there is no increased risk of melanoma.

3.6   Xeroderma pigmentosum

In this dominantly inherited disorder of DNA repair, sunlight-induced damage of the skin develops in exposed areas at an early age. Irregular hyperpigmentation is seen and later, various cutaneous malignant neoplasms develop, of which melanoma is the most important. Histologically, xeroderma pigmentosum is evidenced by epidermal atrophy and hyperkeratosis, focal irregular lentiginous elongation of rete ridges, and irregular epidermal pigmentation. In some lesions, there is an increase in number of melanocytes, in a lentiginous pattern or with the formation of nests (p. 60). The epidermal keratinocytes and melanocytes may exhibit some cytological atypia. Extensive freckling of the skin with similar histological features is rarely produced by PUVA treatment and excessive use of sunbeds (Jones *et al.*, 1987; Williams *et al.*, 1988).

Table 3.5 Reactive hyperpigmentation and melanocyte colonization

---

Cutaneous epithelial lesions
   Solar lentigo
   Seborrhoeic keratosis
   Actinic keratosis
   Melanoacanthoma
   Basal cell carcinoma
   Squamous cell carcinoma
   Hair follicle tumours
   Sweat gland tumours
   Mammary and extramammary Paget's disease
   Clear cell acanthoma
   Keratoacanthoma
Carcinomas of internal organs reaching the epidermis
? Merkel cell carcinoma
? Bednar tumour

3.7 Reactive pigmentation and melanocyte colonization of tumours

Some cutaneous non-melanocytic tumours stimulate pre-existent melanocytes to produce increased amounts of melanin, which may either be transferred to the tumour cells or accumulate in melanocytic dendrites ('pigment transfer block'). This phenomenon is most often seen in coloured patients. In some instances, the melanocytes also proliferate and travel through the tumour itself ('*melanocyte colonization*'; Masson, 1925; Azzopardi and Eusebi, 1977). Such hyperactive and proliferating melanocytes are dendritic and, especially when there is a partial or complete pigment transfer block, the dendrites are engorged with melanin and stand out conspicuously. Apart from the presence of melanin and dendritic melanocytes, these tumours are histologically and biologically identical to their non-pigmented counterparts (Table 3.5).

Of these cutaneous lesions, *solar lentigo* (p. 39), *seborrhoeic keratosis* and *pigmented basal cell carcinoma* (Figure 3.3; Zelickson, 1967; Bleehen, 1975) are perhaps the most common examples. *Dermatosis papulosa nigra* consists of numerous small seborrhoeic keratoses emerging in child-

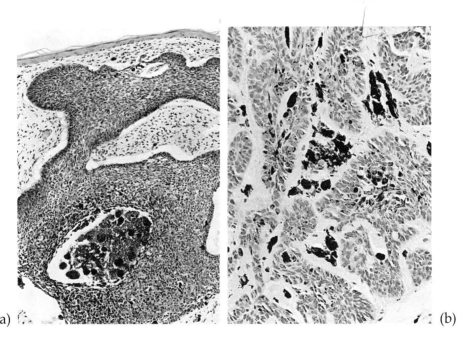

(a)   (b)

Figure 3.3 Pigmented basal cell carcinoma. (a) Melanin accumulates mainly within the necrotic centre of a tumour cell nest (HE, × 90). (b) Melanophages within tumour stroma (HE, × 185).

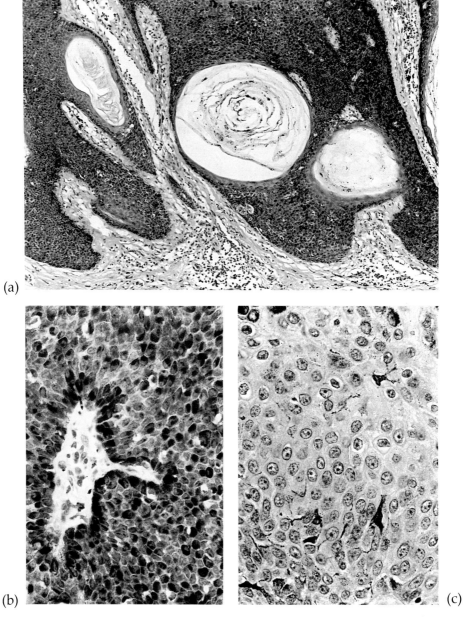

Figure 3.4 Heavily pigmented seborrhoeic keratosis. (a) Varying degrees of pigmentation and characteristic inclusions of horn (HE/Masson Fontana, × 90). (b) In some areas, as in this field, keratinocytes are heavily pigmented, whereas melanocytes are inconspicuous (HE/Masson Fontana, × 370). (c) In other areas of the same lesion, there is a 'pigment transfer block': keratinocytes are not pigmented, whereas dendritic melanocytes engorged with melanin are present throughout the epithelium (HE/Masson Fontana, × 370).

hood, on the face and neck region; it occurs in negroid and some oriental races. *Melanoacanthoma* of the skin (Mishima and Pinkus, 1960; Schlappner *et al.*, 1978) is a pigmented seborrhoeic keratosis, which in addition exhibits markedly increased numbers of dendritic melanocytes, which colonize the epithelial proliferation so that they are present at all levels rather than only in the basal layer. Increased numbers of melanocytes and some degree of migration through the epithelium is very common in heavily pigmented seborrhoeic keratosis, especially in areas where pigment accumulates in melanocytes rather than in keratinocytes (pigment transfer block; Figure 3.4). Therefore, melanoacanthoma appears to be the extreme end of a continuous spectrum rather than constituting a separate entity. *Verrucous naevus, naevus unius lateris, ichthyosis hystrix* and *acanthosis nigricans* show epidermal hyperkeratosis, papillomatosis and acanthosis as well as some degree of epidermal hyperpigmentation.

Other examples of reactive hyperpigmentation occur in *actinic keratosis, squamous carcinoma* (Lund and Chesner, 1953; James *et al.*, 1978), *eccrine poroma, nodular hidradenoma* (Wilson-Jones, 1971; Azzopardi and Eusebi, 1977), *keratoacanthoma* (Figure 3.5) and *hair follicle tumours*, especially *pilomatricoma* where the melanocytic proliferation may be very pronounced indeed (Cazers *et al.*, 1974; Zaim, 1987), and *pigmented follicular cyst* (Mehregan and Medenica, 1982). In *clear cell acanthoma* (Figure 3.6), melanocytes colonize the acanthotic epithelium to varying degrees, which may be associated with increased epithelial pigmentation or with a pigment transfer block (Naeyaert *et al.*, 1987; Fanti *et al.*, 1990). In exceptional cases, *Merkel cell carcinoma* contains some melanin pigment. This tumour shows a diffuse growth pattern or forms ribbons and trabeculae, and is characterized by numerous mitoses, apoptosis and small nucleoli. The nuclei are small or middle-sized, show a finely grained structure or are finely vacuolated, and have a violet tinge. Characteristically, there is a paranuclear dot-like keratin positivity, and chromogranin and neurofilament are positive.

No doubt, this list is not complete since, apparently, a large variety of epithelial proliferations and neoplasms of the skin can at times be pigmented by pre-existent melanocytes.

3.7.1 Mammary and extramammary Paget's disease

The tumor cells in Paget's disease of the nipple and extramammary Paget's disease sometimes contain melanin pigment derived from epidermal dendritic melanocytes (Neubecker and Bradshaw, 1961; Jones *et al.*, 1979), which may have increased in number. Paget's disease of the nipple is caused by a propagation of mammary adenocarcinoma

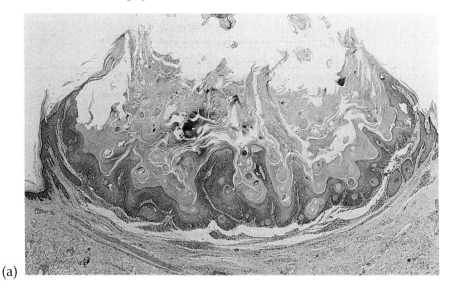

(a)

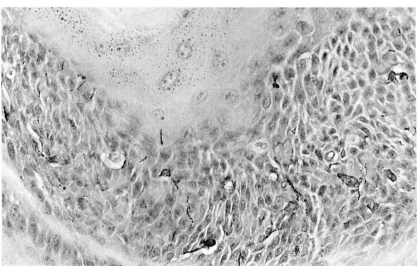

(b)

Figure 3.5   Keratoacanthoma. (a) Characteristic architecture (HE, × 20). (b) Dendritic melanocytes colonizing the epithelium (HE, × 370).

cells which reach the epidermis of the nipple, and therefore indicates the presence of an underlying tumour. In contrast, the large majority of cases of extramammary Paget's disease originate primarily within the skin (Jones *et al.*, 1979); they are most commonly found in vulvar, perianal, penile, scrotal and axillary sites.

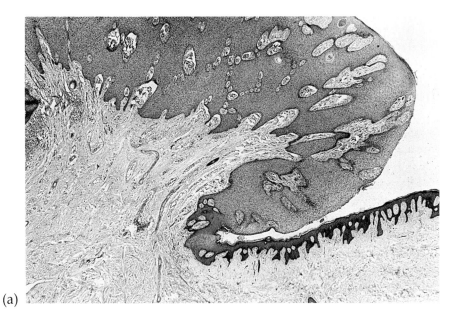

(a)

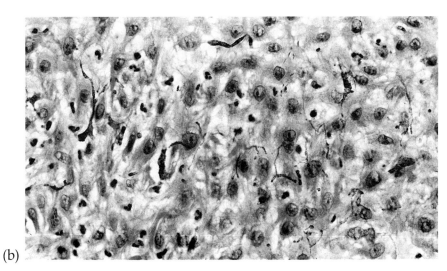

(b)

Figure 3.6 Clear cell acanthoma. (a) Low power view (HE, × 20). (b) Heavily pigmented dendritic melanocytes and also neutrophils are seen between non-pigmented, large, pale keratinocytes (HE, × 370).

It should be realized that melanoma of any type is exceptionally rare in the nipple and even in the areola, a little known fact that has never been explained. Therefore, in the differential diagnosis with melanoma, extramammary Paget's disease is the most important one.

The tumour cells of mammary and extramammary Paget's disease are similar: they are large, with well-developed, pale, sometimes vacuolated cytoplasm, and a usually prominent and often vesicular nucleus, containing a prominent nucleolus. The nucleus may have been pushed to one side by an intracytoplasmic mucin vacuole. These cells are scattered at all levels of the epidermis; this pattern of spread resembles that of many melanomas, where it is known as 'pagetoid spread'. When there is also melanotic pigmentation of the Paget cells, the lesion resembles melanoma *in situ* even more closely.

Usually, the differential diagnosis poses little problems if, for instance, a heavily pigmented superficial spreading melanoma shows invasion into the dermis or, alternatively, when mucin is detected in Paget cells. The features differentiating Paget's disease from melanoma are given in Table 3.6.

In superficial spreading melanoma, solitary cells and nests usually abut the dermis, while in extramammary Paget's disease the basal layer of the epidermis is generally only replaced by tumour cells when there are large sheets or confluent nests; suprabasal localization of solitary cells and nests is more typical of Paget's disease. Nests in Paget's disease are mostly neatly ovoid, and there may be glandular differentiation, whereas in superficial spreading melanoma nests are often somewhat irregularly shaped. Extensive involvement of the cutaneous adnexae is much more characteristic of extracutaneous Paget's disease than of melanoma.

When compared to melanoma cells, the tumour cells of Paget's disease are usually slightly larger, perhaps more consistently polygonal or rounded, and have generally more vesicular nuclei with more prominent nucleoli; however, there is much overlap with the cellular features of melanoma. Mitoses are generally much more numerous in extramammary Paget's disease. The cytoplasm is vacuolated and often distinctly haematoxyphil, and often positive with mucin stains. Classical signet ring cells are seen in over half of cases of extramammary Paget's disease. Any melanin present in Paget cells is of the coarse, refractile granular type, and usually sparse.

Furthermore, one should appreciate the presence of two distinct cell populations; tumour cells and reactive dendritic melanocytes. Finally, immunostains for S-100, EMA, CEA and several anti-keratin antibodies such as CAM 5.2 will reveal the epithelial nature of the tumour cells (Guldhammer and Nørgaard, 1986; Russell Jones *et al.*, 1989; Figure 3.7). It is important to use a panel of antibodies rather than to rely on

Table 3.6 Extramammary Paget's disease *vs* melanoma

Extramammary Paget's disease	Superficial spreading melanoma
Nests and solitary cells characteristically suprabasal; sheets in some areas replace basal layer	Cells at dermoepidermal junction as well as above it
Often more massive epidermal replacement	Less massive replacement of epidermis
Single cells often predominate	Nests usually predominate, even at edge
Glandular differentiation common	No glandular differentiation
Extensive involvement of adnexae	Less adnexal involvement
Clefts between tumour cells and keratinocytes very common	Clefts less common
Nuclei usually vesicular, nucleoli more prominent	Nuclei variably stained, often darker
Mitoses numerous	Mitoses usually less common
Vacuolated or haematoxyphil cytoplasm, mucin-containing, signet ring cells often present	Pale grey-brown cytoplasm, no mucin
Melanin uncommon; when present, few coarse granules	Often dusty melanin
Hyperplasia epidermis usually prominent	Hyperplasia epidermis usually less prominent
Inflammatory infiltrate dermis striking	Inflammatory infiltrate variable
Neutrophils in epidermis common	Neutrophils in epidermis rare

one antibody only; weak S-100 positivity was found in one out of 19 cases of Paget's disease of the nipple, but in this instance, the tumour cells were strongly positive for keratin (Reed *et al.*, 1990).

3.7.2 *Melanocyte colonization of carcinomas invading the skin*

Some degree of melanocyte colonization is seen in the majority of *breast carcinomas* invading through the dermis to reach the overlying epidermis (Azzopardi and Eusebi, 1977); it is present mainly in the vicinity of the epidermis. The melanocytes transfer melanin *via* thin dendrites to adjacent tumour cells. In most cases, pigmentation is only focally present and only apparent when melanin stains are used. The overlying epidermis may show patchy depigmentation. However, markedly increased melanin production may rarely occur, resulting in

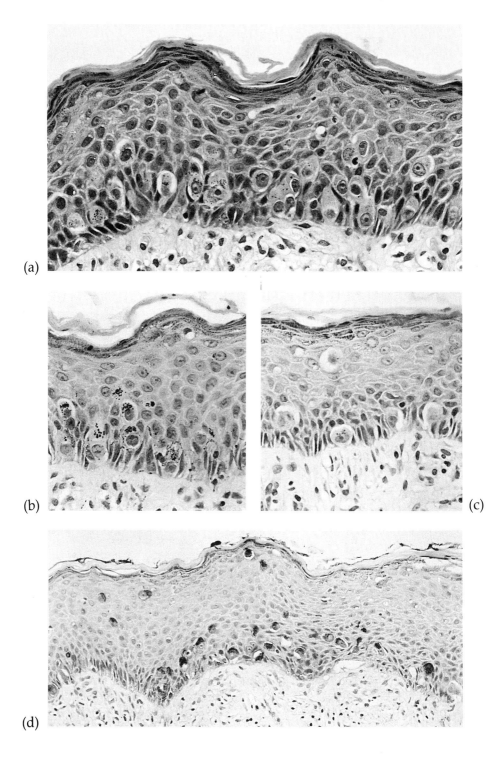

(a)

(b)

(c)

(d)

heavy pigmentation and a close clinical and histological resemblance to melanoma (Sau *et al.*, 1989). In one instance, Azzopardi and Eusebi (1977) found melanocytes in tumour emboli within lymph vessels; this explains why these non-neoplastic melanocytes may occasionally reach metastatic sites (Lund and Chesner, 1953).

Similar pigmentation due to melanocytic colonization may also occur in other carcinomas invading the epidermis, such as adenocarcinoma of the rectum (Chumas and Lorelle, 1981).

3.8   Pigmented dermatofibrosarcoma protuberans (Bednar tumour)

In about 5% of cases, dermatofibrosarcoma protuberans contains a small population of scattered, dendritic pigmented cells. There are no obvious clinicopathological differences between these pigmented tumours and their non-pigmented counterparts, except that they are more common in non-Caucasian patients. The tumour affects both sexes equally and occurs from early childhood to old age, but most commonly arises in early or middle adulthood. There is a predilection for the trunk, especially the shoulder region, and proximal extremities. The tumour grows slowly, with a characteristic combination of exophytic and infiltrative growth. It thus often forms a 'protuberant' nodule or tumour, or several such nodules; alternatively, a plaque-type of growth may be seen. If left untreated, the tumour reaches a large size and eventually ulcerates. The irregular lateral and downward spread is associated with a risk of incomplete excision and recurrence, which occurs in about 30% of cases. Metastasis is, however, exceedingly rare (Bednar, 1957; Dupree *et al.*, 1985; Fletcher *et al.*, 1988).

Macroscopically, the tumour is firm, usually protrudes above the level of the epidermis, and in contrast to the microscopically evident irregular infiltrative spread, often appears well demarcated (Dupree *et al.*, 1985). The tumour is usually grey or white, but some are focally or wholly darkly pigmented. Recurrences may form multiple nodules.

Histologically, the tumour is located in the dermis, usually abutting on the epidermis, often without a subepidermal free 'Grenz' zone, which contrasts with non-pigmented dermatofibrosarcoma, in which sparing of the papillary dermis is not uncommon (Fletcher *et al.*, 1988).

◀ **Figure 3.7**   Pigmented Paget's disease of the nipple. (a) Large, pale, solitary tumour cells are situated mainly above the dermoepidermal junction (HE, × 370). (b) Melanin granules are present in most tumour cells (HE/Masson Fontana, × 370). (c) Tumour cells negative for S-100 protein (Immunoperoxidase, × 370). (d) Tumour cells strongly positive for EMA (Immunoperoxidase, × 185).

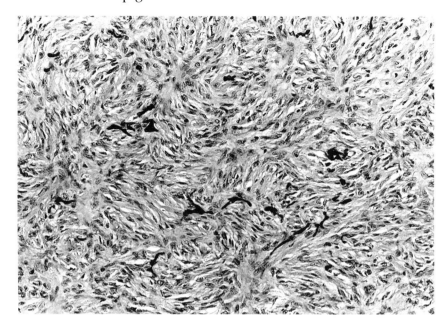

Figure 3.8 Bednar tumour. Heavily pigmented dendritic melanocytes are scattered between fusiform tumour cells arranged in a storiform pattern (HE, × 185).

The tumour spreads laterally and downward, engulfing cutaneous adnexae, and usually extending diffusely into the subcutis. It consists of uniform spindle cells arranged in conspicuous storiform and sometimes fascicular patterns. Mitoses are scarce and there is no necrosis. Foam cells and multinucleate tumour cells are usually absent. Scattered between the tumour cells, pigmented elongated cells, often with branching dendrites, are present (Figure 3.8). These cells vary considerably in number. Immunohistochemically, the tumour cells are negative for S-100 and myelin basic protein, whereas the pigmented cells are S-100 positive (Fletcher *et al.*, 1988) and show the ultrastructural features of melanocytes (Dupree *et al.*, 1985). The overlying epidermis may be hypopigmented, with a decrease in number of melanocytes (Table 3.7).

Several hypotheses as to the histogenesis of this tumour have been put forward: originally, it was considered a pigmented variant of neurofibroma (Bednar, 1957). Dupree and associates (1985) stressed the remarkable clinical and pathological similarities to dermatofibrosarcoma protuberans, but, as they considered the pigmented cells to be neoplastic, they concluded that the tumour is probably of neuroectodermal

Table 3.7 Bednar tumour (pigmented dermatofibrosarcoma protuberans)

Clinical features
  Cutaneous nodule or tumour, usually located on trunk or proximal extremity
  Affects mainly young or middle-aged adults
  More common in non-Caucasians
  Irregular lateral and downward growth, leading to high percentage of
    recurrence; metastasis extremely rare

Histological features
  Conventional features of dermatofibrosarcoma protuberans
  More often direct contact with overlying epidermis: no 'Grenz zone'
  Scattered dendritic pigmented melanocytes, mostly in middle and deeper
    parts of the tumour
  Overlying epidermis may be hypopigmented

Remarks
  Possible pathogenesis: melanocyte colonization of dermatofibrosarcoma
    protuberans

origin. Fletcher and colleagues (1988) raised the alternative possibility that the pigmented dendritic cells are melanocytes, derived from the overlying epidermis, which have colonized the tumour; however, as these workers pointed out, no breaching of the epidermal basal lamina by the tumour was detected, contrasting with melanocytic colonization of mammary carcinoma and, curiously, pigmentation is usually most prominent in the middle and deeper areas of the tumour rather than subepidermally.

References

Azzopardi, J. G. and Eusebi, V. (1977) Melanocyte colonization and pigmentation of breast carcinoma. *Histopathology*, **1**, 21–30.

Becker, S. W. (1949) Concurrent melanosis and hypertrichosis in distribution of nevus unius lateris. *Arch. Dermatol. Syph.*, **60**, 155–60.

Bednar, B. (1957) Storiform neurofibromas of the skin, pigmented and non-pigmented. *Cancer*, **10**, 368–76.

Bleehen, S. S. (1975) Pigmented basal cell epithelioma. Light and electron microscopic studies on tumours and cell cultures. *Br. J. Dermatol.*, **93**, 361–70.

Bolognia, J. L. and Pawelek, J. M. (1988) Biology of hypopigmentation. *J. Am. Acad. Dermatol.*, **19**, 217–55.

Breathnach, A. S. (1957) Melanocyte distribution in forearm epidermis of freckled human subjects. *J. Invest. Dermatol.*, **29**, 253–61.

Cazers, J. S., Okun, M. R. and Pearson, S. H. (1974) Pigmented calcifying epithelioma. Review and presentation of a case with unusual features. *Arch. Dermatol.*, **110**, 773–4.

Chumas, J. C. and Lorelle, C. A. (1981) Melanotic adenocarcinoma of the anorectum. *Am. J. Surg. Pathol.*, **5**, 711–7.

Copeman P. W. M. and Wilson-Jones, E. W. (1965) Pigmented hairy epidermal nevus (Becker). *Arch. Dermatol.*, **92**, 249–51.

Dupree, W. B., Langloss, J. M. and Weiss, S. W. (1985) Pigmented dermatofibrosarcoma protuberans (Bednar tumor). A pathologic, ultrastructural, and immunohistochemical study. *Am. J. Surg. Pathol.*, **9**, 630–9.

Fanti, P. A., Passarini, B. and Varotti C. (1990) Melanocytes in clear cell acanthoma. *Am. J. Dermatopathol.*, **12**, 373–6.

Fletcher, C. D. M., Theaker, J. M., Flanagan, A. and Krausz, T. (1988) Pigmented dermatofibrosarcoma protuberans (Bednar tumour): melanocytic colonization or neuroectodermal differentiation? A clinicopathological and immunohistochemical study. *Histopathology*, **13**, 631–43.

Fulk, C. S. (1984) Primary disorders of hyperpigmentation. *J. Am. Acad. Dermatol.*, **10**, 1–16.

Guldhammer, B. and Nørgaard, T. (1986) The differential diagnosis of intraepidermal malignant lesions using immunohistochemistry. *Am. J. Dermatopathol.*, **8**, 295–301.

James, M. P., Wells, G. C. and Whimster, I. W. (1978) Spreading pigmented actinic keratoses. *Br. J. Dermatol.*, **98**, 373–9.

Jones, R. E., Austin, C. and Ackerman, A. B. (1979) Extramammary Paget's disease. A critical reexamination. *Am. J. Dermatopathol.*, **1**, 101–32.

Jones, S. K., Moseley, H. and MacKie, R. M. (1987) UVA-induced melanocytic lesions. *Br. J. Dermatol.*, **117**, 111–5.

Karo, K. R. and Gange, R. W. (1981) Smooth-muscle hamartoma. Possible congenial Becker's nevus. *Arch. Dermatol.*, **117**, 678–9.

Kopf, A. W., Levine, L J., Rigel, D. S., Friedman, R. J. and Levenstein, M. (1985) Prevalence of congenital nevus-like nevi, and café au lait spots. *Arch. Dermatol.*, **121**, 766–9.

Lund, H. Z. and Chesner, C. (1953) Dendritic melanoblasts in metastatic squamous cell carcinoma. In *Pigment Cell Growth. Proceedings of the Third Conference on the Biology of Normal and Atypical Pigment Cell Growth*, (ed. M. Gordon), New York: Academic Press, pp. 101–7.

Masson, P. (1925) La pigmentation des cancers mammaires envahissant l'epiderme. *Ann. Anat. Pathol.*, **2**, 323–33.

Mehregan, A. H. and Medenica, M. (1982) Pigmented follicular cysts. *J. Cutan. Pathol.*, **9**, 423–7.

Mishima, Y. and Pinkus, H. (1960) Benign mixed tumor of melanocytes and malpighian cells. Melanoacanthoma: its relationship to Bloch's benign non-nevoid melanoepithelioma. *A. M. A. Arch. Dermatol.*, **81**, 539–50.

Naeyaert, J. M., De Bersaques, J., Geerts, M.-L. and Kint, A. (1987) Multiple clear cell acanthomas. A clinical, histological, and ultrastructural report. *Arch. Dermatol.*, **123**, 1670–3.

Neubecker, R. D. and Bradshaw, R. P. (1961) Mucin, melanin and glycogen in Paget's disease of the breast. *Am. J. Clin. Pathol.*, **36**, 49–53.

Person, J. R. and Longcope, C. (1984) Becker's nevus. An androgen-mediated hyperplasia with increased androgen receptors. *J. Am. Acad. Dermatol.*, **10**, 235–8.

Reed, W., Oppedal, B. R. and Egg Larsen, T. (1990) Immunohistology is valuable in distinguishing between Paget's disease, Bowen's disease and superficial spreading malignant melanoma. *Histopathology*, **16**, 583–8.

Russell Jones, R., Spaull, J. and Gusterson, B. (1989) The histogenesis of mammary and extramammary Paget's disease. *Histopathology*, **14**, 409–16.

Sanchez, N. P., Pathak, M. A., Sato, S., Fitzpatrick, T. B., Sanchez, J. L. and Mihm, M. C. (1981) Melasma: a clinical, light microscopic, ultrastructural, and immunofluorescence study. *J. Am. Acad. Dermatol.*, **4**, 698–710.

Sau, P., Solis, J., Lupton, G. P. and James, W. D. (1989) Pigmented breast carcinoma. A clinical and histopathologic simulator of malignant melanoma. *Arch. Dermatol.*, **125**, 536–9.

Schlappner, O. L. A., Rowden, G., Phillips, T. M. and Rahim, Z. (1978) Melanoacanthoma: ultrastructural and immunological studies. *J. Cutan. Pathol.*, **5**, 127–41.

Shapiro, L. and Zegarelli, D. (1971) The solitary labial lentigo: a clinicopathologic study of twenty cases. *Oral Surg. Oral Med. Oral Pathol.*, **31**, 87–92.

Slipman, N., Harrist, T. and Rhodes, A. (1985) Congenital arrector pili hamartoma. A case and review of the spectrum of Becker's melanosis and pilar smooth-muscle hamartoma. *Arch. Dermatol.*, **121**, 1034–7.

Stewart, D. M., Altman, J. and Mehregan, A. H. (1978) Speckled lentiginous nevus. *Arch. Dermatol.*, **114**, 895–6.

Tate, P., Hodge, S. and Owen, L. (1980) A quantitative study of melanocytes in Becker's nevus. *J. Cutan. Pathol.*, **7**, 404–9.

Williams, H. C., Salisbury, J., Brett, J. and Du Vivier, A. (1988) Sunbed lentigines. *Br. Med. J.*, **296**, 1097.

Wilson-Jones, E. (1971) Pigmented nodular hidradenoma. *Arch. Dermatol.*, **104**, 117–23.

Zaim, M. T. (1987) Pilomatricoma with melanocytic hyperplasia: an uncommon occurrence and a diagnostic pitfall. *Arch. Dermatol.*, **123**, 865–6.

Zelickson, A. S. (1967) The pigmented basal cell epithelioma. *Arch. Dermatol.*, **96**, 524–7.

4 Common acquired melanocytic naevi

Practically all Caucasians develop melanocytic naevi at some time during their life. The average number of naevi varies considerably according to age: they are usually absent at birth and emerge during childhood and puberty, to become most numerous in early adulthood. Subsequently, their numbers gradually diminish, so that they are again rare in old age (Nicholls, 1973; Cooke *et al.*, 1985; MacKie *et al.*, 1985). In the study of MacKie and colleagues (1985) the average number of moles in young Caucasian adults living in the United Kingdom was: 33 in females, and 22 in males. However, because of the wide variation in numbers between individuals of the same age group, it is not easy to say what constitutes an excessive number of moles.

There appear to be important *geographic differences in numbers of naevi*. In studies from New Zealand, somewhat lower numbers of naevi were reported and no difference between the sexes was found; interestingly, in a subgroup of Scottish immigrants, moles were again more common in females (Cooke *et al.*, 1985; Cooke, 1988). In an Australian study (Nicholls, 1973), naevi were more common in males and a maximal number was reached at an earlier age; possibly, differences in sunlight exposure may play a role. The emergence of moles in early childhood is associated with increased numbers later in life (MacKie *et al.*, 1985). In a recent study from Queensland, Australia (Green *et al.*, 1989), large numbers of naevi were already present in prepubertal children (an average 28 naevi). A high total number of naevi and the presence of naevi larger than 5 mm were associated with a positive family history of melanoma. Worldwide, Queensland has the highest known incidence rate of cutaneous melanoma; this further strengthens the known epidemiological links between naevi and melanoma. In a systematic study of naevi in adolescents, (Gallagher *et al.*, 1990) naevi in males were most common on the trunk and head and neck area, whereas in females, they were most common on the limbs; furthermore, intermittently exposed body sites contained more naevi. These findings parallel the anatomical distribution of melanoma in males and females and the association between intermittent sun exposure and melanoma (p. 215).

Hereditary factors and exposure to sunlight are not the only factors determining the numbers of moles. For instance, an increased number of moles was found after chemotherapy in childhood (De Wit *et al.*, 1990). Also, *eruptive naevi* and abnormally large naevi may arise after a variety of bullous dermatoses, such as erythema multiforme (Soltani *et al.*, 1979) and Lyell's syndrome (Goetz and Tsambaos, 1978), probably as a result of melanocytic hyperplasia in regenerating epidermis (Kopf *et al.*, 1977; Soltani *et al.*, 1984).

During their natural history, common acquired naevi pass through several phases which can be distinguished histologically, and often recognized clinically. They may start out as simple lentigines which turn into junctional naevi, or they may appear *de novo* as junctional naevi. Later they develop into compound and intradermal naevi, which subsequently involute, so that ultimately they disappear totally or leave a small skin-coloured papule (Maize and Foster, 1979).

In a series of 95 prepubertal melanocytic naevi (Stegmaier and Montgomery, 1953), 14 were lentigines, 47 were junctional naevi, and 34 were compound naevi. Later in life, compound and intradermal naevi are the usual types. Thus it is clear that simple lentigines, junctional naevi, compound naevi and intradermal naevi are not separate entities but constitute phases in the life cycle of one entity, the 'common acquired melanocytic naevus'.

It is generally believed that a melanoma may arise in a junctional or compound naevus, but that origin in an intradermal naevus is exceptional.

4.1 Lentigo simplex (simple lentigo, naevoid lentigo)

This first phase in the evolution of some common acquired naevi consists of a small pigmented macule, corresponding histologically to an increase in number of epidermal melanocytes, which lie as single units along the dermoepidermal junction, and which are associated with an increase in pigmentation of the adjacent and overlying keratinocytes.

4.1.1 Clinical features

Lentigo simplex appears as a small, usually darkly pigmented macule, occurring anywhere on the skin or, less commonly, the mucous membranes. The lesion is completely flat, impalpable, symmetrical, sharply circumscribed and generally does not exceed 4 mm in diameter, except on the palms and soles, external genitalia and mucous membranes, where it may be larger. It is round, oval or slightly angular. Simple lentigines usually arise in childhood, and subsequently turn into junctional, compound and intradermal naevi. However, some arise later in life (Gartmann, 1978). Those located on the palms and soles, the vermilion border of the lip and the genital skin may persist into adulthood.

Many eruptive lentigines may arise after long-term photochemotherapy or intensive use of a UV-solarium (Jones *et al.*, 1987; Williams *et al.*, 1988).

Multiple lentigines may be associated with a variety of clinical syndromes. In the *Peutz-Jeghers syndrome*, an hereditary disorder with autosomal dominant mode of transmission, pigmentation of the skin and mucous membranes in a characteristic distribution is present at birth or appears during infancy, and is associated with gastrointestinal polyposis (Dormandy, 1956). Many lentigines, and some junctional and compound naevi occur around the mouth, and sometimes on the fingers, palms, nostrils, eyes and the periumbilical skin. An important clue to the diagnosis is the presence of pigmentation of the buccal mucosa. The cutaneous pigmentations may fade in adulthood, but the buccal lesions persist. The polyps found in this syndrome occur anywhere in the gastrointestinal tract, and are usually hamartomatous, with a characteristic histology. However, adenomatous change and, occasionally, adenocarcinoma may supervene, in the stomach as well as in the small and large bowel (Narita *et al.*, 1987). Several other malignancies have also been described in the context of this syndrome.

In *centrofacial lentiginosis* (Touraine, 1941), many lentigines appear in infancy, in the infraorbital region and on the nose. In contrast to the Peutz-Jeghers syndrome, there is no involvement of the oral mucosa. In this hereditary condition, defects of the central nervous system (mental retardation, seizures) and skeleton (spina bifida, scoliosis) are common.

In *Moynahan's syndrome* (Moynahan, 1962), the presence of many cutaneous lentigines is associated with congenital mitral stenosis, dwarfism, genital hypoplasia and mental deficiency.

Many thousands of abnormally large lentigines occur in the *LEOPARD syndrome*, a disease with autosomal dominant inheritance; the name is an acronym indicating several of its features: numerous abnormally large Lentigines, Electrocardiographic abnormalities, Ocular hypertelorism, Pulmonary stenosis, Abnormalities (i.e. hypoplasia) of the gonads, Retarded growth, and neural Deafness. However, the spectrum of associated abnormalities is even wider (Voron *et al.*, 1976). Synonyms of the syndrome include 'cardiocutaneous syndrome' and 'progressive cardiocutaneous lentigines'. Development of a melanoma as well as multiple basal cell carcinomas in a 26-year-old patient with the LEOPARD syndrome was recently reported (Yong *et al.*, 1989).

Sporadic cases of large numbers of congenital cutaneous lentigines occur in the absence of other abnormalities: this has been designated *lentiginosis profusa* (Kaufmann *et al.*, 1976).

Recently, Carney (1990) described a familial syndrome including multiple cutaneous lentigines and blue naevi, melanotic schwannoma containing psammoma bodies, myxomas and a variety of endocrine overactivity syndromes (p. 391).

Large numbers of lentigines occur in *xeroderma pigmentosum*, an inherited defect of DNA-repair which leads to a high incidence of UV-induced cutaneous malignancies (Lynch *et al.*, 1977).

4.1.2 *Pathological features*

Simple lentigo consists of a proliferation of solitary melanocytes at the dermoepidermal junction (Figure 4.1). The melanocytes do not ascend into higher levels of the epidermis.

The melanocytes show normal features or exhibit a slight increase in cytoplasm. Melanin within melanocytes is usually granular rather

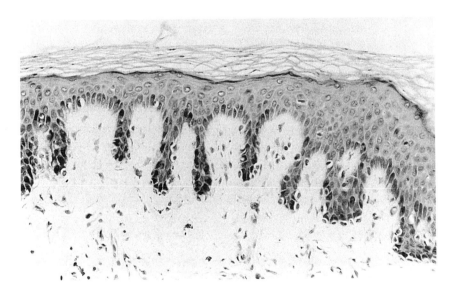

Figure 4.1 Simple lentigo. Regularly spaced, slender, elongated rete ridges; hyperpigmentation, accentuated in rete ridges; slight increase in number of melanocytes without the formation of nests (HE, × 185).

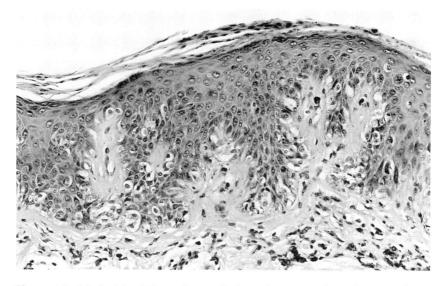

Figure 4.2   Marked lentiginous hyperplasia and some cytological atypia of melanocytes in a case of xeroderma pigmentosum. The patient developed several primary cutaneous melanomas (HE, × 185).

than dusty; very large melanosomes, known as giant melanosomes or melanin macroglobules, are not uncommon (Weiss and Zelickson, 1977; Nakagawa *et al.*, 1984). By definition, there are no nests of melanocytes. Their formation heralds the next step in the evolution of the naevus: the junctional naevus. Lentigo simplex in xeroderma pigmentosum may exhibit a very marked and irregular lentiginous proliferation of melanocytes often associated with some degree of cyto-logical atypia (Figure 4.2).

The rete ridges are elongated, thin, evenly spaced and fairly regular in appearance, with a vertical orientation. Sometimes they are slightly club-shaped. Basal keratinocytes are hyperpigmented, especially in the rete ridges. There is often mild orthokeratosis and a considerable amount of melanin may be present in suprabasal layers, including the cornified layer, resulting in a very dark-brown colour of these lesions.

Often there is a mild degree of subepidermal fibrosis, while a slight perivascular lymphocytic infiltrate with some melanophages is not uncommon.

The main diagnostic features of simple lentigo are listed in Table 4.1. Simple lentigo should be distinguished from solar (senile) lentigo, which is essentially a hyperpigmented keratinocytic proliferation rather than a melanocytic lesion (p. 39; Table 4.2).

Table 4.1 Simple lentigo

Clinical features
 Small pigmented macule, not palpable
 Occurs anywhere on the skin
 Often arises in childhood
 Large numbers of lentigines associated with UV irradiation and a variety of
  clinical syndromes (see text)

Histological features
 Thin, elongated rete ridges
 Increase in melanocytes in basal layer, but no nesting
 Prominent hyperpigmentation of basal keratinocytes
 Often hyperpigmentation of suprabasal keratinocytes; melanin in stratum
  corneum
 Slight perivascular lymphocytic infiltrate with melanophages in upper
  dermis
 Sometimes some subepidermal fibrosis

Table 4.2 Solar lentigo *vs* simple lentigo

	Solar lentigo	*Simple lentigo*
Distribution	sun-damaged skin	anywhere
Age distribution	mostly elderly persons	mostly young persons, but may persist
Rete ridges	irregular elongation, clubbing, branching	more regular elongation
Number of epidermal melanocytes	usually normal	increased
Dermis	elastosis	normal or slight fibrosis
Related lesions	reticulated type seborrhoeic keratosis	common acquired naevus

4.2   Junctional naevus

A junctional naevus, which is characterized by the presence of nests of melanocytes at the dermoepidermal junction, may develop from a lentigo simplex, or may arise *de novo*.

4.2.1   Clinical features

A junctional naevus is a symmetrical, sharply circumscribed, evenly pigmented lesion, generally smaller than 0.8 cm, although it may be somewhat larger on the palms and soles. In contrast to simple lentigo, it is just palpable, but usually not significantly raised. It may be very

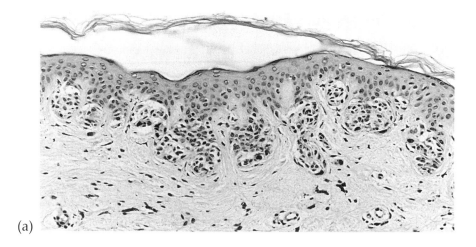

(a)

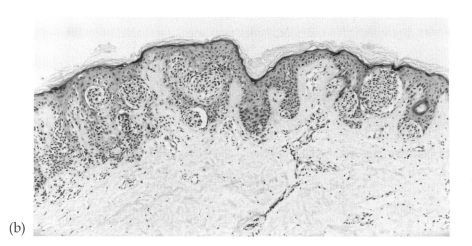

(b)

Figure 4.3   Junctional naevus. (a) Small nests of melanocytes are present, mostly at or near the tips of epidermal rete ridges (HE, × 185). (b) Another case, showing larger nests and slight papillomatosis (HE, × 90).

darkly pigmented (Eng, 1983). It most commonly arises in childhood and early adolescence. Like simple lentigines, those located on the palms and soles may persist in adulthood and such lesions have been regarded with suspicion by some authors. However, in a systematic study, naevi on palms and soles were found in no less than 5.8 and 9% of normal young adults, respectively (Allyn *et al.*, 1963); previously Van Scott and colleagues (1957) had reported an even higher figure of 26.5%. Since acrolentiginous melanoma is a rare tumour, it would appear that volar naevi do not have a clinically significant premalignant potential.

4.2.2 *Pathological features*

The junctional naevus is characterized by the presence of naevus cell nests at the dermoepidermal junction (Figure 4.3). A lentiginous proliferation of solitary melanocytes may be present as well: the hallmark of the transition of a simple lentigo to a junctional naevus is the emergence of nests ('naevus incipiens').

The nests are round or oval; the latter are usually oriented vertically. The nests show some 'rete tip preference', i.e. they are located preferentially, but by no means exclusively, at or near the tips of rete ridges. In each individual lesion, the nests tend to resemble each other in size and shape and are distributed more or less evenly, resulting in a regular and symmetrical architecture.

Table 4.3 Junctional naevus

Clinical features
  Small pigmented macule which is just palpable
  Occurs anywhere on the skin
  Usually found in childhood; junctional naevi are rare in adulthood, except on hands, feet and genital skin

Histological features
  Nests of melanocytes located mainly at the tips of rete ridges
  Increase in solitary melanocytes in basal layer often also present
  Hyperpigmentation of keratinocytes, mainly of the basal layer
  Elongation of rete ridges
  Slight perivascular inflammatory infiltrate and melanophages in upper dermis
  Sometimes subepidermal fibrosis

Remarks
  Junctional naevi may emerge from lentigines, when the proliferating melanocytes start forming nests; the distinction between lentigo and junctional naevus is not always sharp
  The emergence of small groups of melanocytes in the upper dermis marks the transition from a junctional naevus to a compound naevus

---

Generally, dendritic as well as polygonal or rounded melanocytes are seen; both types are present as solitary units as well as in nests. The melanocytes are round or oval and contain varying amounts of melanin pigment. There is only a small or moderate amount of cytoplasm, which may have collapsed against the nucleus during tissue processing. Nuclei are small or moderately sized, and in general do not exceed the size of those of adjacent basal keratinocytes. A small nucleolus may be visible. Mitoses are uncommon. Ascent of melanocytes into the upper epidermis, as seen in many melanomas, is absent or exceedingly rare (Table 4.3).

As in simple lentigo, there may be some subepidermal fibrosis, especially when there is also a lentiginous type of melanocytic proliferation. Lymphocytes and some melanophages are often seen near the superficial vascular plexus. When marked fibrosis is present, together with an uneven distribution and irregular shape of melanocytic nests, one should look for cytological atypia of melanocytes; when this is unequivocally present, the lesion is classified as a dysplastic junctional naevus (Chapter 8).

4.3   Compound naevus

At this next stage in the evolution of the common acquired naevus, nests, strands and sheets of melanocytes are present within the dermis; they are largely confined to the thickened papillary dermis. These intradermal melanocytes are derived from the junctional component, from which they bulge downward, and subsequently become surrounded wholly by increasing amounts of loose connective tissue of the papillary dermis.

4.3.1   Clinical features

Compound naevi are symmetrical, round or oval, elevated lesions, usually smaller than 0.8 cm, but occasionally slightly over 1 cm in diameter. They may be smooth-surfaced or verrucous; most are sessile but they may be pedunculated. Coarse, pigmented, terminal hairs are sometimes present. There is considerable variation between different compound naevi but the individual lesions show a similar morphology throughout the lesion.

4.3.2   Pathological features

At this stage of its development, there is still a junctional component similar to that of the junctional naevus, but part of the melanocytes, solitary as well as nests, lose their junctional location and become entrapped wholly within the thickened papillary dermis. The junctional component is often referred to as *'junctional activity'*, since the proliferating compartment of the naevus is commonly thought to be localized to that part of the naevus. However, thymidine-labelling studies (Piérard and Piérard-Franchimont, 1984) and Ki-67 immuno-staining (Smolle *et al.*, 1989) indicate that proliferating cells are also present in the dermal compartment.

The gradual loss of contact with the overlying epidermis has been called *'Abtropfung'* ('dropping off'; Unna, 1896). However, increased collagen production in the papillary dermis with entrapment of mel-anocytes of the overlying dermoepidermal junction is more likely. Intradermal melanocytes, lying as solitary units or arranged in nests, are often enveloped by a distinct basement membrane, especially in superficial parts, as visualized by immunostaining for collagen type IV.

In many compound naevi, rete tip preference of junctional nests is not very apparent; some nests lying at the sides of rete ridges, or even at the suprapapillary plate. In thick, papillomatous compound naevi particularly, which have greatly elongated and sometimes branched rete ridges with irregular outline, rete tip preference is no longer demonstrable. The nests are round or oval, the latter often with a vertical or almost vertical orientation. Nests may be closely juxtaposed, but fusion of nests, resulting in irregular conglomerates of melanocytes, as seen in many dysplastic naevi, pigmented spindle cell naevi and some Spitz naevi, is absent. Some lentiginous proliferation of individ-ual melanocytes may still be seen but it is usually not a conspicuous feature.

The epidermis shows elongation of rete ridges and often some degree of basket-weave type hyperkeratosis (Figure 4.4) and may form papillary projections. In such *papillomatous compound naevi*, the supra-papillary plates are often thinned. When epidermal hyperplasia and orthokeratosis are marked, the histology of seborrhoeic keratosis may be mimicked (Figure 4.5); rarely, a *'cutaneous horn'* consisting of a very thick and compact horn mass overlying the naevus may be formed (Figure 4.6). Suprabasal clefting and acantholytic dyskeratosis in the epidermis overlying the naevus have been described (Weedon, 1982).

A variety of *epidermal* and *adnexal epithelial proliferations* and *tumours* have been described in association with naevi: the latter include syringoma, basal cell carcinoma, trichoepithelioma and desmo-plastic trichoepithelioma (Weedon, 1982). The latter especially shows a frequent association with naevi: in a series of 76 such tumours, 10 were associated with an intradermal naevus (Starink and Brownstein, 1986).

The intradermal component consists of nests, strands and sheets of melanocytes, the latter being basally located. In many compound and intradermal naevi, the cells and their nuclei are smaller at the base of the lesion than subepidermally, a phenomenon known by the in-appropriate term *'maturation'*.

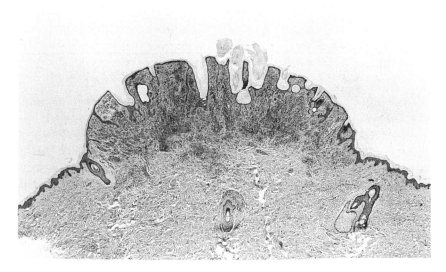

Figure 4.4 Largely intradermal compound naevus. Note symmetry and sharp lateral demarcation. Some epidermal papillomatosis and basket-weave hyperkeratosis is commonly present in compound naevi (HE, × 20).

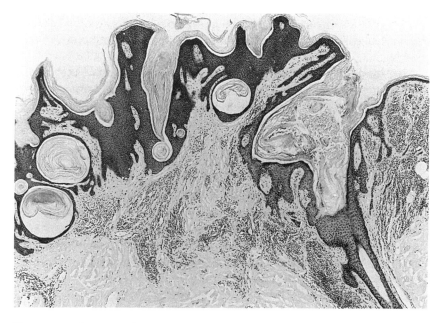

Figure 4.5 Compound naevus associated with epidermal proliferative changes resembling seborrhoeic keratosis (HE, × 35).

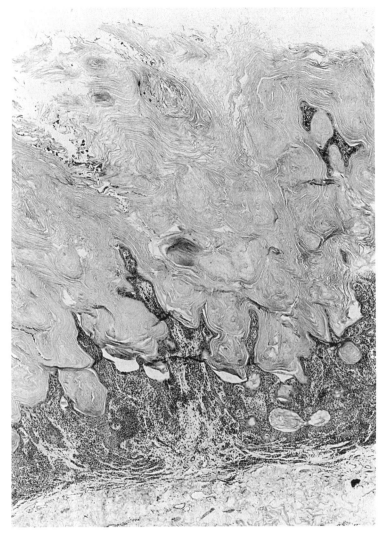

Figure 4.6 Compound naevus with marked epidermal papillomatosis and an extreme degree of hyperkeratosis, resulting in a 'cutaneous horn' (HE, × 45).

Maturation indicates a state of differentiation in which the cells are optimally equipped to perform their function. The function of melanocytes is to produce melanin, and since the 'matured' cells in the deeper parts of a naevus are generally devoid of melanin, the term 'maturation' is hardly warranted. Indeed, on the basis of a light and electron microscopical morphometrical study, Goovaerts and Buyssens

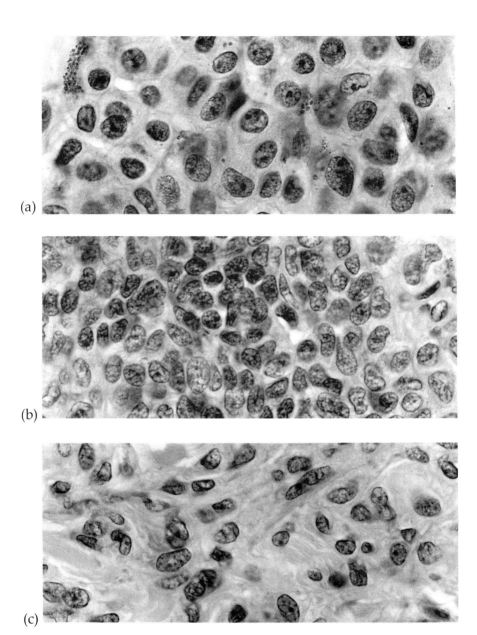

Figure 4.7 Naevus cell types A, B and C. Three fields from the same naevus. (a) Superficially, large, polygonal or round type A cells, some of which are pigmented. (b) In the middle area, small, usually non-pigmented type B cells with smaller, dark nuclei are present. (c) At the base, elongated, non-pigmented type C cells are found between an increased amount of collagen (HE, × 920).

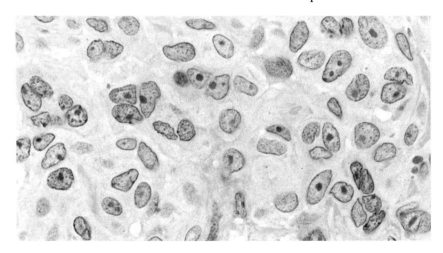

Figure 4.8   Intradermal naevus cells, plastic section. Nucleoli are much more conspicuous than in paraffin sections (HE, × 920).

(1988) indicated that 'atrophy' would be a more accurate term to describe this particular change in the melanocytes. The melanocytes deep in the naevus were found to be smaller, with smaller nuclei, and had fewer and less well-developed organelles, except for mitochondria and microfilaments. Importantly, such melanocytic 'maturation' may not be readily apparent in compound naevi, especially when they are small and thin.

The different cytological appearances of melanocytes at different levels of the naevus have led to a division into three subtypes, designated types A, B and C (Figure 4.7; Miescher and Von Albertini, 1935; Mishima, 1967). Type A cells are largest, often contain melanin pigment and are found in the superficial parts. These cells are round or oval and possess a moderate amount of pale amphophilic cytoplasm, which often contains some melanin granules. The nuclei are round or oval, and show a diffuse or very finely stippled chromatin pattern, or may be vacuolated due to tissue-processing artifacts. A centrally placed nucleolus is often present and may be striking in plastic sections (Figure 4.8). Type B cells are smaller and rounded, commonly non-pigmented, with darkly staining nuclei; these cells show some resemblance to lymphocytes. Type C cells are oval or spindled, usually non-pigmented, and are present at the base of the naevus. These cells show some resemblance to Schwann cells (Aso *et al.*, 1988), but, as will be discussed below, there are also important differences, so that it seems unlikely that this cell type represents true metaplasia to a

Schwann cell phenotype (Van Paesschen *et al.*, 1990). Mitoses are very rare indeed in intradermal naevus cells.

The pigment in common acquired naevi is generally granular in character and is usually confined to the upper parts of the naevus; although in some instances there may be some diffuse or focal pigmentation in deeper parts. This appears to be more common in females, especially during pregnancy or in association with the use of oral contraceptives, and in negroid persons.

Even in larger naevi, the intradermal component is largely confined to the expanded papillary dermis, but may extend along the adventitial dermis of the skin appendages. This occurs in the form of compact nests and strands rather than as single cells or 'Indian files', which is commonly the pattern of dermal invasion of congenital naevi and Spitz naevi. Between melanocytic nests and strands, a finely fibrillar stroma is formed. It should be noted that the intradermal component of common acquired naevi does not involve the reticular dermis to any substantial extent.

The main features of compound naevi are summarized in Table 4.4.

Various morphological variants of intradermal melanocytes may be encountered in compound and intradermal naevi. *Multinucleated cells* (Figure 4.9) are regularly seen, most often in superficial parts. These cells often have somewhat smaller and darker nuclei, which are tightly crowded together, while the cytoplasm is inconspicuous ('mulberry-type giant cells'), or the nuclei are arranged in a rosette surrounding a centre of slightly granular eosinophilic cytoplasm, while the periphery of the cell is pale and often finely vacuolated.

Table 4.4 Compound naevus

Clinical features
  Raised symmetrical pigmented or non-pigmented papule or nodule,
    generally ≤ 6 mm in diameter
  Sometimes papillomatous or polypoid

Histological features
  Epidermal component similar to junctional naevus
  Dermal component consists of nests, strands and aggregates of melanocytes
  'Maturation': decreased cellular and nuclear size towards the base
  Dermal component generally limited to widened papillary dermis and
    superficial reticular dermis
  Sometimes marked elongation of rete ridges and papillary projections of
    epidermis

Remark
  No 'rete ridge preference' of junctional nests in papillomatous compound
    naevi

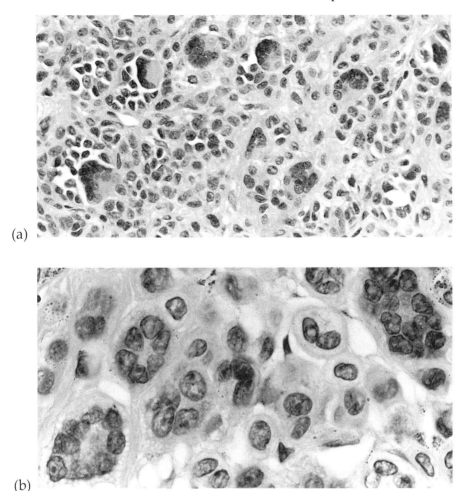

(a)

(b)

Figure 4.9 Binucleated and 'mulberry-type' multinucleated naevus cells in compound naevus. (a) Giant cells with closely adjacent hyperchromatic nuclei. (b) Nuclei of multinucleated melanocytes are often arranged in an irregular circle or crescent (HE, × 920).

Naevus cells may show small intracytoplasmic *clear vacuoles* (Figure 4.10): this change is not uncommon. It is different from balloon cell change (see below), which consists of a more conspicuous increase in cell size and a much finer type of cytoplasmic vacuolization.

At the base of the naevus, the cells often attain an elongated shape, with fibrillary cytoplasm, and form short bundles. Such so-called *neurotization* or *neuroid change* is in fact an exaggeration of the

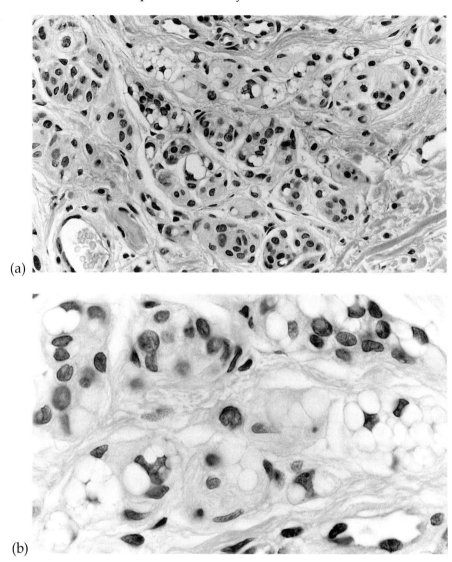

Figure 4.10   Naevus cells with multivacuolated cytoplasm are found scattered singly or grouped together in some compound and intradermal naevi, expecially in the subepidermal region. ((a) HE, × 370. (b) HE, × 920).

type C phenotype of naevus cell commonly present in compound or intradermal naevi. Structures strongly resembling tactile corpuscles (Wagner-Meissner corpuscles) may be formed, and have been de-signated *'lames foliacées'* (Masson, 1951), or 'foliate laminae' (Figure

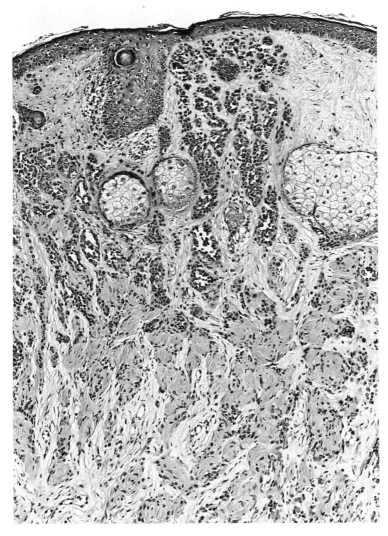

Figure 4.11   Neuroid change in intradermal naevus. Finely fibrillar 'neuroid' structures are present in deeper parts of the naevus (HE, × 115).

4.11). This phenomenon probably does not represent a true metaplasia to a schwannian phenotype, at least not to a mature one recognizable immunologically. There are important differences between the cells of neurotized naevi and Schwann cells: the latter are positive for myelin basic protein, Leu-7 and glial fibrillary acidic protein, while 'neurotized' type C naevus cells are negative for these markers (Nickoloff *et al.*,

1986; Van Paesschen *et al.*, 1990; Gray *et al.*, 1990a), but may be positive for EMA (Cramer, 1990). Immunostaining for the markers mentioned above is of help in the distinction between completely neurotized naevi and cutaneous neurofibromas (Gray *et al.*, 1990a). In addition, neurofibromas are positive for Factor XIIIa, whereas neurotized naevi are negative (Gray *et al.*, 1990b). At the ultrastructural level, neurotized naevi exhibit stacks of cytoplasmic processes surrounded by basal laminae, but no features of neurilemmal differentiation (Van Paesschen *et al.*, 1990).

Irregular clefts are sometimes formed in the dermal component of some naevi (Figure 4.12): they are probably the result of tissue shrinkage during histological processing, and poor intercellular cohesion within sheets of dermal naevus cells. They are easily distinguished from vascular spaces: the latter are more regular in contour and are lined by flattened endothelial cells. Rarely, the whole naevus shows such pseudovascular spaces, and it has been claimed that it may occasionally be well-nigh impossible to distinguish such a lesion from a cutaneous haemangioma (Söderström, 1987).

Groups of naevus cells bulging into lumina of dermal lymphatics have been described (Bell *et al.*, 1979; Levene, 1980) and may be relevant to the histogenesis of naevus cell aggregates sometimes found in lymph nodes (p. 362). They are more common in congenital naevi and in Spitz naevi.

Focal 'balloon cell change' (p. 90) is not very rare. Small, Congo red-positive, eosinophilic, amorphous amyloid deposits occur rarely subepidermally or between naevus cells; they probably represent remnants of apoptotic naevus cells (MacDonald and Black, 1980). The relationship of such amyloid to deposits found more frequently in lesions of keratinocytes is not clear.

In the majority of naevi there is some increase in dermal elastin (Mehregan and Staricco, 1962), especially at the periphery; in 0.5% of naevi there is a conspicuous coarsening of elastin fibres around the naevus (Weedon, 1982). Increase of elastin within the naevus itself is more prominent in congenital naevi (p. 146).

4.4   Intradermal naevus

During the further evolution of the naevus, the junctional component is gradually lost. The palms, soles and external genitalia constitute an exception in that a proportion of naevi at these sites tend to maintain a junctional (lentiginous and/or nested) component throughout life.

When all the naevus cells are localized within the dermis, the naevus is designated as an intradermal naevus. This name is preferable to

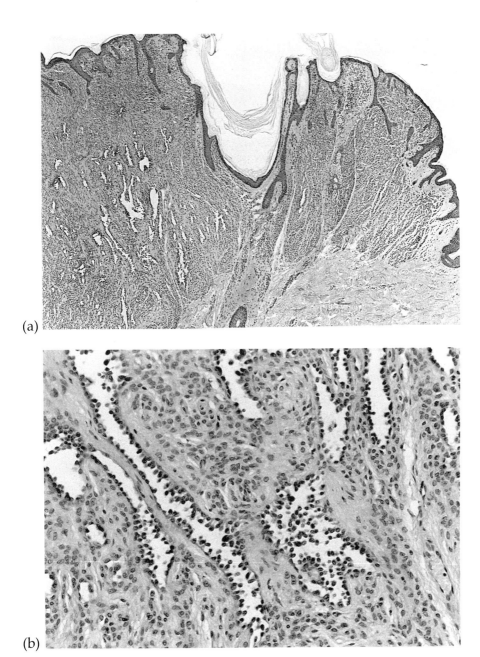

Figure 4.12 'Pseudovascular spaces' in intradermal naevus. (a) Irregular clefts are formed within sheets of naevus cells (HE, × 35). (b) These clefts are lined by dissociating naevus cells rather than endothelial cells (HE, × 185).

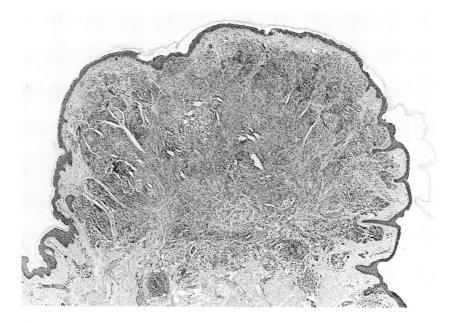

Figure 4.13 Intradermal naevus. There are no junctional nests; the surface is relatively smooth, when compared to compound naevi, and rete ridges are partly lacking (HE, × 35).

'dermal naevus', in order to avoid drawing an inappropriate parallel to epidermal naevus, which is not a melanocytic lesion.

4.4.1 Clinical features

Intradermal naevi are skin-coloured or slightly pigmented dome-shaped, polypoid or papillomatous lesions; they are most common in adulthood. The large majority are smaller than 1 cm; most do not exceed 6 mm. Ageing intradermal naevi decrease in size and often disappear gradually, or they may become pendulous and eventually dislodge from the skin (Stegmaier, 1959).

4.4.2 Pathological features

At this stage, the junctional component of the naevus has disappeared completely, so that only the intradermal part remains (Table 4.4). On serial section, some junctional foci may be detected in a proportion of naevi which, on a single section, qualify as intradermal naevi; however, since the distinction between intradermal naevus and

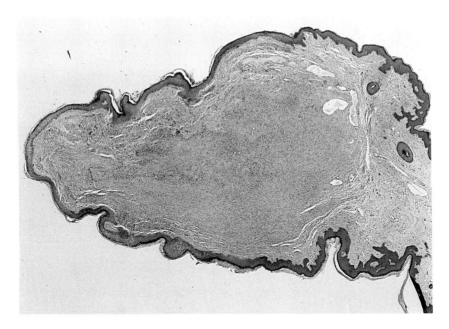

Figure 4.14   Polypoid, pendulous intradermal naevus. Such ageing intradermal naevi, which are usually not pigmented, clinically resemble soft fibromas (HE, × 20).

compound naevus with a minimal residual junctional component is not important clinically, such serial sections are not required.

Most intradermal naevi show a smooth contour of the epidermis and rete ridges are often shallow and few in number (Figure 4.13). Some are pedunculated (Figure 4.14). If a given naevus has a papillomatous surface and there is marked elongation of rete ridges, there is usually still a junctional component.

Several factors are probably instrumental in bringing about the transition from compound to intradermal naevus. Of these, cessation of 'junctional activity' of melanocytes, followed by the incorporation of junctional melanocytes in the thickened papillary dermis, is probably by far the most important.

Transepithelial elimination of naevus cell nests (Rupec and Vakilzadeh, 1974; Yuki *et al.*, 1984; Kantor and Wheeland, 1987), i.e. upward movement of nests through the epidermis or skin appendages and subsequent loss *via* the cornified layer, may also play a minor role. Of the various forms of transepithelial elimination (i.e. elimination *via* the epidermis, sweat glands, and hair follicles), Yuki and colleagues (1984) only observed elimination *via* the epidermis, but they pointed to

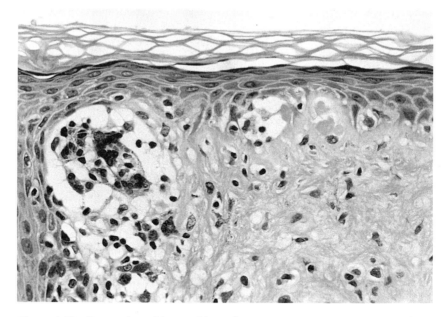

Figure 4.15   Regression of intraepidermal naevus component; apoptosis of melanocytes, fibrosis of the papillary dermis. This is not a common finding (HE, × 370).

earlier descriptions of naevus cell nests within sebaceous glands (Shitara *et al.*, 1977; Kawamura *et al.*, 1982) which may also constitute examples of transepithelial elimination. Massive transepidermal elimination of melanocytes leading to spontaneous regression of a giant congenital naevus has been described (Hasegawa *et al.*, 1987).

Apoptosis of naevus cells (Figure 4.15) may perhaps also contribute to the loss of the junctional component of compound naevi.

4.4.3   Regressive phenomena in ageing intradermal naevi

A variety of regressive changes may occur in ageing naevi. Not uncommonly, groups of fat cells (Figure 4.16) emerge between the naevus cells. It is unclear whether these fat cells result from accumulation of fat within naevus cells, or whether they develop from the stroma; the latter seems more likely, since no convincing evidence of transition of naevus cells into fat cells is seen. Soft fibromas may contain many fat cells within the dermis; it is likely that at least some of these lesions represent involuted dermal naevi. They should not be confused with naevus lipomatosus, which is an altogether different lesion, usually

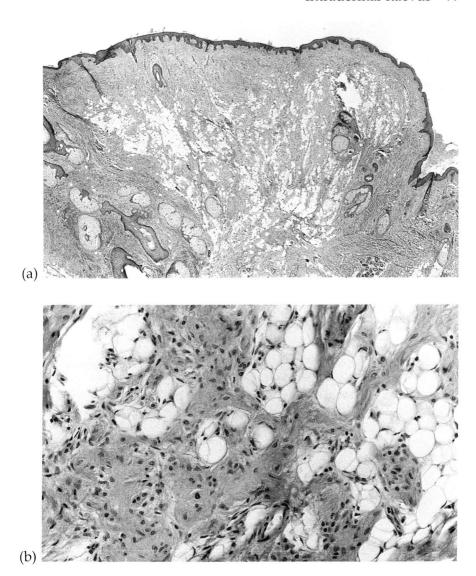

(a)

(b)

Figure 4.16   Adipocytes scattered throughout an intradermal naevus. ((a) HE, × 20; (b) HE, × 185).

developing as multiple small papules on the buttock during childhood or adolescence (Wilson Jones *et al.*, 1975).

In ageing naevi, increasing *fibrosis* or, less commonly, *myxoid change* of the stroma, together with atrophy and subsequent dis-

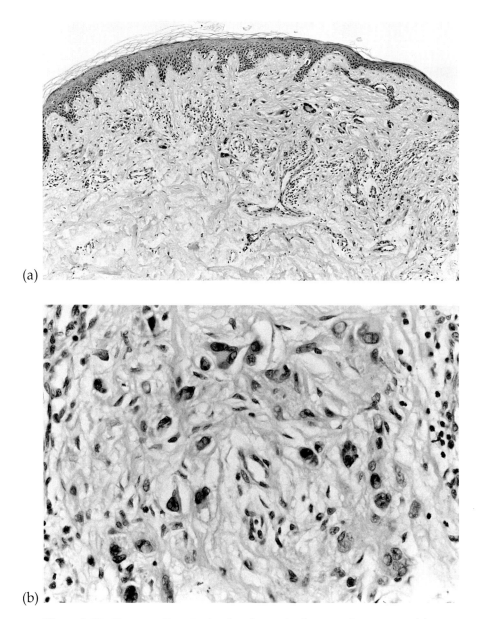

Figure 4.17 Degenerative atypia of melanocytes in an ageing naevus. (a) Scattered giant naevus cells with hyperchromatic nuclei are seen in the fibrotic upper dermis; mild vascular proliferation and perivascular lymphocytic infiltrates are present (HE, × 90). (b) Melanocytes possess one or more variably hyperchromatic nuclei, with a vacuolated or smudged chromatin pattern. Mitoses are absent. There is some fibrosis and inflammation (HE, × 370).

appearance of the naevus cells may lead to clinical disappearance of the naevus (Maize and Foster, 1979), or may result in a residual small fibrotic intradermal nodule or small soft fibroma (Stegmaier, 1959). Also, some degree of *inflammatory response*, as in halo naevi, is not uncommon.

Some of the so-called fibrous papules of the face have been regarded as regressing melanocytic naevi (McGibbon and Wilson Jones, 1979). However, it is more likely that they represent angiofibromas or, less commonly, perifollicular fibromas.

Hitherto, little attention has been paid to a specific type of *cytological atypia* in ageing naevi, which we interpret as a degenerative pheno-menon rather than as evidence of malignant transformation. In such naevi, a considerable amount of fibrous tissue is present, in which scattered large atypical naevus cells are seen (Figure 4.17). These naevus cells have hyperchromatic nuclei with a smudged chromatin pattern and usually possess a generous amount of poorly defined amphophilic cytoplasm. Binucleated and multinucleated naevus cells are commonly seen; mitoses are always absent. These cells lie singly or in small groups within the fibrotic tissue which may be loosely textured or sclerotic. There may be perivascular accentuation of sclerosis. The cytological appearace suggests 'degenerative cytological atypia' rather

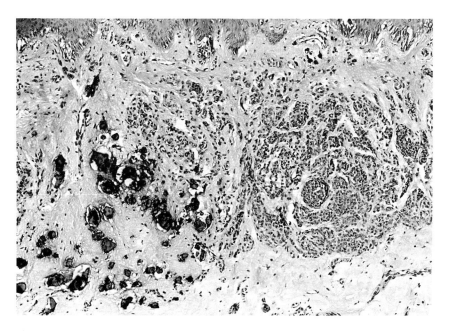

Figure 4.18   Fibrosis and calcification in a compound naevus (HE, × 90).

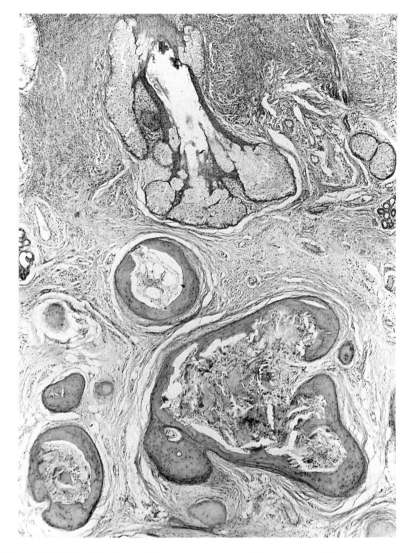

Figure 4.19   Ossification subjacent to compound naevus. Small, slightly irregular foci of ossification are seen within the reticular dermis underlying the naevus (HE, × 45).

than atypia associated with malignant transformation; the histological appearance calls to mind the features of ancient schwannoma, the cytological atypia of which has a similar character and, possibly, a similar pathogenesis. The changes described may rarely be focal, leading to asymmetry of the naevus.

Calcification (Figure 4.18), sometimes with the characteristic concentric layering of *psammoma bodies*, and formation of cartilage and bone (Figure 4.19; 'osteonaevus of Nanta') occurs in about 1 to 1.5% of intradermal naevi, usually at or just below the base of the naevus (Salm and Swinburne, 1963; Rupeck and Huck, 1976; Weedon, 1982), which is usually located on the face. Involution, trauma and infection are probably responsible for dystrophic calcification and metaplastic bone formation.

Plugging of hair follicles entrapped within a naevus is not uncommon, and may lead to suppurating *folliculitis* (Figure 4.20),

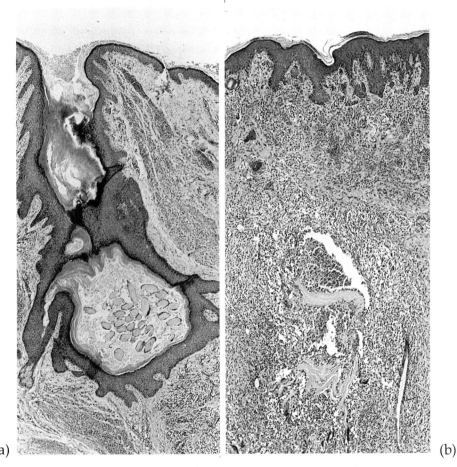

(a)

(b)

Figure 4.20 (a) Dilated hair follicle containing multiple hair shafts, in an intradermal naevus (HE, × 35). (b) Folliculitis with foreign-body giant-cell response in the reticular dermis underlying a compound naevus. This may lead to enlargement and tenderness of the naevus and cause clinical suspicion of melanoma (HE, × 45).

bringing the naevus to clinical attention (Salm and Swinburne, 1963). Usually the histological diagnosis is easy; inflammatory destruction of the hair follicle leads to a foreign-body giant-cell reaction, in which remnants of hair shaft are usually still demonstrable. A trichilemmal cyst within the dermis underlying a compound naevus (Requena *et al.*, 1990) and two cases of follicular mucinosis in naevi (Jordaan, 1987) have been reported.

Focal necrosis in a benign naevus is exceedingly rare, and may be related to trauma or ischaemia (Figure 4.21).

Various aspects of intradermal naevi are summarized in Table 4.5.

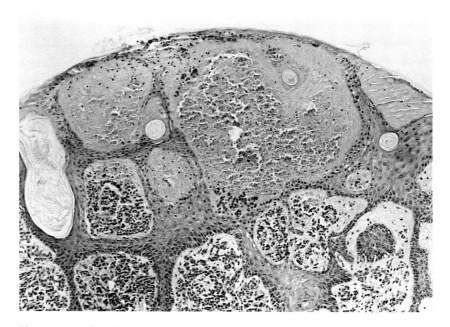

Figure 4.21   Small area of necrosis, possibly due to ischaemia, in an otherwise unremarkable compound naevus. This is a very rare finding (HE, × 90).

Table 4.5 Intradermal naevus

Clinical features
  Raised symmetrical pigmented or non-pigmented papule or nodule,
    generally ≤ 6 mm in diameter
  Sometimes polypoid

Histological features
  As in compound naevus, but without intraepidermal component

---

4.5 Halo naevus (Sutton's naevus, leukoderma acquisitum centrifugum)

The halo naevus, or Sutton's naevus (Sutton, 1916) is characterized by an active immune response against the naevus, usually causing depigmentation of the surrounding skin, and subsequently leading to disappearance of the naevus, leaving a depigmented spot. More rarely, the formation of a depigmented halo occurs in the absence of a lymphocytic inflammatory response (Berger and Voorhees, 1971; Gauthier et al., 1978) or, conversely, a lymphocytic response is present while a halo is absent. Patients with halo naevi have been shown to produce antibodies against melanocyte-associated antigens (Mitchell et al., 1980). A classical paper on halo nevi, providing a review of the early literature together with a detailed clinical and histological description of 108 cases, was published by Wayte and Helwig (1968).

A lesser degree of the same change, resulting in a very faint ring of cutaneous hypopigmentation, more easily detected with a Wood's lamp, not uncommonly surrounds acquired and congenital naevi (Berger and Voorhees, 1971), dysplastic naevi and blue naevi (Barnes and Nordlund, 1987). Such haloes are commonest soon after the highest numbers of naevi have been reached, suggesting that the decline in numbers of naevi during adulthood may be in part due to an immunological response similar to that seen in halo naevi (Nicholls, 1973).

Other changes of perinaeval skin of unknown significance include eczematous change (Meyerson, 1971) and, in the case of naevi of the scalp, a rim of alopecia (Yesudian and Thambiah, 1976).

It should be noted that a depigmented halo may also surround some non-melanocytic lesions, including fibrous histiocytoma, seborrhoeic keratosis, angioma and verruca plana (Berman, 1978).

4.5.1 Clinical features

Halo naevus occurs in Caucasians, most commonly on the trunk, especially the back; it is uncommon on the extremities. Most cases are seen in childhood and adolescence; they are rare after the age of 50 (Kopf et al., 1965; Wayte and Helwig, 1968). Although vitiligo patients are not exempt from the development of halo naevi, most halo naevi occur in persons without disorders of pigmentation. Multiple halo naevi are found in about 25–50% of the patients.

In the earliest phase, a rim of depigmentation develops around a naevus which has often been present for many years, and which is symmetrical, usually red-brown in colour and a few millimetres in diameter. The surrounding depigmentation is more or less symmetrical, although the naevus may be situated somewhat off-centre. This contrasts with the often irregularly distributed depigmentation seen in and adjacent to regressing melanomas. The ring of depigmentation of a halo naevus grows centripetally, so that finally, a round or oval depigmented macule is all that remains. Finally the depigmented macule may repigment again, so that it becomes indistinguishable from the surrounding skin.

4.5.2 *Pathological features*

The naevus is usually a compound naevus, which is symmetrical and sharply demarcated. In the early phases, a dense infiltrate consisting of lymphocytes, histiocytes and sometimes a small number of plasma cells and mast cells, is seen throughout the intradermal part of the lesion (Figure 4.22). It is largely confined to the widened papillary dermis, sometimes with a minor degree of involvement of the peri-adnexal dermis, so that the basal demarcation is usually rather sharp. The infiltrate disrupts naevus cell nests and aggregates; in some lesions, residual naevus cells are difficult to identify. S-100 immunostaining may then be of help. The naevus cells may show slight nuclear atypia (Ainsworth *et al.*, 1979), including some enlargement, hyperchromasia, a mild degree of coarsening of the chromatin pattern and prominence of nucleoli. Mitoses are rare and usually confined to the upper parts. Because of the close intermingling of different cell types, it is often difficult to decide that a mitosis indeed concerns a melanocyte. Some melanocytes show increased cytoplasmic eosinophilia. Melanin pigment is usually confined to the upper parts of the naevus but in some cases it is present also deep within the lesion. There is often proliferation of dermal capillaries, and endothelial cells may be prominent (Table 4.6).

Importantly, there are no abrupt changes in architecture or cytological features, and compact nodules or aggregates of cells at the base of the lesion are absent. The process is more or less in the same phase throughout the naevus; *there is no irregular mixture of scarring and active inflammation.*

Figure 4.22   Halo naevus. (a) Note small size, symmetry and diffuse   ▶
infiltration by inflammatory cells (HE, × 35). (b) Intradermal nests are
disrupted by a diffuse, predominantly lymphocytic infiltrate (HE, × 185).
(c) Intermingling of naevus cells and predominantly lymphocytic infiltrate,
virtually devoid of plasma cells (HE, × 370).

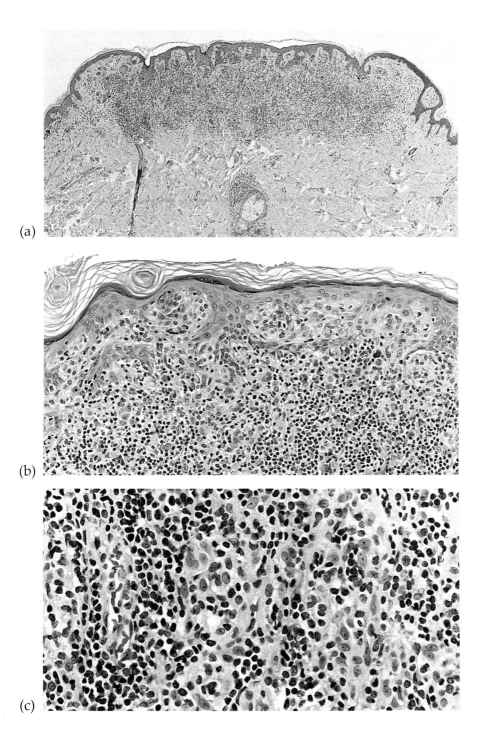

(a)

(b)

(c)

Table 4.6 Halo naevus

Clinical features
  Most common on the trunk of children and adolescents
  Multiple in 25–50% of cases
  Rim of depigmentation around the naevus
  Gradual centripetal growth of depigmentation associated with disappearance
    of the naevus

Histological features
  Heavy lymphohistiocytic infiltrate throughout the naevus, disrupting dermal
    naevus cell nests
  Slight scarring of the superficial dermis in late phase
  Sometimes slight cytological atypia of intradermal melanocytes

The overlying epidermis is often unremarkable, or shows a mild degree of hyperkeratosis with plugging of follicles, and mild acanthosis. Suprabasal or subepidermal clefting may occasionally be seen (Lambert, 1986). Ulceration and ascent of melanocytes are absent. There is no exocytosis of inflammatory cells. Junctional melanocytic nests usually consist of prominent pigmented epithelioid-type cells with vesicular nuclei.

In later stages, the inflammatory infiltrate and melanocytes disappear, leaving slight superficial scarring, and scattered melanophages in the dermis (Figure 4.23). At the final stage, the histological picture is no longer distinguishable from postinflammatory cutaneous scarring from other causes or from completely regressed melanoma, except that the latter may cover a larger area.

The depigmented skin surrounding the naevus is usually histologically normal, except for the absence of melanin in the epidermis and the presence of slightly increased numbers of intraepidermal Langerhans cells (Wayte and Helwig, 1968).

Because of its distinct clinical features, the halo naevus is usually diagnosed correctly by the clinician. However, depending on its stage of development, its histology may resemble other cutaneous diseases, both melanocytic and non-melanocytic. Therefore, *adequate clinical data* accompanying the specimen are *vital*. Halo naevus can be confused with various forms of dermatitis, lichenoid keratosis and even cutaneous lymphoma (Wayte and Helwig, 1968). In this respect, S-100 immunostaining aids in the recognition of melanocytes amidst a heavy inflammatory infiltrate (Penneys *et al.*, 1985).

The main histological differential diagnosis, however, is regressing

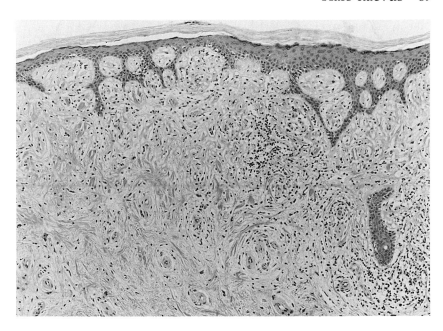

Figure 4.23   Halo naevus, late, fibrosing phase. Within the greatly thickened, fibrotic papillary dermis, increased numbers of blood vessels and a sparse lymphocytic infiltrate are seen (HE, × 90).

Table 4.7 Differential diagnosis of halo naevus *vs* regressing melanoma

Diagnostic feature	Halo naevus	Regressing melanoma
Shape	symmetrical	often asymmetrical
Lateral demarcation	sharp	often not sharp
Ascent of atypical melanocytes	absent	often present
Compact intradermal melanocytic nodules	absent	often present
Atypia	slight, same degree throughout lesion	often varying from area to area
Infiltrate	throughout lesion	basal and band-like or patchy and irregular
Phase of inflammatory process	same throughout lesion	areas of active inflammation and scarring often occur simultaneously

melanoma (p. 227); this distinction may occasionally prove difficult (Reed *et al.*, 1990). The most important distinguishing features are listed in Table 4.7.

4.6   Balloon cell naevus

Balloon cell naevus, first described by Miescher (1935), and later more extensively by Schrader and Helwig (1967), is characterized by the presence of many greatly enlarged, pale naevus cells, which possess copious, microvacuolar cytoplasm. The cytoplasmic vacuolation is caused by a defect of melanosome formation (Nordlund *et al.*, 1974) and also occurs in some melanomas and blue naevi (Schrader and Helwig, 1967). A case of halo balloon cell naevus, combining the clinical and histological features of halo naevus and balloon cell naevus, was reported by Côté and colleagues (1986).

4.6.1   Clinical features

Balloon cell naevus occurs mainly in Caucasians under the age of 30; there is no obvious sex predilection. It is most often located on the trunk and the head and neck region, and is uncommon on the extremities. The clinical appearance is that of a conventional naevus; there are no clinical distinguishing features. Most often the naevus is under 6 mm in diameter, but very rarely it exceeds 1 cm (Schrader and Helwig, 1967). It is most often lightly pigmented (Schrader and Helwig, 1967). There is no history of recent change.

4.6.2   Pathological features

Histologically, balloon cell naevus is a compound or intradermal naevus, in which the majority of melanocytes are greatly enlarged and possess a large amount of pale, finely vacuolated cytoplasm (Figure 4.24). These cells are found in the junctional as well as the intradermal component, and form abnormally large nests, often merging with nests and sheets of conventional naevus cells. This may result in a somewhat

Figure 4.24   Balloon cell naevus. (a) The dermal part of the naevus consists largely of strands and nests of large, pale 'balloon' cells (HE, × 35). (b) Conventional naevus cells (upper left) as well as balloon cells are present (HE, × 185). (c) Balloon cells exhibit a large amount of pale, finely vacuolated cytoplasm, conspicuous cells borders, and centrally placed, dark, slightly indented nuclei (HE, × 920).

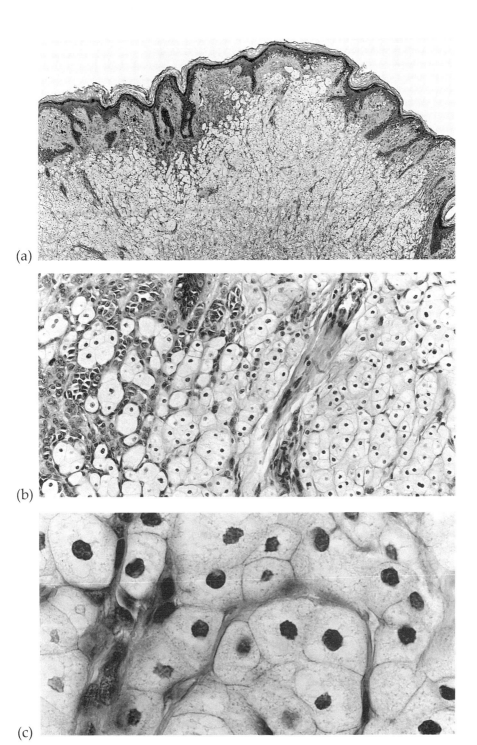

(a)

(b)

(c)

worrisome architectural appearance. Especially when there is one focus of balloon cell change, 'intralesional transformation' may be suggested. Rarely, a naevus is composed entirely of balloon cells (Goette and Doty, 1978).

The intracytoplasmic vacuoles vary in size: most are very small, but larger vacuoles are usually also present. They are PAS-negative and do not contain fat. Ultrastructurally, vacuolar degeneration and confluence of melanosomes is found (Hashimoto and Bale, 1972; Okun *et al.*, 1974); the abnormal melanosomes can be transmitted to epidermal keratinocytes. Balloon cells usually contain a small amount of melanin pigment, detected more easily with special stains, and mainly located at the periphery of the cytoplasm.

Isolated balloon cells are not uncommonly seen in otherwise unremarkable naevi; Gartmann (1960) found a prevalence of slightly less than 2%. It is unclear whether the much more common multivacuolated melanocytes occurring subepidermally in some compound and intradermal naevi (p. 71) bear any relation to the larger and more finely vacuolated balloon cells.

The most important differential diagnosis is balloon cell melanoma (p. 271). Irregular lateral pagetoid spread and ascent of atypical melanocytes is absent in balloon cell naevus, but they may also be lacking in melanoma. The cytological features are probably the most important in the differential diagnosis. In balloon cell naevi, the nuclei are small, centrally located, and may be slightly scalloped due to adjacent cytoplasmic microvacuoles. There may be a small central eosinophilic nucleolus. Nuclear enlargement and pleomorphism is absent, and is variably present in balloon cell melanoma. Mitoses are absent, whereas they are usually present in balloon cell melanoma (p. 271; Su *et al.*,

Table 4.8 Balloon cell naevus

Clinical features
   Most common under age of 30
   Trunk and head and neck region preferred sites
   Usually lightly pigmented; no distinguishing macroscopical features

Histological features
   Majority of naevus cells greatly enlarged, with finely vacuolar cytoplasm
   Small, monomorphic central nuclei
   Sometimes apparently irregular architecture due to large naevus cell nests
      and aggregates (because of large size of balloon cells)

Remarks
   Focal balloon cell change not uncommon in naevi
   Differential diagnosis with balloon cell melanoma (Table 9.4, p. 271)

1985). The cells and their nuclei tend to diminish in size in deeper parts of the lesion. Multinucleated mulberry-type or ballooned giant naevus cells are usually found and may be a striking feature. The main features of balloon cell naevus are listed in Table 4.8.

4.7   Cockarde naevus

Cockarde naevus, or cockade naevus (Mehregan and King, 1972; James and Wells, 1980; Guzzo *et al.*, 1988) is an unusual clinical variant of common acquired naevus showing concentric variation of pigmentation. It occurs, often as multiple lesions, in children and young adults. Clinically, a central pink to darkly pigmented papule is surrounded at a distance of several millimetres by a stippled pigmented circle. Histologically, the centre consists of a junctional or compound naevus. No inflammation is seen. The stippled periphery shows multiple junctional melanocytic nests; the skin between the central naevus and the peripheral pigmented rim is generally devoid of naevus cells or shows a few junctional nests.

The lesion should be distinguished from halo naevus (p. 85) and target blue naevus (p. 125) both of which also show concentric variations in pigmentation; very rarely, melanoma may exhibit a target-like appearance (Champion, 1964).

4.8   Deep penetrating naevus

Recently, Seab and colleagues (1989) described an important new entity which they designated 'deep penetrating naevus'. It consists of a compound naevus in which the dermal component extends deeply into the reticular dermis and may even reach the subcutaneous fat. Since there may also be some cytological atypia, there is a danger of overdiagnosis of these lesions.

According to Seab and his colleagues (1989), the deep penetrating naevus usually takes the form of a symmetrical and darkly pigmented nodule, up to 9 mm in diameter, most often on the face, neck or upper trunk. It occurs most often between the ages of 10 and 30 years, although there is a wide age range.

Histologically, the lesion is usually a compound naevus, in which the junctional component is usually not prominent, and consists of a few well-defined nests. The dermal part consists of nests or fascicles of pigmented cells, which extend into the deep dermis, preferentially along the adventitial dermis surrounding skin appendages (Figures 4.25, 4.26). The architecture of the dermal collagen bundles and adnexae is not disturbed. Pilar muscles may be infiltrated by naevus cells.

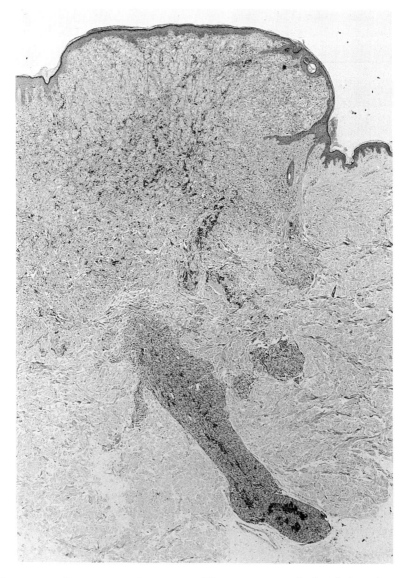

Figure 4.25 Deep penetrating naevus. The naevus extends deeply into the reticular dermis. Note pigment production at the base (HE, × 25).

Figure 4.26 Deep penetrating naevus. (a) Tightly packed intradermal naevus ▶ cell nests (HE, × 370). (b) Extension into the reticular dermis; the dermal architecture is not disturbed (HE, × 370). (c) A compact, pigmented nodule reaches the subcutaneous fatty tissue (HE, × 185).

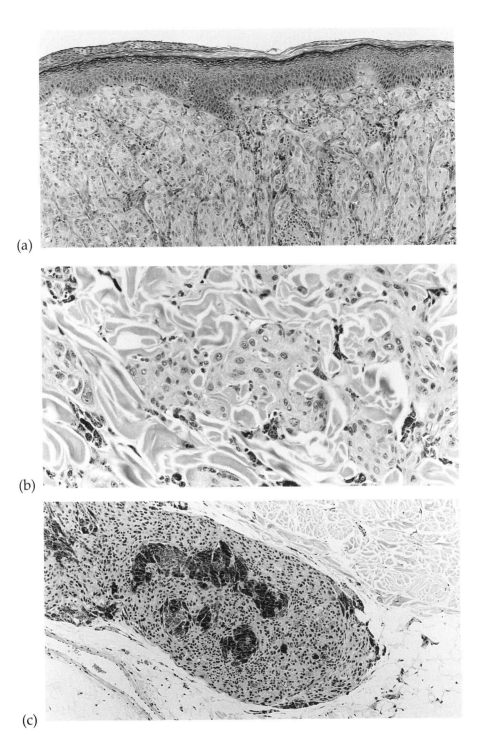

(a)

(b)

(c)

Table 4.9 Deep penetrating naevus

Clinical features
  Symmetrical darkly pigmented nodule ≤ 9 mm
  Most often on face, neck and upper trunk
  Wide age range; most cases between 10 and 30 years

Histological features
  Unusual compound naevus with deep penetration of reticular dermis,
      sometimes extending into subcutis
  Vertical extension often exceeds horizontal extension
  Cells in strands, usually vertically orientated
  Abundant melanin, also at the base
  Some cytological atypia, nuclear pseudoinclusions
  Mitoses absent or very scarce
  No or very little inflammatory infiltrate

Remarks
  At present it is unclear whether some might actually be congenital naevi;
      possibly also a relation to blue and combined naevi

Usually, the vertical extension is greater than the lateral extension, resulting in a wedge shape of the lesion.

Nuclear pleomorphism and anisochromasia is conspicuous in some lesions; however, the chromatin appears smudged and mitoses are absent or very scarce. The cytoplasm often contains some melanin granules, also in deep parts of the lesion. There is an admixture of melanophages. There is no or very little inflammatory infiltrate (Table 4.9). Intranuclear vacuoles and pseudoinclusions are often seen and may be conspicuous.

It is possible that some of the deep penetrating naevi represent small congenital naevi because of the known extension of this type of naevus into the deep reticular dermis and subcutaneous fat. Also, extension along adnexae and invasion of arrector pili muscles is seen far more often in congenital than in acquired naevi (Mark *et al.*, 1973). However, the pigment distribution in deep penetrating naevus differs from that of most congenital naevi. Furthermore, Seab and colleagues (1989) found no clinical evidence to support a congenital origin. Deep penetrating naevus has apparently been diagnosed at times as combined ('true and blue') naevus, presumably in part because of the presence of melanin in the deep parts of the lesion. There is a possibility that some lesions may be related to cellular blue naevi. Clearly this enigmatic lesion requires further study.

The most important differential diagnosis is melanoma; in deep penetrating naevus there are none of the hallmarks of malignancy like asymmetry, intraepidermal ascent, the presence of more than a very few mitoses, a destructive growth pattern in the dermis, a heavy lymphocytic infiltrate, a plasmocellular infiltrate and prominent fibrosis, although these features may also be missing in melanoma, at times causing considerable differential diagnostic difficulty. This is accentuated by the fact that deep penetrating naevus is a recently described and relatively little known entity.

4.9 Recurrent naevus after incomplete removal ('pseudomelanoma')

After incomplete removal, especially by way of shave biopsy and electrodesiccation, some naevi recur, often within a few weeks but sometimes after several months or even years (Schoenfeld and Pinkus, 1958; Kornberg and Ackerman, 1975; Park *et al.*, 1987).

Although the majority of such recurrent naevi will not give rise to clinical or histological suspicion of malignancy (Park *et al.*, 1987), *a minority take the form of a larger, irregularly shaped pigmentation, which may be confused with melanoma both clinically and histologically.* Kornberg and Ackerman (1975) reported eight such cases, seven females and one male, ranging in age from 16 to 37 years. Histologically, such lesions show an irregular intraepidermal proliferation of partly atypical melanocytes, with marked variation and sometimes confluence of nests. Solitary melanocytes are also increased in numbers and some may be located above the basal layer. Some cells are enlarged due to an increased amount of cytoplasm which may contain granular melanin pigment; a few melanocytes also show mild nuclear atypia. There is, however, a sharp lateral demarcation of the intraepidermal component and mitoses are absent or rare. Scarring

Table 4.10 Recurrent naevus after incomplete excision ('pseudomelanoma')

Clinical features
    Recurrence of pigmentation, often within a few weeks after incomplete
        excision of naevus (shave biopsy, electrodesiccation)
    Flat, sometimes irregularly pigmented and irregularly shaped

Histological features
    Irregular proliferation of intraepidermal melanocytes
    Occasional melanocytes above basal layer
    Sometimes mild cytological atypia of melanocytes
    Sharp lateral demarcation
    No or very few mitoses
    Scarring of subjacent dermis, often remnant of naevus at the base of scar

Remarks
    Histological re-evaluation of first biopsy very important

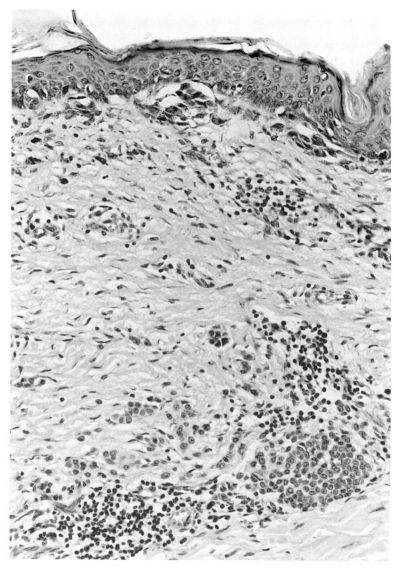

Figure 4.27 Recurrent naevus after shave biopsy. Irregular proliferation of melanocytes within the flattened epidermis overlying the scar tissue. Note remnants of intradermal naevus at the base (HE, × 230).

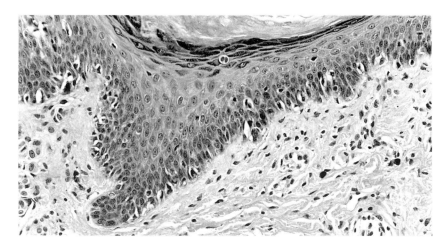

Figure 4.28 Recurrent naevus after shave biopsy. Lentiginous proliferation of melanocytes with hyperchromatic nuclei and ascent of two melanocytes. Note small remnant of intradermal naevus (extreme left) (HE, × 185).

of the dermis takes the shape of thick, often horizontally orientated bundles of collagen in the upper dermis; some perivascular lympho-histiocytic infiltrate is often present. An intradermal remnant of the pre-existent naevus can usually be detected under the scar tissue (Figures 4.27, 4.28; Table 4.10). S-100 immunostaining often reveals scattered elongated melanocytes within the scar tissue (Estrada *et al.*, 1990), which are presumably derived from the deep unremoved portion of the naevus.

To distinguish such lesions from recurrent incompletely removed melanoma, histological reassessment of the initial lesion is very important.

4.10   'Active' naevi (so-called 'hot naevi')

Several exogenous and endogenous factors have been found to be associated with proliferative activity and melanogenesis in naevi. Such stimulated naevi have been referred to collectively as 'activated naevi' or, colloquially, as 'hot naevi'. Sunshine, pregnancy, the contraceptive pill, the presence of a cutaneous melanoma at another site, and situation on the vulva are the main factors implicated.

Holman and colleagues (Holman *et al.*, 1983; Armstrong *et al.*, 1984) made the interesting observation that *naevi excised during the summer months* more often show junctional activity, have a higher mitotic count and a more pronounced inflammatory response. In some cases there was some cytological atypia of melanocytes, but this did not reach statistical significance in their study. The observations of these authors point to a direct, short-latency effect of sunlight, inducing increased junctional activity of naevi, together with some features which have been incriminated as features of dysplastic naevi.

During *pregnancy* or with the use of *oral contraceptives*, naevi may become larger and/or darker. Histologically, such naevi may show lentiginous proliferation of melanocytes, with or without a slight degree of cytological atypia (Ainsworth *et al.*, 1979). Initial studies indicated that naevi might be oestrogen-sensitive, but later studies have shed doubt on this (Jemec *et al.*, 1988). In a systematic study no increase in numbers of naevi was found in women using oral contraceptives or in multiparous women (MacKie *et al.*, 1985). Foucar and colleagues (1985) compared 128 naevi from pregnant patients with naevi from age-matched male and female controls. The histological differences found in this study were minor; the diagnostically important conclusion of these authors is that *prominent cytological atypia and architectural irregularity in a naevus from a pregnant female should not be dismissed as 'pregnancy effect'.*

In some *melanoma patients*, similar 'activation' of naevi may occur, which may be noticed clinically as darkening of naevi. The reported increase of activated naevi in the lymphatic drainage area of melanomas (Tucker *et al.*, 1980) is an interesting phenomenon which requires confirmation and further study. Such changes, which are presumably reactive in nature, might lead to an overestimation of the prevalence of dysplastic naevi in melanoma patients.

In conclusion, naevi are apparently subject to various exogenous or endogenous stimuli which may influence their clinical and histological appearance. Importantly, *this phenomenon complicates the distinction between common and dysplastic naevi*, a distinction which will be discussed in Chapter 8.

4.11   Vulvar naevi

Naevi located on the vulvar skin show basically the same features as those located elsewhere, but not uncommonly junctional nests are larger, irregularly spaced and may have an irregular shape. In addition, there may be lentiginous melanocytic hyperplasia. Cytological atypia of melanocytes is absent, which is important in the distinction from dysplastic naevus, which may also occur on the vulva (Christensen *et al.*, 1987), and melanoma. Pigmented lesions of the vulvar and vaginal mucous membranes are discussed in Chapter 11 (p. 359).

References

Ainsworth, A. M., Folberg, R., Reed, R. J. and Clark, W. H. (1979) Melanocytic nevi, melanocytomas, melanocytic dysplasias, and uncommon forms of melanoma. In *Human malignant Melanoma* (eds W. H. Clark, L. I. Goldman and M. J. Mastrangelo) New York: Grune & Stratton pp. 167–208.

Allyn, B., Kopf, A. W., Kahn, M. and Witten, V. H. (1963) Incidence of pigmented nevi. *J. Am. Med. Assoc.*, **186**, 890–3.

Armstrong, B., Heenan, P., Caruso, V., Glancy, R. and Holman, C. D. J. (1984) Seasonal variation in the junctional component of pigmented naevi. *Int. J. Cancer*, **34**, 441–2.

Aso, M., Hashimoto, K., Eto, H. *et al.* (1988) Expression of Schwann cell characteristics in pigmented nevus. Immunohistochemical study using monoclonal antibody to Schwann cell associated antigen. *Cancer*, **62**, 938–43.

Barnes, L. M. and Nordlund, J. J. (1987) The natural history of dysplastic nevi. A case history illustrating their evolution. *Arch. Dermatol*, **123**, 1059–61.

Bell, M. E. A., Hill, D. P. and Bhargava, M. K. (1979) Lymphatic invasion in pigmented nevi. *Am. J. Clin. Pathol.*, **72**, 97–100.

Berger, R. S. and Voorhees, J. J. (1971) Multiple congenital giant nevocellular nevi with halos. *Arch. Dermatol.*, **104**, 515–21.

Berman, A. (1978) Halo around a histiocytoma. *Arch. Dermatol.*, **114**, 1717–8.

Carney, J. A. (1990) Psammomatous melanotic schwannoma: a distinctive heritable tumor with special associations, including cardiac myxoma and the Cushing syndrome. *Am. J. Surg. Pathol.*, **14**, 206–22.

Champion, R. H. (1964) An unusual melanoma: 'malignant Sutton's naevus'. *Br. J. Dermatol.*, **76**, 347.

Christensen, W. N., Friedman, K. J., Woodruff, J. D. and Hood, A. F. (1987) Histologic characteristics of vulvar nevocellular nevi. *J. Cutan. Pathol.*, **14**, 87–91.

Cooke, K. R. (1988) Frequency of benign pigmented naevi in the general population. *Pigment Cell*, **9**, 8–26.

Cooke, K. R., Spears, G. F. S. and Skegg, D. C. G. (1985) Frequency of moles in a defined population. *J. Epidem. Comm. Health*, **39**, 48–52.

Côté, J., Watters, A. K. and O'Brien, E. A. (1986) Halo balloon cell nevus. *J. Cutan. Pathol.*, **13**, 123–7.

Cramer, S. F. (1990) Epithelial membrane staining of melanocytic nevi. *Hum. Pathol.*, **21**, 121–2.

De Wit, P. E. J., De Vaan, G. A. M., De Boo, Th. M., Lemmens, W. A. J. G. and Rampen, F. H. J. (1990) Prevalence of naevocytic naevi after chemotherapy for childhood cancer. *Med. Pediatr. Oncol.*, **18**, 336–8.

Dormandy, T. L. (1956) Gastrointestinal polyposis with mucocutaneous pigmentation (Peutz-Jeghers syndrome). *New Engl. J. Med.*, **256**, 1093–1103, 1141–6, 1186–90.

Eng, A. M. (1983) Solitary small active junctional nevi in juvenile patients. *Arch. Dermatol.*, **119**, 35–38.

Estrada, J. A., Piérard-Franchimont, C. and Piérard, G. (1990) Histogenesis of recurrent nevus. *Am. J. Dermatopathol.*, **12**, 370–2.

Foucar, E., Bentley, T. J., Laube, D. W. and Rosai, J. (1985) A histologic evaluation of nevocellular nevi in pregnancy. *Arch. Dermatol.*, **121**, 350–4.

Gallagher, R. P., McLean, D. I., Young, C. P. *et al.* (1990) Anatomic distribution of acquired menalocytic nevi in white children. A comparison with melanoma: the Vancouver mole study. *Arch. Dermatol.*, **126**, 466–71.

Gartmann, H. (1960) Ueber blasige Zellen im Naevuszellnaevus. *Z. Haut. Geschlechtskrankh.*, **28**, 148–59.

Gartmann, H. (1978) Zur Dignität der naevoiden Lentigo. *Z. Hautkr.*, **53**, 91–100.

Gauthier, Y., Surlève-Bazeille, J. E. and Texier, L. (1978) Halo nevi without dermal infiltrate. *Arch. Dermatol.*, **114**, 1718.

Goette, D. K. and Doty, R. D. (1978) Balloon cell nevus. Summary of the clinical and histologic characteristics. *Arch. Dermatol.*, **114**, 109–11.

Goetz, G. and Tsambaos, D. (1978) Eruptive nevocytic nevi after Lyell's syndrome. *Arch. Dermatol.*, **114**, 1400–1.

Goovaerts, G. and Buyssens, N. (1988) Nevus cell maturation or atrophy? *Am. J. Dermatopathol.*, **10**, 20–27.

Gray, M. H., Smoller, B. R., McNutt, N. S. and Hsu, A. (1990a) Neurofibromas and neurotized melanocytic nevi are immunohistochemically distinct neoplasms. *Am. J. Dermatol.*, **12**, 234–41.

Gray, M. H., Smoller, B. R., McNutt, N. S. and Hsu, A. (1990b) Immunohisto-chemical demonstration of Factor XIIIa expression in neurofibromas. A practical means of differentiating these tumours from neurotized melanocytic nevi and schwannomas. *Arch. Dermatol.*, **126**, 472–6.

Green, A., Siskind, V., Hansen, M.-E., Hanson, L. and Leech, P. (1989) Melanocytic nevi in schoolchildren in Queensland. *J. Am. Acad. Dermatol.*, **20**, 1054–60.

Guzzo, C., Johnson, B. and Honig, P. (1988) Cockarde nevus: a case report and review of the literature. *Pediatr. Dermatol.*, **4**, 250–3.

Hasegawa, J. I., Maeda, N., Kanzaki, T. and Mizuno, N. (1987) Spontaneous regression of congenital giant cell pigmented nevus with malignant melanoma. In *Clinical Dermatology. The CMD Case Collection* (eds D. S. Wilkinson, J. M. Mascaró and C. E. Orfanos), Stuttgart: Schattauer, pp. 46–47.

Hashimoto, K. and Bale, G. (1972) An electron microscopic study of balloon cell nevus. *Cancer*, **30**, 530–40.

Holman, C. D. J., Heenan, P. J., Caruso, V., Glancy, R. J. and Armstrong, B. K. (1983) Seasonal variation in the junctional component of pigmented naevi. *Int. J. Cancer*, **31**, 213–5.

James, M. P. and Wells, R. S. (1980) Cockade naevus: an unusual variant of the benign cellular naevus. *Acta Derm. Venereol. (Stockh.)*, **60**, 360–3.

Jemec, G. B., Bhogal, B. S. and Wojnarowska, F. (1988) Are acquired nevi oestrogen-dependent tumours? *Acta Derm. Venereol. (Stockh.)*, **67**, 451–3.

Jones, S. K., Moseley, H. and MacKie, R. M. (1987) UVA-induced melanocytic lesions. *Br. J. Dermatol.*, **117**, 111–5.

Jordaan, H. F. (1987) Follicular mucinosis in association with a melanocytic nevus. A report of two cases. *J. Cutan. Pathol.*, **14**, 122–6.

Kantor, G. R. and Wheeland, R. G. (1987) Transepidermal elimination of nevus cells. A possible mechanism of nevus involution. *Arch. Dermatol.*, **123**, 1371–4.

Kaufmann, J., Eichmann, A., Neves, C. *et al.* (1976) Lentiginosis profusa. *Dermatologica*, **153**, 116.

Kawamura, T., Shishiba, T. and Horie, N. (1982) The involvement of the sebaceous gland by nevus cells. Pathogenesis of the involvement and the fate of the involved gland. *J. Dermatol. (Tokyo)*, **9**, 185–8.

Kopf, A. W., Morrill, S. D. and Silberberg, I. (1965) Broad spectrum of leukoderma acquisitum centrifugum. *Arch. Dermatol.*, **92**, 14–35.

Kopf, A. W., Grupper, C., Baer, R. L. and Mitchell, J. C. (1977) Eruptive nevocytic nevi after severe bullous disease. *Arch. Dermatol.*, **113**, 1080–4.

Kornberg, R. and Ackerman, A. B. (1975) Pseudomelanoma: recurrent melanocytic nevus following partial surgical removal. *Arch. Dermatol.*, **111**, 1588–90.

Lambert, W. C. (1986) Focal transient acantholytic dermatosis in sites of regression in melanocytic lesions. *J. Cutan. Pathol.*, **13**, 452.

Levene, A. (1980) On the histological diagnosis and prognosis of malignant melanoma. *J. Clin. Pathol.*, **33**, 101–24.

Lynch, H. T., Frichot, B. C. and Lynch, J. F. (1977) Cancer control in xeroderma pigmentosum. *Arch. Dermatol.*, **113**, 193–5.

MacDonald, D. M. and Black, M. M. (1980) Secondary localized cutaneous amyloidosis in melanocytic naevi. *Br. J. Dermatol.*, **103**, 553–6.

MacKie, R. M., English, J., Aitchison, T. C., Fitzsimons, C. P. and Wilson, P. (1985) The number and distribution of benign pigmented moles (melanocytic naevi) in a healthy British population. *Br. J. Dermatol.*, **113**, 167–74.

Maize, J. C. and Foster, G. (1979) Age-related changes in melanocytic nevi. *Clin. Exp. Dermatol.*, **4**, 49–58.

Mark, G. J., Mihm, M. C., Liteplo, M. G., Reed, R. J. and Clark, W. H. (1973) Congenital melanocytic nevi of the small and garment type. Clinical, histologic and ultrastructural studies. *Hum. Pathol.*, **4**, 395–418.

Masson, P. (1951) My conception of cellular nevi. *Cancer*, **4**, 9–38.

McGibbon, D. H. and Wilson Jones, E. (1979) Fibrous papule of the face (nose). Fibrosing nevocytic nevus. *Am. J. Dermatopathol.*, **1**, 345–8.

Mehregan, A. H. and King, J. R. (1972) Multiple target-like pigmented nevi. *Arch. Dermatol.*, **105**, 129–30.

Mehregan, A. H. and Staricco, R. G. (1962) Elastic fibers in pigmented nevi. *J. Invest. Dermatol.*, **38**, 271–6.

Meyerson, L. B. (1971) A peculiar papulosquamous eruption involving pigmented nevi. *Arch. Dermatol.*, **103**, 510–2.

Miescher, G. (1935) Umwandlung von Naevuszellen in Talgdrüsenzellen? *Arch. Derm. Syph.*, **171**, 119–24.

Miescher, G. and Von Albertini, A. (1935) Histologie de 100 cas de naevi pigmentaires d'après les mèthodes de Masson. *Bull. Soc. Fr. Dermatol. Syphil.*, **42**, 1265–73.

Mishima, Y. (1967) Melanotic tumors. In *Ultrastructure of Normal and Abnormal Skin* (ed. A. S. Zelickson), Philadelphia: Lea & Febiger, pp. 388–424.

Mitchell, M. S., Nordlund, J. J. and Lerner, A. B. (1980) Comparison of cell-mediated immunity to melanoma cells in patients with vitiligo, halo nevi or melanoma. *J. Invest. Dermatol.*, **75**, 144–7.

Moynahan, E. J. (1962) Multiple symmetrical moles with psychic and somatic infantilism and genital hypoplasia: first male case of a new syndrome. *Proc. Royal Soc. Med.*, **55**, 959–60.

Nakagawa, H., Hori, Y., Sato, S. *et al.* (1984) The nature and origin of the melanin macroglobule. *J. Invest. Dermatol.*, **83**, 134–9.

Narita, T., Eto, T. and Ito, T. (1987) Peutz-Jeghers syndrome with adenomas and adenocarcinomas in colonic polyps. *Am. J. Surg. Pathol.*, **11**, 76–81.

Nicholls, E. M. (1973) Development and elimination of pigmented moles, and the anatomical distribution of primary malignant melanoma. *Cancer*, **32**, 191–5.

Nickoloff, B. J., Walton, R., Pregerson-Rodan, K., Jacobs, A. H. and Cox, A. J.

(1986) Immunohistologic patterns of congenital nevocellular nevi. *Arch. Dermatol.*, **122**, 1263–8.

Nordlund, J. J., Kirkwood, J., Forget, B. M. *et al.* (1974) An ultrastructural study of balloon cell nevus. Relationship of mast cells to nevus cells. *Cancer*, **34**, 615–25.

Okun, M. R., Donellan, B. and Edelstein, L. (1974) An ultrastructural study of balloon cell nevus. *Cancer*, **34**, 615–25.

Park, H. K., Leonard, D. D., Arrington III, J. H. and Lund, H. Z. (1987) Recurrent melanocytic nevi: clinical and histologic review of 175 cases. *J. Am. Acad. Dermatol.*, **17**, 285–92.

Penneys, N. S., Mayoral, F., Barnhill, R., Ziegels-Weissman, J. and Nadji, M. (1985) Delineation of nevus cell nests in inflammatory infiltrates by immunohistochemical staining for the presence of S100 protein. *J. Cutan. Pathol.*, **12**, 28–32.

Piérard, G. E. and Piérard-Franchimont, C. (1984) The proliferative activity of cells of malignant melanomas. *Am. J. Dermatopathol.*, **6**, 317S–23S.

Reed, R. J., Webb, S. V. and Clark, W. H. (1990) Minimal deviation melanoma (halo nevus variant). *Am. J. Surg. Pathol.*, **14**, 53–68.

Requena, L., Ambrojo, P. and Sánchez Yus, E. (1990) Trichilemmal cyst under a compound melanocytic nevus. *J. Cutan. Pathol.*, **17**, 185–8.

Rupec, M. and Huck, H. J. (1976) Zur Frage des sogenannten Osteo-Naevus Nanta. *Dermatol. Monatsschr.*, **162**, 730–7.

Rupec, M. and Vakilzadeh, F. (1974) Zur Frage der Transepidermalen Ausscheidung von Nävuszellnestern. *Dermatologica*, **148**, 61–64.

Salm, R. and Swinburne, L. M. (1963) Bone formation in pigmented naevi. *J. Pathol. Bacteriol.*, **85**, 297–303.

Schoenfeld, R. J. and Pinkus, H. (1958) The recurrence of nevi after incomplete removal. *Arch. Dermatol.*, **78**, 30–35.

Schrader, W. A. and Helwig, E. B. (1967) Balloon cell nevi. *Cancer*, **20**, 1502–14.

Seab, J. A., Graham, J. H. and Helwig, E. B. (1989) Deep penetrating nevus. *Am. J. Surg. Pathol.*, **13**, 39–44.

Shitara A., Sato, Y. and Morohashi, M. (1977) Nevus cells observed in the sebaceous glands. *J. Dermatol.*, **4**, 141–5.

Smolle, J., Soyer, H. -P. and Kerl., H. (1989) Proliferative activity of cutaneous melanocytic tumors defined by Ki-67 monoclonal antibody. A quantitative immunohistochemical study. *Am. J. Dermatopathol.*, **11**, 301–7.

Söderström., K. O. (1987) Angiomatous type of intradermal nevi. *Am. J. Dermatopathol.*, **9**, 549–51.

Soltani, K., Bernstein, J. E. and Lorinez, A. L. (1979) Eruptive nevocytic nevi following erythema multiforme. *J. Am. Acad. Dermatol.*, **1**, 503–5.

Soltani, K., Pepper, M. C., Simjee, S. and Apatoff, B. R. (1984) Large acquired nevocytic nevi induced by the Koebner phenomenon. *J. Cutan. Pathol.*, **11**, 296–9.

Starink, T. M. and Brownstein, M. H. (1986) Desmoplastic trichoepithelioma with intradermal nevus: a combined malformation. *J. Cutan. Pathol.*, **13**, 464.

Stegmaier, O. C. (1959) Natural regression of the melanocytic nevus. *J. Invest. Dermatol.*, **32**, 413–9.

Stegmaier, O. C. and Montgomery, H. (1953) Histopathologic studies of pigmented nevi in children. *J. Invest. Dermatol.*, **20**, 51–64.

Su, W. P. D., Goellner, J. R. and Peters, M. S. (1985) Unusual histopathologic variants of malignant melanoma. In *Pathology of Unusual Malignant Cutaneous Tumors* (ed. M. R. Wick), New York: Marcel Dekker, pp. 281–98.

Sutton, R. L. (1916) An unusual variety of vitiligo (leukoderma acquisitum centrifugum). *J. Cutan. Dis.*, **34**, 797–800.

Touraine, A. (1941) Lentiginose centrofaciale et dysplasies associées. *Bull. Soc. Fr. Dermatol. Syphil.*, **48**, 518.

Tucker, S. B., Horstmann, J. P., Hertel, B., Aranha, G. and Rosai, J. (1980) Activation of nevi in patients with malignant melanoma. *Cancer*, **46**, 822–7.

Unna, P. G. (1896) *Histopathology of the Diseases of the Skin*. New York: Macmillan Publ., p. 1129.

Van Paesschen, M.-A., Goovaerts, G. and Buyssens, N. (1990) A study of the so-called neurotization of nevi. *Am. J. Dermatopathol.*, **12**, 242–8.

Van Scott, E. J., Reinertson, R. P. and McCall, C. B. (1957) Prevalence, histological types, and significance of palmar and plantar nevi. *Cancer*, **10**, 363–7.

Voron, D. A., Hatfield, H. H. and Kalkhoff, D. K. (1976) Multiple lentigines syndrome, case report and review of the literature. *Am. J. Med.*, **60**, 447–56.

Wayte, D. M. and Helwig, E. B. (1968) Halo nevi. *Cancer*, **22**, 69–90.

Weedon, D. (1982) Unusual features of nevocellular nevi. *J. Cutan. Pathol.*, **9**, 284–92.

Weiss, L. W. and Zelickson, A. S. (1977) Giant melanosomes in multiple lentigines syndrome. *Arch. Dermatol.*, **113**, 491–4.

Williams, H. C., Salisbury, J., Brett, J. and Du Vivier, A. (1988) Sunbed lentigines. *Br. Med. J.*, **296**, 1097.

Wilson Jones, E., Marks, R. and Pongsehirun, D. (1975) Naevus superficialis lipomatosus. *Br. J. Dermatol.*, **93**, 121–33.

Yesudian, P. and Thambiah, A. S. (1976) Perinevoid alopecia. An unusual variant of alopecia areata. *Arch. Dermatol.*, **112**, 1432–4.

Yong, S. L., Lozinski, A. Z., McLean, D. I. and Worth, A. J. (1989) *Second International Conference on Melanoma*, Poster Session, Venice, 16–19 October, 1989.

Yuki, N., Shitara, A., Ito, M. and Sato, Y. (1984) Transepithelial elimination of nevus cell nests. *J. Dermatol.*, **11**, 149–54.

5 Cutaneous blue naevi and related lesions

Blue naevi are proliferations of dendritic and/or fusiform melanocytes, located entirely within the dermis, and sometimes extending into the subcutis. In contrast to common acquired naevi, blue naevi are thought to originate within the dermis rather than the epidermis; a migratory arrest of melanocytes travelling from the neural crest to the epidermis has been postulated by some (Levene, 1980). However, the occurrence of naevi combining the histology of common acquired naevus and blue naevus (p. 126), points to a close histogenetic relationship between the two and indicates that the theory of migratory arrest may not be the entire story.

Blue naevi are usually divided into 'common' and 'cellular' variants, although the histological spectrum of these lesions is considerable, so that it is sometimes difficult to assign an individual lesion to one of these two subtypes. Common and cellular blue naevi were described by Tièche (1906), and Darier (1925), but a detailed, classical description of their histological appearances was given in 1968 by Rodriguez and Ackerman.

Cutaneous blue naevi are mainly located within the reticular dermis, and because of the relatively deep location and marked pigmentation, they appear somewhat bluish when viewed through the opaque layers of epidermis and upper dermis. This bluish colour results from the fact that the *Tyndall phenomenon* (light scattered in the opaque overlying layers and partly reflected back) is strongest with short wavelengths, while light of longer wavelengths is scattered backwards to a lesser extent, and is absorbed more in the pigmented deeper dermal layers. This results in a colour shift towards blue, when the lesion is viewed through the overlying epidermis and upper dermis, a phenomenon not called into play when the lesion is viewed on cross-section.

Related lesions, some of which are congenital, include the mongolian spot, Ota's naevus (naevus fuscocoeruleus ophthalmomaxillaris), Ito's naevus (naevus fuscocoeruleus acromiodeltoideus), Sun's naevus (naevus fuscocoeruleus zygomaticus), and intradermal melanocytic hamartoma. Because of their histological similarities with blue naevus, these will be discussed here rather than in the next chapter dealing with congenital naevi.

Blue naevi have been reported in a variety of extracutaneous sites, such as the sclera, oral mucosa, vagina, uterine cervix, prostate, spermatic cord and lymph node; these lesions are dealt with in Chapter 11.

5.1   Common blue naevus

5.1.1   Clinical features

The common blue naevus is usually a symmetrical, slightly raised, smooth-surfaced papule or nodule with a bluish grey, black or dark brown colour and often indistinct borders. It usually occurs singly, with a predilection for the scalp, face and distal extremities, especially the dorsum of the hand and foot (Dorsey and Montgomery, 1954). The common blue naevus is usually smaller than 1 cm, but exceptional cases exceed 3 cm in diameter (Rodriguez and Ackerman, 1968). There is a broad age range: it may be present at birth, but most often comes to clinical attention in the third to fifth decade. It appears to be about twice as common in females as in males. Rarely, a perilesional depigmented halo is present.

Malignancy developing in a common blue naevus is exceedingly rare; recently, a case was reported as such by Modly and colleagues (1989). However, the data presented leave room for some doubt. For example, the lesion was located on the buttock, a rare site for a common blue naevus, but a predilection site for cellular blue naevus. The pre-existent lesion showed features of common rather than cellular blue naevus, but this may have been due to destruction of much of the pre-existent lesion by the melanoma; cellular blue naevi may exhibit areas indistinguishable from common blue naevus.

5.1.2   Pathological features

On section, the cut surface shows an area of brown or black pigmentation with indistinct borders located within the thickened dermis.

Microscopically, a poorly circumscribed proliferation of elongated melanocytes is seen within the dermis, usually mainly the reticular dermis (Figure 5.1). The lesion often involves the entire thickness of the dermis and may reach the subcutaneous fat. The growth pattern is infiltrating rather than pushing; compact, well-demarcated groups of

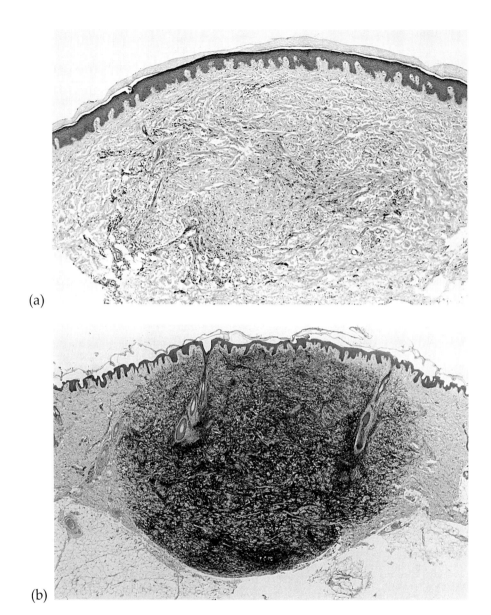

(a)

(b)

Figure 5.1 Common blue naevus. (a) An ill-defined proliferation of pigmented dendritic melanocytes, with accompanying fibrosis, is situated in the reticular dermis (HE, × 35). (b) Heavily pigmented blue naevus occupying the entire thickness of the dermis (HE, × 20).

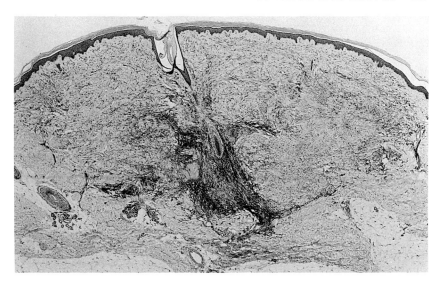

Figure 5.2   Common blue naevus; increased cellularity and pigmentation around a hair follicle (HE, × 20).

melanocytes are absent. However, as indicated above, some lesions may combine the histological features of common and cellular blue naevus. A large proportion of melanocytes are pigmented, both superficially and deeply within the lesion. Melanocytes infiltrate between the thick collagen fibres of the reticular dermis, sometimes accompanied by a small amount of finely fibrillar amphophilic stroma. In other cases there is a marked fibrotic response, and perivascular lymphocytic infiltrates may be present. There is often an increased cellularity and pigmentation in the vicinity of skin appendages entrapped within the naevus (Figure 5.2). Melanocytes may also aggregate preferentially along nerves and vessels. Often there is a preferential horizontal orientation of the melanocytes, or a storiform architecture resembling a dermatofibroma is seen. However, especially in cases located on the head and neck, where the skin may contain numerous well-developed hair follicles, vertical orientation of bundles of melanocytes along these adnexal structures may result in a varied and somewhat irregular architecture.

The melanocytes of a common blue naevus are slender, fusiform or elongated and bipolar, or may possess long, branching dendrites, which are most apparent in cells engorged with melanin (Figure 5.3) and when melanin stains are used. The cells vary somewhat in size, and contain an oval or elongated nucleus, which may be grooved longitudinally or may show irregular wrinkles and folds. These elon-

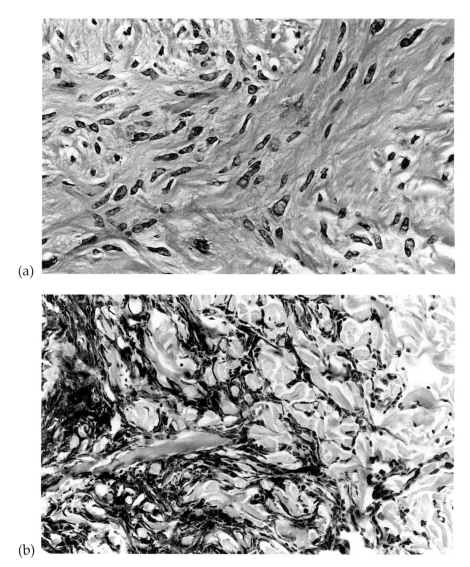

(a)

(b)

Figure 5.3 Common blue naevus. (a) The melanocytes exhibit slightly irregular, oval or elongated nuclei and a small amount of poorly defined pale cytoplasm (HE, × 370). (b) Heavily pigmented elongated melanocytes (HE, × 185).

gated nuclei may exhibit a mild degree of nuclear pleomorphism and anisochromasia. Mitoses are, however, rare. The nuclear chromatin is usually finely dispersed, or the nucleus is vacuolated, and there may be a small or moderately sized central nucleolus, which is, however, often obscured by the chromatin. Scattered melanocytes possess larger nuclei with a less finely stippled chromatin pattern. Mostly the melanocytes have only a small amount of pale cytoplasm, hardly visible on HE-stained sections except when it contains melanin granules. In darkly pigmented blue naevi, the melanin may be so abundant that it obscures the nucleus. *There is no 'maturation' or zoning: melanocytes at the base of the lesion are similar to those in the upper parts.* Rarely, ballooning of melanocytes (p. 90) may be seen (Schrader and Helwig, 1967; Gardner and Vazquez, 1970).

Varying numbers of melanophages, studded with coarse melanin granules, are present between the melanocytes. On HE-stained sections, heavily pigmented melanocytes may be difficult to distinguish from melanophages. The latter are generally plumper and contain coarser, irregular clumps of melanin (secondary melanosomes) rather than the more regularly shaped melanosomes present in melanocytes (Figure 5.4). They are negative with the DOPA reaction, but melanocytes may be negative as well. Immunocytochemically, dermal melanocytes and macrophages can be distinguished by S-100 and HAM-56 (antimacrophage) immunostaining (Fleming and Bergfeld, 1990). Furthermore, the melanocytes of blue naevi are positive for monoclonal antibody HMB-45 (p. 23; Sun *et al.*, 1990).

There is often a thin uninvolved zone immediately beneath the overlying epidermis, which may exhibit some hyperpigmentation and melanocytic hyperplasia (Ainsworth *et al.*, 1979). Usually, at least part

Table 5.1 Common blue naevus

Clinical features
  Symmetrical bluish grey, brown or black nodule with smooth surface,
    usually <1 cm
  Congenital, or acquired with broad age range (peak incidence in 3rd–5th
    decade)
  Scalp, face, distal extremities preferred sites
  Female preponderance (2:1)

Histological features
  Intradermal poorly circumscribed proliferation of fusiform, bipolar or
    dendritic melanocytes with varying degrees of pigmentation
  Often free subepidermal Grenz zone
  Sclerotic stromal response often present

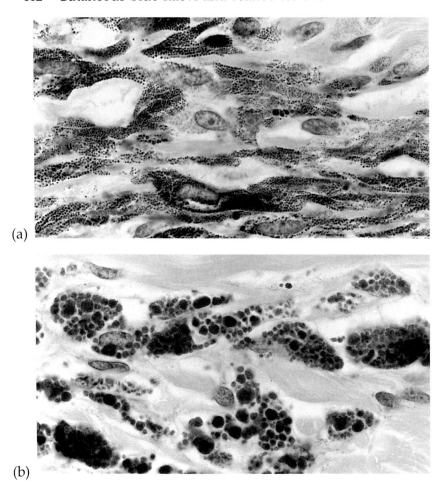

Figure 5.4   Common blue naevus. (a) Melanocytes exhibit slender processes laden with small, round melanin granules. (b) Melanophages are laden with irregular clumps of melanin ('secondary melanosomes'), varying greatly in size and shape (HE, × 920).

of these junctional melanocytes are heavily pigmented, and they may possess long dendritic processes.

The main features of common blue naevus are summarized in Table 5.1.

5.1.3   Differential diagnosis

The diagnosis usually poses no great difficulties. Common blue naevus should be distinguished from mongolian spot, Ito's naevus, Ota's naevus, desmoplastic Spitz naevus and dermatoses leading to incontinentia pigmenti, such as lichen planus, lupus erythematosus and fixed drug eruption, as well as from lesions containing iron rather than melanin, such as dermatofibroma and cutaneous histiocytoma. In some instances, desmoplastic melanoma enters the differential diagnosis.

Desmoplastic Spitz naevus (p. 175) consists of larger cells, especially in the superficial portion; there may be a junctional component, or the papillary dermis contains compact nests or strands of amelanotic or lightly pigmented melanocytes.

Occasionally, a *dermatofibroma* with prominent haemosiderin deposition and little fat may resemble a blue naevus; however, the different appearance of the golden-brown, strongly refractile iron pigment granules, the absence of long pigmented dendrites, and especially stains for melanin and iron will establish the correct diagnosis. *Formalin pigment* deposition in dermal macrophages may occur when formalin is not buffered and the pH drops below 6; the resulting picture may sometimes resemble a blue naevus. However, formalin pigment is birefringent and does not accept melanin stains (Ackerman and Penneys, 1970). *Tattoos* may also mimic common blue naevus; however, the pigment does not stain as melanin, pigmented dermal macrophages are usually more widely scattered, and dendritic melanocytes are absent.

In some instances, common blue naevus has to be distinguished from *desmoplastic melanoma* (p. 253). Importantly, lesions exhibiting preferential vertical orientation of long, broad and densely cellular bundles of melanocytes should be viewed with much suspicion. Especially when present in sun-damaged skin of elderly patients, one should search for the features of lentigo maligna of the overlying epidermis, mitotic activity and neurotropism (p. 256). Desmoplastic melanoma shows a greater degree of nuclear enlargement and pleomorphism, so that attention to the cytology is very important in this respect. Furthermore, at the time it comes to clinical attention, desmoplastic melanoma is usually larger than most blue naevi.

5.2 Cellular blue naevus

Like the common blue naevus, the cellular blue naevus consists of an intradermal proliferation of melanocytes, but with a more varied, often characteristically biphasic architecture. It is often larger and more densely cellular than the common blue naevus, and confusion with melanoma is more likely to occur, both clinically and histologically. Early pathological descriptions of this tumour were provided by Darier (1925) and Masson (1950).

5.2.1   Clinical features

Cellular blue naevus occurs in a wide age range. Some are congenital or form part of a congenital naevus (Iemoto and Kondo, 1984), or arise in early childhood. About two-thirds arise before the fifth decade, but they may occur even in old age (Temple-Camp *et al.*, 1988). Some workers report a female predominance of about 2:1 (Rodriguez and Ackerman, 1968), while others found a roughly equal distribution among the sexes (Temple-Camp *et al.*, 1988). The majority occur in Caucasians. In contrast to common blue naevi, the buttocks and sacrococcygeal region are favoured sites. There is also a preference for the scalp, face and distal parts of the limbs, but they may occur in a wide variety of sites.

Cellular blue naevus presents as a bluish black, slate-grey or, rarely, skin-coloured nodule. Sometimes, there is a dark centre and a greyish surrounding zone. Cystic change is present in some cases and may occasionally be noted clinically. Rarely, the tumour is polypoid. Ulceration is seen in a minority of cases. In Rodriguez and Ackerman's series of 45 cases (1968), the average size was 1.76 cm, as opposed to 0.57 cm for common blue naevi. In a later series, 19 out of 26 cases were smaller than 1 cm (Temple-Camp *et al.*, 1988). Sizes over 3 cm are occasionally seen; because of their size, intense pigmentation and, occasionally, rapid growth, ulceration and bleeding, cellular blue naevi may be misdiagnosed clinically as melanoma (Epstein and Pinkus, 1969). In rare instances, cellular blue naevi reach giant sizes (Upshaw *et al.*, 1947; Sterchi *et al.*, 1987). Sudden increase in size and pigmentation during pregnancy has been reported (Sterchi *et al.*, 1987), a phenomenon which may also occur in common acquired naevi and melanomas.

Malignant transformation is a rare but well-documented occurrence: 'malignant blue naevus' is discussed in Chapter 9 (p. 274).

5.2.2   Pathological features

Macroscopically, the cellular blue naevus presents as an intradermal tumour, sometimes extending into the subcutis, and with an often irregularly distributed pigmentation, ranging from light brown to jet-black. Rarely, it is almost devoid of pigment.

Histologically, cellular blue naevi exhibit a very varied spectrum of histological appearances. The most important common denominators are their *primary location within the dermis, the presence of fusiform, bipolar and/or dendritic melanocytes, and a high cellularity.*

The melanocytes usually form compact nodules, masses and/or sheets, which generally alternate with a second component of more

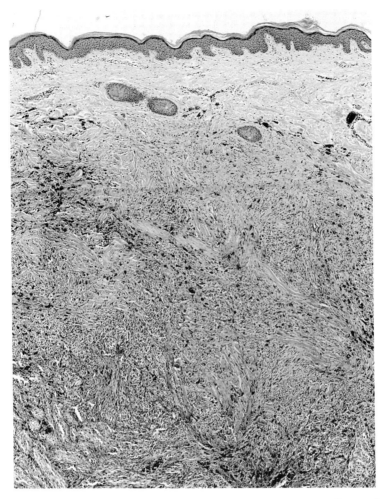

Figure 5.5   Cellular blue naevus. Low power view, with partly diffuse and partly biphasic growth pattern (HE, × 45).

heavily pigmented elongated or dendritic melanocytes, which form less compact aggregates, and which are embedded in a fibrotic or sclerotic tissue (Figure 5.5). These two cell types may be closely intermingled and merge with one another, or they may contrast sharply, resulting in a characteristic biphasic pattern (Figure 5.6).

This architecture contrasts with that of common blue naevi, in which compact nodules and aggregates of melanocytes are absent. The 'biphasic' picture may be somewhat reminiscent of neural differentiation, hence the former name of 'neuro-naevus' (Masson, 1950).

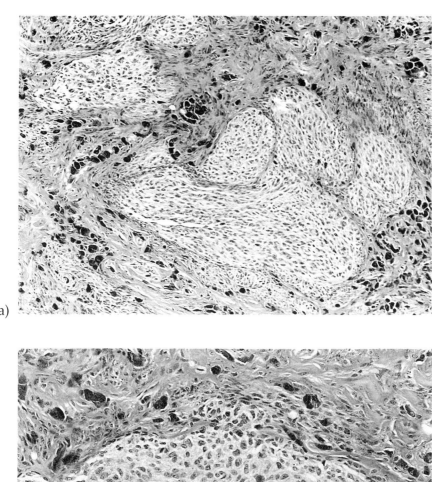

(a)

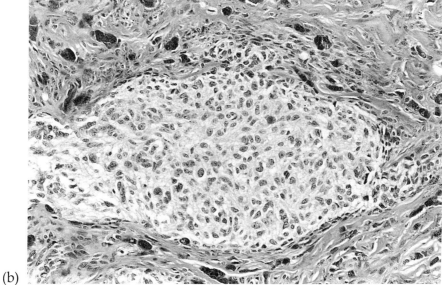

(b)

Figure 5.6 Cellular blue naevus. Slightly irregular nodules of pale melanocytes alternate with sclerotic tissue containing pigmented elongated melanocytes and melanophages (a) (HE, × 90). (b) (HE, × 185).

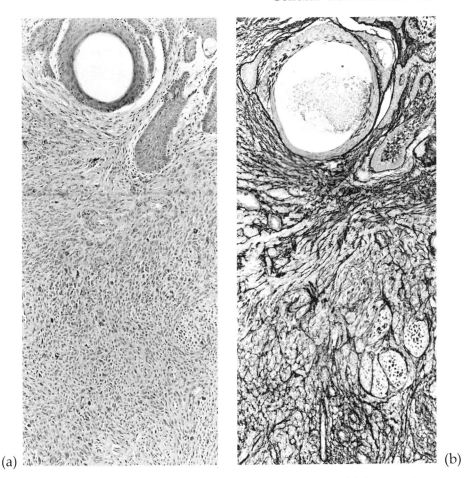

(a)   (b)

Figure 5.7   Cellular blue naevus. Even when on HE sections (a) the growth pattern appears diffuse, a reticulin stain (b) often reveals a conspicuously nested pattern (HE, × 90).

However, *in rare instances a biphasic pattern is absent*, the lesion consisting largely or wholly of the oval cell type, forming closely adjacent compact nests, or exhibiting a diffuse growth pattern (Figures 5.7–5.9). Temple-Camp and colleagues (1988) subdivided cellular blue naevi into mixed biphasic, alveolar, fascicular-neuronaevoid and 'atypical' subtypes. Several of their cases showed more than one architectural pattern of growth, so that such a subdivision is more indicative of the histological variability of these lesions rather than that it constitutes a separation into distinct subtypes.

The epidermis overlying a cellular blue naevus is usually intact, but

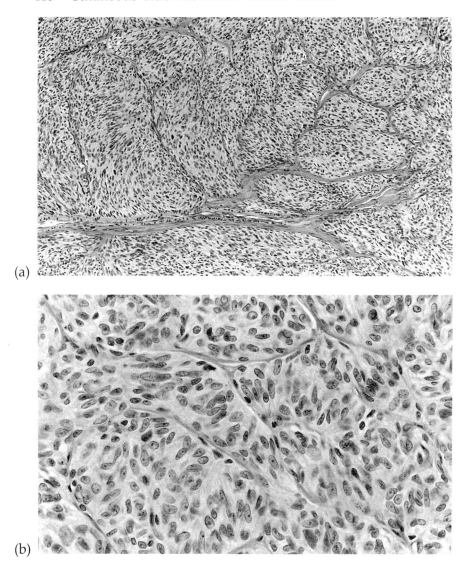

Figure 5.8   Cellular blue naevus. Compact nodules and trabeculae of non-pigmented oval melanocytes; very little intervening stroma. (a) HE, × 90; (b) HE, × 370.

ulceration occurs in a minority of cases. The proliferation often *engulfs cutaneous adnexae* (Figure 5.10); there may be follicular stasis or widening of entrapped sweat glands. Arrector pili muscles may also be invaded

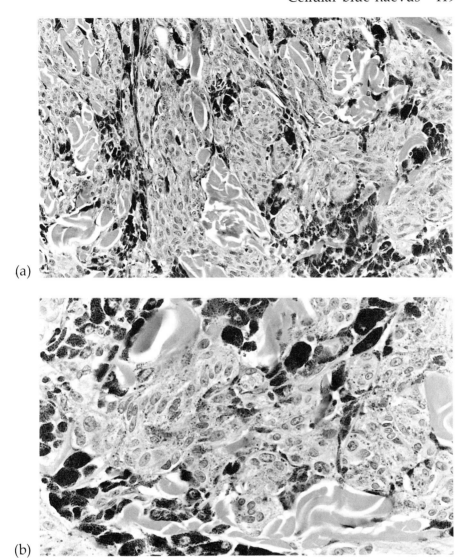

(a)

(b)

Figure 5.9   Cellular blue naevus. Strands and nests of oval or elongated, lightly pigmented melanocytes, surrounded by heavily pigmented melanophages, are closely intermingled with pre-existent dermal collagen. (a) HE, × 185; (b) HE, × 370.

by the melanocytes. In some instances, perivascular hyalinization is seen; there may be some perivascular lymphocytic infiltrate.

The lesion *often extends into the subcutaneous fatty tissue* (Figure 5.11), *which may be associated with an abrupt change to a 'pushing' growth pattern:*

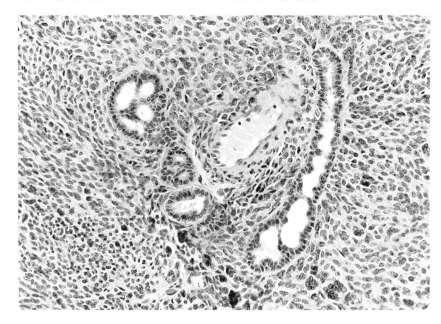

Figure 5.10   Cellular blue naevus. Sweat gland engulfed by fusiform melanocytes. A few tumour giant cells are present (HE, × 185).

this may look alarming to those unfamiliar with this feature. Sometimes, perineural growth and invasion of lymph vessels is detected. *Necrosis is very rarely present, which contrasts with malignant blue naevus, which shows an early tendency to necrosis* (p. 123).

Table 5.2 Cellular blue naevus

Clinical features
  Cutaneous pigmented or skin-coloured nodule, usually under 2 cm
  Ulceration uncommon, sometimes cystic change
  Wide age range, most occur before age 40
  Female predominance 2:1
  Predilection sites: buttocks, sacrococcygeal region, distal limbs, scalp, face

Histological features
  Intradermal location, often extension into subcutis
  Proliferation of oval, elongated, bipolar, or dendritic melanocytes
  Usually 'biphasic' pattern of compact nodules intermingled with more
    heavily pigmented dendritic cells
  Mitoses often present, usually less than 1 per mm^2
  Necrosis very rare

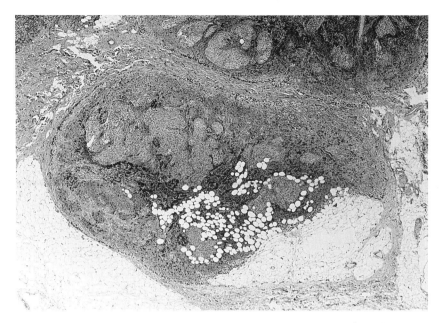

Figure 5.11   Cellular blue naevus, extending into subcutaneous fatty tissue (HE, × 20).

Cytologically, cellular blue naevi also present a more varied spectrum of appearances than common blue naevi. Within the compact nodules and aggregates, the melanocytes are usually plump, oval or fusiform, and contain little or no melanin. The nuclei are oval, sometimes mildly pleomorphic, and may show some anisochromasia. Small or moderate numbers of mitoses are often present, but atypical mitoses are very rare. The melanocytes between these nodules are usually elongated, slender, bipolar or dendritic, and contain a moderate or large amount of melanin (Figure 5.12). As indicated above, there may be a gradual merging of different cell types and growth patterns, whereas in other areas different cell types may appear as separate and distinct populations. *Melanocytic giant cells* (Figure 5.13) are not uncommon.

The features of cellular blue naevus are summarized in Table 5.2.

Tschen and colleagues (1989) described a cellular blue naevus in which the melanocytes contained conspicuous eosinophilic, PAS-positive, intracytoplasmic globules, measuring up to 15 μm in diameter. They were often surrounded by a clear halo. Melanin stains often revealed some central positivity. Electron microscopy indicated that these globules represented large, abnormal melanosomes.

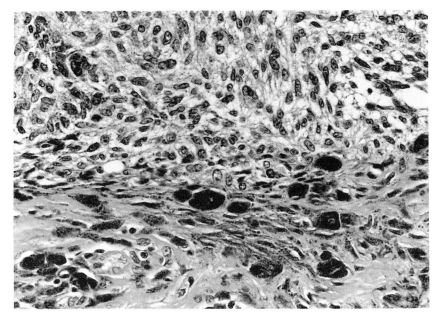

Figure 5.12 Cellular blue naevus. Compact nodule of pale non-pigmented melanocytes (top) and heavily pigmented dendritic melanocytes and melanophages in sclerotic stroma (bottom) (HE, × 370).

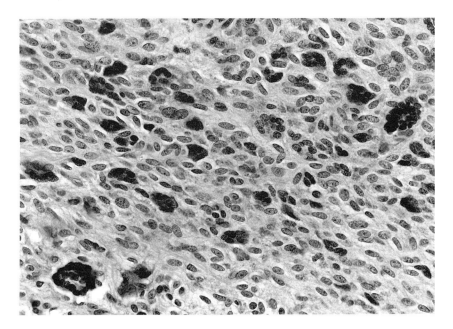

Figure 5.13 Giant cells in cellular blue naevus (HE, × 370).

Table 5.3 Cellular blue naevus *vs* malignant blue naevus

	Cellular blue naevus	*Malignant blue naevus*
Size	usually less than 2 cm (but may be over 3 cm)	most over 3 cm
Involvement of skeletal muscle	rare	not uncommon
Widespread necrosis	rare	common
Cystic change	sometimes	sometimes
Nuclear atypia	moderate, seldom marked	often marked
Mitoses	usually less than 1 per mm^2	may be numerous

5.2.3   *Differential diagnosis*

Because of their size, the extension into the subcutis, the presence of mitoses and some cytonuclear atypia, cellular blue naevi may be mis-diagnosed as *melanoma* or *malignant blue naevus* (Avidor and Kessler, 1977). Indeed, seven out of the 45 cellular blue naevi reported by Rodriguez and Ackerman (1968) had been originally diagnosed as melanoma. Importantly, an intraepidermal component is generally present in primary melanoma and melanoma cells within the dermis are seldom dendritic. *Malignant blue naevus* is very rare and usually shows necrosis even in small tumours, as well as many mitoses, including atypical ones (Table 5.3; p. 274).

Cellular blue naevus should also be distinguished from *melanoma of soft parts* (clear cell sarcoma; p. 366). The latter arises practically always in the deep soft tissues of the extremities, usually from tendons and aponeuroses, but may involve the overlying skin. Histologically, melanoma of soft parts lacks the biphasic pattern usually present in cellular blue naevus: strands and fascicles of pale tumour cells with vesicular nuclei containing a prominent nucleolus are seen within a usually paucicellular sclerotic stroma.

The recently described *cellular neurothekeoma* (Barnhill and Mihm, 1990), occurring mainly on the head and neck of young adults, exhibits fascicles of pale polygonal, oval or spindled cells, lying within the reticular dermis. The architecture of the lesion may superficially resemble that of a cellular blue naevus. However, a biphasic pattern and melanin are both absent. The cells are S-100 negative, although this needs confirmation since S-100 positivity has been reported by some workers in conventional neurothekeoma.

5.2.4 'Atypical blue naevus'

Avidor and Kessler (1977) described three cases of a lesion which they designated 'atypical blue naevus'. Two of these occurred in young children. They were characterized by the presence of a nodule of large, pleomorphic melanocytes deep within the dermis, associated with an inflammatory response. One case showed an additional intradermal naevus component, so that this lesion would appear to qualify as a combined naevus (p. 126). In one lesion, mitoses were present within the melanocytic nodule. No statement was made as to the complete-ness of the resections, and the follow-up time of the latter case was only one year, which does not provide conclusive evidence that these lesions were benign.

A further case of this currently ill-defined and still debatable entity, occurring in the paravertebral muscles of a 9-year-old girl, was reported by Temple-Camp and colleagues (1988). In the latter case, there was a 2.5-year disease-free follow-up period. Evidently, more such cases and longer follow-up will be necessary to substantiate claims that such lesions are indeed benign and that they constitute an identifiable and distinct subgroup of blue naevus.

5.2.5 Involvement of regional lymph nodes

Occasionally a blue naevus of the skin is associated with small aggregates of similar melanocytes situated in regional lymph nodes (Allen and Spitz, 1953; Dorsey and Montgomery, 1954; Rodriguez and Ackerman, 1968; Lambert and Brodkin, 1984; Sterchi et al., 1987). This appears to be far more commonly seen in lymph nodes draining cellular blue naevi than in those draining common blue naevi (Rodriguez and Ackerman, 1968; Lambert and Brodkin, 1984). The aggregates are often located in the subcapsular sinus and lymph node parenchyma, as opposed to the more common naevus cell aggregates and blue naevi of lymph nodes (p. 362, 364) which are located within the lymph node capsule. Such nodal aggregates of blue naevus cells are highly suggestive of metastatic tumour. This phenomenon is prob-ably not infrequent in view of the relative rarity of cellular blue naevi, and poses an obvious diagnostic challenge to the histopathologist.

The underlying mechanisms are poorly understood; some authors envisaged an arrest of migration of melanoblasts from the neural crest, but it is unclear why such melanoblasts would localize specifically in lymph nodes. Others have favoured a process of spread from the skin lesion via afferent lymph vessels.

The important practical point is that *these lymph node deposits do not adversely affect the prognosis*. When these intranodal nests of cellular blue naevus conform to the histological appearance of benign cellular blue naevus, they do not indicate the presence of potentially life-threatening disease, and treatment should accordingly be conservative.

Metastatic malignant blue naevus is dealt with in Chapter 9 (p. 274).

5.3   Plaque-type blue naevus

Occasionally blue naevi form large plaques, which sometimes invade into underlying tissues. Such lesions have measured up to 17 cm in largest diameter (Upshaw *et al.*, 1947) and may occur anywhere on the body. Some are congenital, but others appear later in life, even in adulthood (Tsoïtis *et al.*, 1983). There is no familial clustering of cases. Reported numbers are small, but there appears to be a male preponderance. A case occurring several years after severe sunburn was described in a 14-year-old boy (Hendricks, 1981).

Rarely, destructive invasive growth has been reported in large congential blue naevi: in one case, occurring on the thorax of a 9-year-old boy, there was ingrowth into the pectoral muscle (Upshaw *et al.*, 1947). Similar cases have been described by others (McWhorter and Woolner, 1954; Silverberg *et al.*, 1971; Findler *et al.*, 1981).

Histologically, the features of the common (Pittman and Fisher, 1976) or cellular type of blue naevus are seen. The overlying and adjacent epidermis may show lentiginous hyperplasia and hyperpigmentation (Ishibashi *et al.*, 1990). Often there is peri-appendageal accumulation of spindled melanocytes (Tuthill *et al.*, 1982), sometimes with an additional epithelioid component associated with increased cellular atypia (Upshaw *et al.*, 1947; Hendricks, 1981). The histology of such cases resembles that of so-called equine melanotic disease, which occurs in ageing grey horses (Levene, 1980).

5.4   Target blue naevus

Rarely, a common or cellular blue naevus shows a concentrically arranged variation in pigmentation, the pigmented centre being surrounded by a less pigmented rim, which in turn is surrounded by a circle of increased pigmentation. This lesion, which is often sufficiently distinctive to be recognized clinically, has been designated 'target blue naevus' (Bondi *et al.*, 1983). It occurs especially on the dorsum of the hand and foot, but very occasionally on the back or the perianal region. The striking pattern of pigmentation often evolves from an evenly pigmented lesion *via* a process of depigmentation, which may have caused alarm (Bondi *et al.*, 1983).

Histologically, the dark centre and outer ring contain closely aggregated, heavily pigmented dermal dendritic melanocytes, with or without the focal aggregates of plump spindle cells seen in cellular blue naevus, whereas the less pigmented area shows far fewer melanocytes. (Gartmann, 1965; Bondi *et al.*, 1983; Gartmann, 1987). The histogenesis of the striking architecture of this lesion remains obscure. For practical purposes, it is important to know of this type of blue naevus, in order to avoid confusion with regressing melanoma. The lesion should also be distinguished from cockade naevus (p. 93) and from halo naevus (p. 85).

5.5   Combined naevus

In combined ('true and blue') naevus, first described by Dubreuilh and Petges (1912), *two components are present: a common acquired naevus* (junctional, compound or intradermal, rarely Spitz) *and a blue naevus* (common or cellular).

Leopold and Richards (1968) observed foci of common naevus cells in many blue naevi, especially of the cellular variety. This occurrence should now be regarded as a little less common than was indicated by them, in view of the fact that giant naevus cells are now interpreted as an integral part of blue naevi, without signifying a mixture with common naevus. Because of the relative frequency of such combined naevi, especially on the face, they considered the possibility that blue naevi are derived from epidermal melanocytes, perhaps hair follicle-associated, as previously suggested by Lund and Kraus (1962). They rejected this origin, despite some suggestive evidence, but hypothesized that blue naevi arise from 'pools' of dermally situated melanocytes that have failed to complete the embryonic migration from the neural crest to the epidermis.

Several other authors have also drawn attention to the occurrence of a very minor and inconspicuous common acquired naevus component in many blue naevi (Figure 5.14; Stout, 1953; Leopold and Richards, 1968), so that *probably the combined naevus represents an exaggeration of a phenomenon commonly occurring in blue naevi*. In the series of 29 cellular blue naevi of Temple-Camp and colleagues (1988), four were associated with a common acquired naevus component. An extensive systematic study of this type of naevus was reported in the German

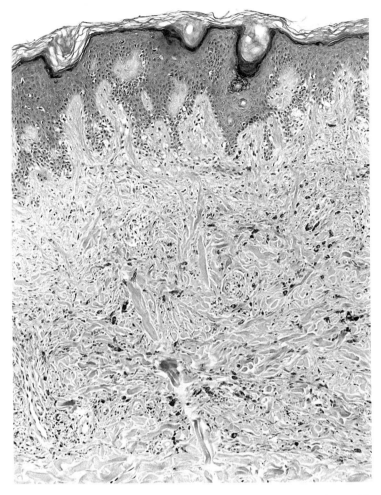

Figure 5.14   Common blue naevus, associated with elongation of rete ridges of the overlying epidermis and an increased number of melanocytes at the dermoepidermal junction (HE, × 115).

literature by Gartmann and Müller (1977). As indicated above, the common acquired naevus component possibly represents a remnant of the initial melanocytic proliferation from which the blue naevus developed; indeed, a transition in time of dermal naevus cells in a congenital naevus to a histological picture of blue naevus was reported by Nickoloff and colleagues (1986). Alternatively, the epidermal melanocytes may somehow have been stimulated to proliferate by the

Table 5.4 Combined naevus

Clinical features
   Bluish or black papule or nodule, sometimes with slightly irregular contour
   Most common on face, less common on extremities, rare on the trunk
   Female preponderance 2 : 1

Histological features
   Combined histological features of common acquired naevus or one of its
      variants (such as Spitz naevus) and blue naevus (common or cellular type)
   Architecture of the common acquired component may be unusual, with large
      pigmented cells deeper in the dermis

---

melanocytes constituting the blue naevus. Another hypothesis is, that one developmental abnormality leads to partial failure of migration of melanocytes and also to disturbances of epidermal melanocytes resulting in an ordinary naevus. Thus, although the two types of naevus have a different immediate histogenesis, there might thus be a shared embryological defect. It is very unlikely that the combined naevus represents a coincidential combination of a common acquired and blue naevus. The features of combined naevus are summarized in Table 5.4.

Maize and Ackerman (1987) use the term 'combined naevus' in a quite different and less restricted sense: all naevi showing more than one type of naevus cell, except for the combination of banal and multinucleated naevus cell, are designated combined naevus. For instance, these authors include naevi exhibiting 'banal' naevus cells as well as naevus cells with neuroid differentiation in the group of combined naevi. The combination of Spitz naevus and common naevus has also been designated combined naevus (Weedon, 1985). However, this would make combined naevus a very heterogeneous group of lesions, so that this usage of the term is not advocated.

5.5.1   Clinical features

Combined naevi occur in a wide age range, from early childhood to old age; some are congenital. Females appear to be affected about twice as often, and about half the cases occur on the face, most others being located on the extremities. Both the sex difference and the common occurrence on the face may in part be related to cosmetic considerations as the reason for their removal (Gartmann and Müller, 1977).

Generally, a combined naevus appears as a raised bluish or black papule or nodule, which may sometimes have a slightly irregular contour; one-quarter of cases in the series cited above were diagnosed clinically as melanoma.

5.5.2   Pathological features

Histologically, the common acquired naevus component consists of a junctional, compound or intradermal naevus; curiously, this component sometimes shows an abnormal architecture, with larger, pigmented ('type A') naevus cells situated deep within the dermis instead of being restricted to a subepidermal location (Mihm and Imber, 1989). The blue naevus component is of the common or cellular type. Usually, the two

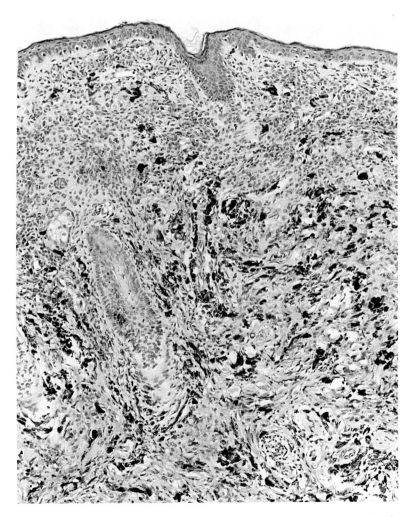

Figure 5.15   Combined naevus. The upper dermis contains a conventional intradermal naevus, which merges with the blue naevus occupying the reticular dermis (HE, × 115).

components are arranged in vertical tiers (Figure 5.15), but occasionally they are situated side-by-side, or are closely intermingled.

5.6   Mongolian spot, Ota's and Ito's naevus, and related lesions

A number of cutaneous pigmentations exhibit intradermally located pigmented bipolar or dendritic melanocytes but are distinct from blue naevi, both clinically and histologically. These include the mongolian spot, Ota's naevus, Ito's naevus, Sun's naevus (Table 5.6) and the intradermal melanocytic hamartoma. In these, the intradermal melanocytes are scattered more widely apart than those of blue naevi, and the area of skin involved is usually larger. They occur especially in mongolian races; Ota's, Ito's and Sun's naevus may have a brownish rather than bluish or slate-grey tinge, in keeping with the location of melanocytes mainly in the upper dermis.

5.6.1   Mongolian spot

The mongolian spot consists of an ill-defined area of diffuse bluish discolouration of the skin, up to several centimetres in size, usually located in the lumbosacral region, but sometimes also at other sites, including the hand (Mevorah et al., 1977) and the face (Inoue et al., 1982) where it may be associated with a cleft lip. It is common in mongoloid and negroid races but rare in Caucasians. It is usually present at birth or appears shortly afterwards, and may occur together with Ota's naevus. Usually it disappears in early childhood, but occasionally it persists, especially when it is multiple or associated with Ota's naevus (Kikuchi and Inoue, 1980).

Histologically, a thin scatter of markedly elongated, often bipolar and dendritic pigmented melanocytes is seen in the deeper parts of the reticular dermis (Table 5.5). This contrasts with Ota's and Ito's naevus, in which the dendritic melanocytes are slightly more numerous and are located mainly in the upper parts of the reticular dermis (Table 5.6).

Table 5.5 Mongolian spot

Clinical features
  Ill-defined area of bluish discolouration
  Lumbosacral region, sometimes other sites, including face
  Usually present at birth; most disappear in early childhood
  Common in mongoloid and some negroid races

Pathological features
  Thinly scattered bipolar/dendritic melanocytes
  Location in deep reticular dermis

Table 5.6 Naevus of Ota, naevus of Ito, naevus of Sun

	Ota's naevus	Ito's naevus	Sun's naevus
Location	ophthalmo-maxillary area	shoulder region	zygomatic region
Uni/biláteral	usually unilateral	usually unilateral	bilateral
Shape	confluent patches	confluent patches	scattered speckles
Onset	often at birth	often at birth	after 1st decade
Female:male ratio	4:1		6:1
Familial clustering	rare		not uncommon
Melanocytes	mainly in upper reticular dermis	mainly in upper reticular dermis	upper dermis
Areas with blue naevus histology	often	often	none

5.6.2   Ota's naevus

Ota's naevus (naevus fuscocoeruleus ophthalmomaxillaris; Ota, 1939) consists of a poorly circumscribed area of confluent slate-grey to bluish black patches, occurring in the skin area corresponding to the first two, and sometimes also the third, branches of the trigeminal nerve. Small papules or nodules with increased pigmentation may be present. The lesion is usually unilateral but may occur bilaterally. Associated pigmentation of the sclera and conjunctiva is seen in about two-thirds of cases, and the uvea and optic nerve may also be involved; sometimes, pigmentation of the nasal mucosa, palate, auditory canal and tympanic membrane is also present. Ota's naevus is congenital in the majority of cases, most others appearing either in early childhood or in adolescence. There is a 4:1 female preponderance. During childhood the naevus may fade somewhat, but often the pigmentation increases again after puberty (Kopf and Weidman, 1962; Hidano et al., 1967).

Cutaneous melanoma develops very rarely in Ota's naevus (Dorsey and Montgomery, 1954; MacKie, 1985); it shows the histological features of malignant blue naevus. Associated uveal and leptomeningeal melanosis occasionally gives rise to primary uveal and meningeal melanoma (Hartmann et al., 1989).

Histologically, Ota's naevus exhibits scattered dendritic melanocytes mainly located in the upper part of the reticular dermis. Extension into the lower dermis or even the subcutis is occasionally seen. The papular and nodular areas of the lesion contain larger numbers of melanocytes, together with a fibrotic response, so that these areas are indistinguishable from common blue naevus.

5.6.3 Ito's naevus

Ito's naevus (naevus fuscocoeruleus acromiodeltoideus; Ito, 1954) is located in the region of the supraclavicular and lateral branchial cutaneous nerves, i.e. the scapular, supraclavicular and shoulder region. Otherwise, it is indistinguishable from Ota's naevus. The two may occur together (Hidano *et al.*, 1965). In contrast to the mongolian spot, which may occasionally also occur at this site, the lesion persists in adulthood. A cutaneous melanoma developing in Ito's naevus has been reported (Van Krieken *et al.*, 1988).

5.6.4 Sun's naevus

Sun and colleagues (1987) described a bilateral, speckled pigmentation of the zygomatic region occurring in Chinese people. For reasons of convenience, the term 'naevus fuscocoeruleus zygomaticus' proposed by these authors could be replaced by Sun's naevus, in parallel with the other convenient eponyms.

In the original series of 110 cases from Taiwan, all patients were Chinese, and a 6:1 female preponderance was found in the general population. The lesion appears mainly in or after the second decade of life and there may be a familial clustering of cases. There is no associated ocular or oral melanosis. Histologically, scattered slender, elongated pigment-bearing melanocytes are seen between the collagen fibres of the upper dermis.

The features of Ota's, Ito's and Sun's naevus are summarized in Table 5.6.

5.6.5 Intradermal melanocytic hamartoma

Intradermal melanocytic hamartoma consists of a congenital, large, grey-bluish area of pigmentation, or of a number of coalescing similar but smaller patches; there may be a dermatomal distribution. Histologically, there is a scattering of dendritic melanocytes in the upper dermis, which contrasts with the deep dermal location of melanocytes in the mongolian spot (Burkhart and Gohara, 1981).

References

Ackerman, A. B. and Penneys, N. S. (1970) Formalin pigment in skin. *Arch. Dermatol.*, **102**, 318–21.

Ainsworth, A. M., Folberg, R., Reed, R. J. and Clark, W. H. (1979) Melanocytic nevi, melanocytomas, melanocytic dysplasias, and uncommon forms of melanoma. In *Human Malignant Melanoma* (eds W. H. Clark, L. I. Goldman and M. J. Mastrangelo). New York: Grune & Stratton, pp. 167–208.

Allen, A. C. and Spitz, S. (1953) Malignant Melanoma. *Cancer*, **6**, 1–45.

Avidor, I. and Kessler, E. (1977) 'Atypical' blue nevus — a benign variant of cellular blue nevus. Presentation of three cases. *Dermatologia*, **154**, 39–44.

Barnhill, R. L. and Mihm, M. C. (1990) Cellular neurothekeoma. A distinctive variant of neurothekeoma mimicking nevomelanocytic tumors. *Am. J. Surg. Pathol.*, **14**, 113–20.

Bondi, E. E., Elder, D., Guerry IV, D. P. and Clark, W. H. (1983) Target blue nevus. *Arch. Dermatol.*, **119**., 919–20.

Burkhart, C. G. and Gohara, A. (1981) Dermal melanocyte hamartoma. *Arch Dermatol.*, **117**, 102–4.

Darier, J. (1925) Le melanome malin mesenchymatieux ou melanosarcome. *Bull. Assoc. Fr. Cancer*, **14**, 221–49.

Dorsey, C. S. and Montgomery, H. (1954) Blue nevus and its distinction from Mongolian spot and the nevus of Ota. *J. Invest. Dermatol.*, **22**, 225–36.

Dubreuilh, W. and Petges, G. (1912) Le naevus bleu. *Ann. Dermatol.*, **2**, 552.

Epstein, E. and Pinkus, H. (1969) Giant blue nevus: cellular blue nevus as a clinical concept. *Cutis*, **5**, 309–12.

Findler, G., Hoffman, H. J., Thomson, H. G. and Becker, L. (1981) Giant nevus of the scalp associated with intracranial pigmentation. *J. Neurosurg.*, **54**, 108–12.

Fleming, M. G. and Bergfeld, W. F. (1990) A simple immunochemical technique for distinguishing melanocytes and melanophages in paraffin-embedded tissue. *J. Cutan. Pathol.*, **17**, 77–81.

Gardner, W. A. and Vazquez, M. D. (1970) Balloon cell melanoma. *Arch. Pathol.*, **89**, 470–2.

Gartmann, H. (1965) Neuronaevus bleu Masson: cellular blue nevus *Allen. Arch. Klin. Exp. Dermatol.*, **221**, 109–24.

Gartmann, H. (1987) Target blue nevi. *Arch. Dermatol.*, **123**, 18.

Gartmann, H. and Müller, H.-D. (1977) Ueber das gemeinsame Vorkommen von blauem Naevus und Naevuszellnaevus in ein und derselben Geschwulst ('combined nevus'). *Z. Hautkr.*, **52**, 389–98.

Hartmann, L. C., Oliver, G. F., Winkelmann, R. K., Colby, T. V., Sundt, T. M., Jr. and O'Neill, B. P. (1989) Blue nevus and nevus of Ota associated with dural melanoma. *Cancer*, **64**, 182–6.

Hendricks, W. M. (1981) Eruptive blue nevi. *J. Am. Acad. Dermatol.*, **4**, 50–53.

Hidano, A., Kajima, H. and Endo, Y. (1965) Bilateral nevus Ota associated with nevus Ito. *Arch. Dermatol.*, **91**, 357–9.

Hidano, A., Kajima, H., Ikeda, S., Mizutani, H., Miyasato, H. and Niimura, M. (1967) Natural history of nevus of Ota. Arch. Dermatol., **95**, 187–95.

Iemoto, Y. and Kondo, Y. (1984) Congenital giant cellular blue nevus resulting in dystocia. *Arch. Dermatol.*, **120**, 798–9.

Inoue, S., Kikuchi, I. and Ono, T. (1982) Dermal melanocytosis associated with cleft lip. *Arch. Dermatol.*, **118**, 443–4.

Ishibashi, A., Kimura, K. and Kukita, A. (1990) Plaque-type blue nevus combined with lentigo (nevus spilus). *J. Cutan. Pathol.*, **17**, 241–5.

Ito, M. (1954) Nevus fusco-caeruleus acromio-deltoideus. *Tohoku Exp. Med.*, **60**, 10.

Kikuchi, I. and Inoue, S. (1980) Natural history of the Mongolian spot. *J. Dermatol.*, **7**, 449–50.

Kopf, A. W. and Weidman, A. (1962) Nevus of Ota. *Arch. Dermatol.*, **85**, 195–208.

Lambert, W. C. and Brodkin, R.H. (1984) Nodal and subcutaneous cellular blue nevi. A pseudometastasizing pseudomelanoma. *Arch. Dermatol.*, **120**, 367–70.

Leopold, J. G. and Richards, D. B. (1968) The interrelationship of blue and common naevi. *J. Pathol. Bacteriol.*, **95**, 37–46.

Levene, A. (1980) On the natural history and comparative pathology of the blue naevus. *Ann. Rep. Coll. Surg. Engl.*, **62**, 327–34.

Lund, H. Z. and Kraus, J. M. (1962) *Melanotic Tumors of the Skin. Atlas of Tumor Pathology*. Washington: Armed Forces Institute of Pathology.

MacKie, R. M. (1985) Malignant melanocytic tumours. *J. Cutan. Pathol.*, **12**, 251–65.

Maize, J. C. and Ackerman, A. B. (1987) *Pigmented Lesions of the Skin. Clinico-pathologic Correlations*. New York: Lea & Febiger, p. 152.

Masson, P. (1950) Neuro-nevi 'bleu'. *Arch. De Vecchi Anat. Pathol.*, **14**, 1–28.

McWhorter, H. E. and Woolner, L. B. (1954) Pigmented nevi, juvenile melanomas, and malignant melanomas in children. *Cancer*, **7**, 564–85.

Mevorah, B., Frenk, E. and Delacrétaz, J. (1977) Dermal melanocytosis. Report of an unusual case. *Dermatologica*, **154**, 107–14.

Mihm, M. C. and Imber, M. J. (1989) Melanocytic lesions. In *Diagnostic Surgical Pathology* (ed. S. S. Sternberg). New York: Raven Press, pp. 103–18.

Modly, C., Wood, C. and Horn, T. (1989) Metastatic malignant melanoma arising from a common blue nevus in a patient with subacute cutaneous lupus erythematosus. *Dermatologica*, **178**, 171–5.

Nickoloff, B. J., Walton, R., Pregerson-Rodan, K., Jacobs, A. H. and Cox, A. J. (1986) Immunohistologic patterns of congenital nevocellular nevi. *Arch. Dermatol.*, **122**, 1263–8.

Ota, M. (1939) Nevus fusco-coeruleus ophthalmo-maxillaris. *Jap. J. Dermatol.*, **46**, 369.

Pittman, J. L. and Fisher, B. K. (1976) Plaque-type of blue nevus. *Arch. Dermatol.*, **112**, 1127–8.

Rodriguez, H. A. and Ackerman, L. V. (1968) Cellular blue naevus. Clinico-pathologic study of forty-five cases. *Cancer*, **21**, 393–405.

Schrader, W. A. and Helwig, E. B. (1967) Balloon cell nevi. *Cancer*, **20**, 1502–14.

Silverberg, G. D., Kadin, M. E., Dorfman, R. F. *et al.* (1971) Invasion of the brain by a cellular blue nevus of the scalp. A case report with light and electron microscopic studies. *Cancer*, **27**, 349–55.

Sterchi, J. M., Muss, H. B. and Weidner, N. (1987) Cellular blue nevus simulating metastatic melanoma: report of an unusually large lesion associated with nevus-cell aggregates in regional lymph nodes. *J. Surg. Oncol.*, **36**, 71–5.

Stout, A. P. (1953) *Tumors of the Soft Tissues. Atlas of Tumor Pathology*. Washington: Armed Forces Institute of Pathology, p. 65.

Sun, C.-C., Lü, Y.-C., Lee, E. F. and Nakagawa, H. (1987) Naevus fusco-caeruleus zygomaticus. *Br. J. Dermatol.*, **117**, 545–53.

Sun, J., Morton, T. H. and Gown, A. M. (1990) Antibody HMB-45 identifies the cells of blue nevi. An immunohistochemical study on paraffin sections. *Am. J. Surg. Pathol.*, **14.**, 748–51.

Temple-Camp, C. R. E., Saxe, N. and King, H. (1988) Benign and malignant cellular blue nevus. A clinicopathological study of 30 cases. *Am. J. Dermatopathol.*, **10**, 289–96.

Tièche, M. (1906) Ueber benigne Melanome ('Chromatophorome') der Haut 'blaue Naevi'. *Virchows Arch. Pathol. Anat.*, **186**, 212–29.

Tschen, J. A., Cartwright, J. and Font, R. L. (1989) Nonmelanized macro-melanosomes in a cellular blue nevus. *Arch. Dermatol.*, **125**, 809–12.

Tsoïtis, G., Kanitakis, C. and Kapetis, E. (1983) Naevus bleu multinodulaire en plaque, superficiel et neuroïde. *Ann. Dermatol. Venereol.*, **110**, 231–5.

Tuthill, R. J., Clark, W. H. and Levene, A. (1982) Pilar neurocristic hamartoma. Its relationship to blue nevus and equine melanotic disease. *Arch. Dermatol.*, **118**, 592–6.

Upshaw, B. Y., Ghormley, R. K. and Montgomery, H. (1947) Extensive blue nevus of Jadassohn-Tièche. Report of a case. *Surgery*, **22**, 761–5.

Van Krieken, J. H. J. M., Boom, B. W. and Scheffer, E. (1988) Malignant transformation in a naevus of Ito. A case report. *Histopathology* **12**, 100–2.

Weedon, D. (1985) Borderline melanocytic tumors. *J. Cutan. Pathol.*, **12**, 266–70.

6 Congenital melanocytic naevi

By definition, congenital melanocytic naevi are present at birth; all other naevi are acquired. However, some congenital naevi only become clinically apparent in early infancy rather than at birth (Kopf *et al.*, 1985a). When compared to acquired naevi, congenital naevi are usually larger, are more frequently centred around cutaneous adnexae, more often penetrate the reticular dermis, sometimes exhibit more complex differentiation, e.g. a greater degree of neurotization and occasional blue naevus-like areas, and manifest a greater propensity to malignant change, which can assume unusual forms. Therefore, distinction between the two is of practical importance.

Some of the lesions discussed in the previous chapter may be congenital, but were dealt with there because of the histological similarities with acquired blue naevi. Here we shall discuss the other types of congenital melanocytic lesions, which most probably originate in the epidermis and its appendages rather than in the dermis.

6.1 Clinical features

As compared to acquired naevi, congenital naevi are more variable in size and appearance. Most are under 1.5 cm in diameter, but they are usually larger than acquired naevi. There is a predilection for the trunk, especially the upper back and chest, and the limbs. Some paraxial congenital naevi stop abruptly at the midline, whereas others seem to originate at the posterior midline (Reed *et al.*, 1965); the latter may be associated with spina bifida and myelomeningocele. Other congenital malformations which are sometimes associated with congenital naevi are club foot and vascular malformations. An association with neurofibromatosis has been proposed but, although the two may rarely occur together, it is very likely that reported cases represent extensive neuroid change in large congenital naevi rather than a genuine combination with neurofibromatosis; the two entities are clearly distinct (Solomon *et al.*, 1980).

Congenital naevi of the head and neck region may be associated with melanocytosis of the meninges (p. 369). Giant congenital naevi may occur in the context of *melanophakomatosis*, a syndrome in which, apart from the giant naevus, multiple 'satellite naevi' are often present. As is the case with congenital naevi examined in early infancy (p. 139), the histology of such satellite naevi in early stages of their development may show pagetoid intraepidermal proliferation of melanocytes, very similar to that seen in *in situ* melanoma (Hundeiker, 1987). In *neurocutaneous melanosis*, the cutaneous changes of melanophakomatosis are combined with similar melanocytic proliferations within the central nervous system, leading to various neurological symptoms and usually causing death before the patient reaches adulthood.

Large congenital naevi are often disfiguring and result in important psychological and social problems for the patient. Also, there is a distinct *risk of malignant transformation*, which has been estimated to lie in the range of a few percent. In small congenital naevi the potential for malignant transformation has not yet been adequately quantitated, but it is certainly much less.

Very rarely, the remarkable phenomenon of spontaneous regression of intermediate-sized or large congenital naevi has been reported (Kikuchi *et al.*, 1984; Hasegawa *et al.*, 1987).

6.1.1   Size

For practical purposes congenital naevi are usually subdivided into three groups: small naevi (smaller than 1.5 cm), intermediate-sized naevi (up to 20 cm in largest diameter) and large or giant naevi, which are larger still (Consensus Conference, 1984). Others have divided congenital naevi into small ($\leq$10 cm) and large ($>$10 cm) lesions (Ainsworth *et al.*, 1979; Illig *et al.*, 1985). Size by itself, unrelated to body surface area, is not a very satisfactory parameter, and Enhamre (1986, 1987) therefore proposed using a 'relative area index' (RAI) which equals 100 $\times$ Naevus Area/Body Surface Area. In this way, relative changes in size of the naevus during growth of the patient can be assessed accurately.

Giant congenital naevus has also been defined less precisely as a congenital naevus covering a 'major part' of trunk, head or extremity. Synonyms include *garment naevus, giant hairy naevus,* or *bathing trunk naevus*, although it is not always covered with hairs, and it may not be located on the trunk.

Estimates of the prevalence of small, intermediate-sized and giant congenital naevi in neonates are: 1 in 100, 1 in 170, (Walton *et al.*, 1976) and 1 in 20 000 (Castilla *et al.*, 1981), respectively. In an adult population, however, intermediate-sized 'congenital naevus-like naevi' were found in no less that 2.5% of subjects (Kopf *et al.*, 1985b), possibly because many of these lesions, recognizable as congenital naevi from their size and clinical appearance, become apparent only some time after birth.

6.1.2   *Morphology*

At birth, congenital naevi are usually flat, lightly pigmented and sharply defined, but in larger lesions especially the borders may be irregular; they may closely resemble café-au-lait spots (Mark *et al.*, 1973). It should be realized that not all pigmented cutaneous lesions present at birth are melanocytic in origin (Walton *et al.*, 1976).

During postnatal development, small congenital naevi usually retain a regular appearance, often becoming slightly raised to form a papule or nodule; they may become covered by hairs. Larger congenital naevi may develop multiple darkly pigmented macules or papules.

At puberty the whole or part of the naevus often becomes raised, sometimes verrucous, and more darkly pigmented, resulting in an irregular plaque. Larger naevi especially may be covered with fine or coarse, pale or darkly pigmented hairs, leading to their German designation of 'Tierfell-Naevus' (animal coat-naevus). Hypopigmented nodules are sometimes present. The margins of the naevi are generally sharp, even when they are irregular. At the margins perifollicular sparing may be noted. There may be 'satellite lesions' in the vicinity or at a distance, especially in the case of a giant congenital naevus. Occasionally, congenital naevi are surrounded by a depigmented halo (Mark *et al.*, 1973; Langer and Konrad, 1990).

6.2   Pathological features

During their evolution, the histology of congenital naevi changes significantly, and the differential diagnosis changes accordingly.

In the postnatal period and in early infancy the emergence of a nodule or 'satellite lesion' may raise a clinical suspicion of malignancy, and the histology may show disquieting features, such as (a minor degree of) pagetoid spread of melanocytes within the epidermis, and the presence of mitotic activity in deeper parts of the naevus. In this situation, one should be conservative with the diagnosis of melanoma for reasons discussed in the following subsection.

In adulthood, the differential diagnosis is often between congenital and acquired naevus: in view of the discussion on the premalignant potential of congenital naevus, much attention has been paid to its histological features in adulthood and its distinction from acquired naevus. Since it is often impossible to assess in retrospect whether a naevus was present at birth, it would be valuable if a congenital naevus could be distinguished histologically from an acquired one. Several systematic studies comparing the histology of congenital and acquired naevi have been reported (Mark *et al.*, 1973; Rhodes *et al.*, 1985; Nickoloff *et al.*, 1986; Walsh and MacKie, 1988).

6.2.1   Histology in early infancy

The histology of congenital naevi in neonates has been well documented. In a study by Walton and colleagues (1976), 11 of 34 biopsied pigmented lesions in newborn infants were found to represent melanocytic naevi, the others being lentigines, café-au-lait spots and various entities unrelated to melanocytes. In the melanocytic naevi, junctional nests of melanocytes were seen with or without an intradermal naevus component located in the papillary or upper reticular dermis. Deep reticular dermal involvement, as characteristically seen in congenital naevi at a later age, was present in only two cases. In a study by Silvers and Helwig (1981), melanocytes in early congenital naevi were also located largely within the epidermis (Figure 6.1) and especially the pilosebaceous units and sweat glands; when present, the dermal component was often located in the immediate vicinity of skin appendages. At this very early age, the predilection of naevus cells for the eccrine sweat glands and pilosebaceous units was more striking than in congenital naevi in adolescence and adulthood. Likewise, Nickoloff *et al.* (1986) found that the naevus cells in 23 of 29 congenital naevi examined during the first year of life were located in the epidermis, upper dermis and periadnexal adventitial tissue only. In this respect it is of interest that Mishima (1973) illustrated dendritic melanocytes within sweat gland walls in a 4-month-old fetus, indicating that migration of melanocytes to the skin may lead to colonization of sweat glands at an early stage of fetal development.

These studies suggest that involvement of the deep reticular dermal tissue usually occurs after the first year of life, presumably due to penetration of the reticular dermis by naevus cells initially located within the epidermis and adnexae, especially the sweat glands, and in the superficial dermis.

However, Zitelli and colleagues (1984) drew attention to the importance of naevus size in determining the extent of dermal involvement in the early postnatal period: in their material, small congenital naevi showed features very similar to common acquired naevi, whereas large

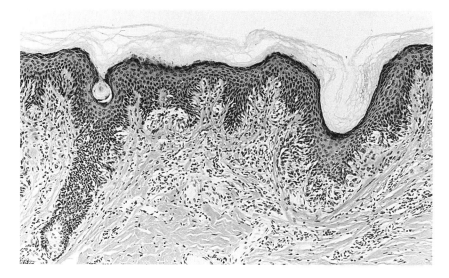

Figure 6.1 Congenital naevus in a 2-year-old child. This congenital naevus in early childhood is largely confined to the dermoepidermal junction and hair follicle (HE, × 90).

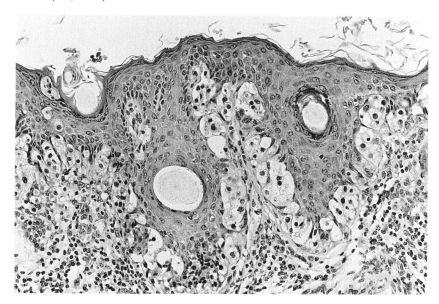

Figure 6.2 Congenital naevus in an 18-month-old child. Extensive proliferation of melanocytes along the dermoepidermal junction and, focally, also above it (left). Melanocytic nuclei are small; there is some ballooning of the cytoplasm. Note lymphocytic infiltrate and naevus cells in the upper dermis (HE, × 370).

congenital naevi already exhibited full-thickness involvement of the dermis and often also reached the subcutis. Consequently, superficial dermabrasion at an early age may produce a much improved cosmetic result but does not eradicate the naevus. Kuehnl-Petzoldt and colleagues (1984) also found that large congenital naevi in the first year of life often involve deeper parts of the dermis: these authors distinguished two distinct cell types: large and round cells located at or near the dermoepidermal junction, and small nonpigmented cells scattered between the collagen bundles of the reticular dermis.

In early infancy, the intraepithelial component of congenital naevi may exhibit a somewhat irregular architecture. Ascent of a few solitary cells or nests of cells into the upper epidermis is occasionally seen (Figure 6.2; Hundeiker, 1987; Kerl *et al.*, 1989). Ainsworth and colleagues (1979) reported a congenital naevus of a 5-week-old infant, in which pagetoid intraepidermal distribution of atypical melanocytes was strongly suggestive of melanoma; however, at biopsies taken after 7 and 13 months, the intraepidermal component showed less atypia and a more regular architecture. These authors warned explicitly against overdiagnosis of congenital naevi examined during early infancy. In the dermal component, foci of increased mitotic activity associated with increase in cell size and some nuclear atypia may also raise a suspicion of malignancy (Figure 6.3); however, in early infancy, one should be hesitant with the diagnosis of melanoma and reserve it for those rare cases where malignancy is evidenced by necrosis, atypical mitoses and marked nuclear atypia. This conclusion recently received support from the study of Mancianti and co-workers (1990) who, investigating tumours simulating melanoma histologically and arising in congenital naevi during early infancy, found normal karyotypes and *in vitro* growth properties indicative of benign melanocytes rather than melanoma cells.

However, in contrast to the previous studies, Nickoloff and associates (1986) reported no cytological atypia or architectural irregularity in a series of 29 congenital naevi investigated in the first year of life. According to Rhodes (1986), this apparent discrepancy may be related to referral bias: clinically atypical congenital naevi are probably biopsied more often at an early age, leading to a relatively high prevalence of histologically irregular features, which cannot therefore be regarded as representative of congenital naevi in general. This bias may be even more pronounced when referral slides are concerned, as in the series of Silvers and Helwig (1981).

In summary, it appears that some but not all congenital naevi in early infancy exhibit some degree of architectural irregularity and cytological atypia.

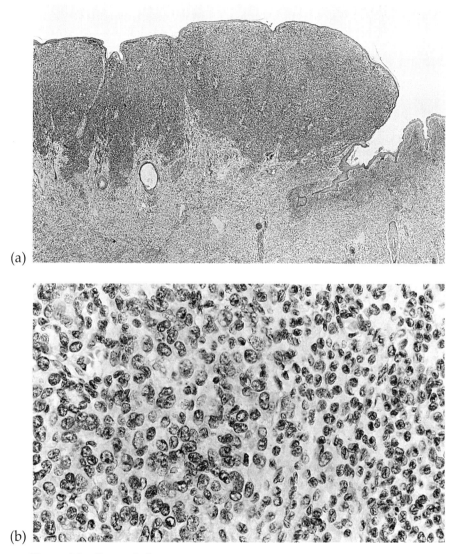

Figure 6.3 Congenital naevus in a 2-month-old infant, with cytological variability. (a) There were several nodules, one of which is illustrated here (upper left). (HE, × 20). (b) The nodules consist of a larger cell type (left). Transitions to a smaller cell type seen in the remainder of the naevus are abrupt. Abnormal mitoses, necrosis and ulceration are absent (HE, × 370).

Table 6.1 Congenital naevus

Clinical features
   Usually apparent at birth
   Division into small (<1.5 cm), medium (1.5–20 cm) and large (>20 cm) naevi
   Large lesions may be irregular in contour and often become covered by hairs

Histological features
   Small lesions may be indistinguishable from common acquired naevus
   Often involvement of lower third of reticular dermis
   Growth along sweat glands, hair follicles (including lower part), sebaceous
      glands
   Growth within arrector pili muscles and the walls of lymph vessels and
      blood vessels
   Single cell or Indian-file pattern of growth between collagen bundles of the
      reticular dermis
   Sometimes involvement of reticular dermis only
   Neurotization often present, not only at the base but also in superficial
      portions of the naevus

Remarks
   Risk of malignant change in large congenital naevi probably a few percent;
      risk in small lesions much smaller
   Associated meningeal melanocytic lesions in some congenital naevi involving
      scalp and neck

6.2.2   Histology in adolescence and adult life

The histological characteristics of congenital naevi include the variable patterns of distribution of naevus cells in the dermis, extension into the subcutaneous fatty tissue and certain cytological features of the naevus cells (Mark *et al.*, 1973). The main features are summarized in Table 6.1.

   In adolescence and adulthood, congenital naevi are usually compound or intradermal. The epidermis is sometimes acanthotic, rarely atrophic. In some cases there is pronounced papillomatosis with follicular plugging and formation of keratin-pseudocysts between epidermal papillae (Figure 6.4).

   The intraepidermal component of the naevus usually shows a nested architecture, with or without an associated lentiginous proliferation of single cells. Ascent of melanocytes is absent. The melanocytic proliferation often extends deeply along hair follicles and sweat glands, within the epithelium as well as the surrounding adventitial dermis, resulting in a characteristic scattering of naevus cell aggregates throughout the thickness of the dermis (Figure 6.5).

   The pattern of dermal involvement may vary considerably between cases (Stenn *et al.*, 1983). In some, the melanocytes are largely confined to the papillary dermis (Figure 6.6), even though there is peri-

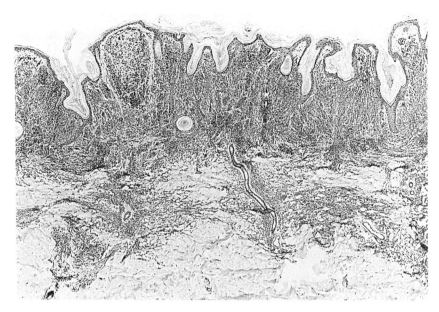

Figure 6.4 Marked papillomatosis and hyperkeratosis in a congenital compound naevus. Such surface irregularities often become more pronounced at puberty. Note the characteristic involvement of periappendageal adventitial dermis, from which naevus cells extend into the reticular dermis (HE, × 35).

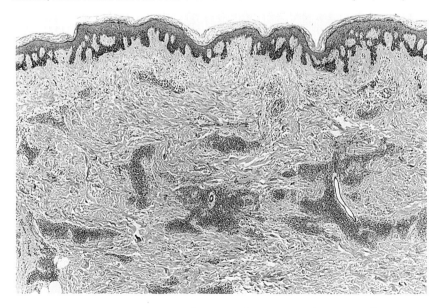

Figure 6.5 Congenital compound naevus. Aggregates of naevus cells are seen around skin appendages and some blood vessels in the deep dermis. This pattern is virtually diagnostic of congenital naevus (HE, × 35).

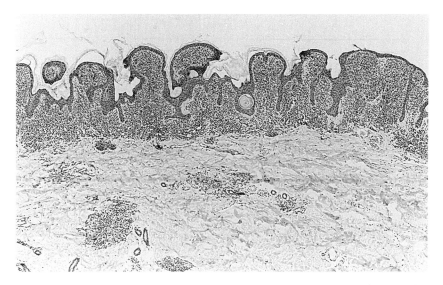

Figure 6.6 Congenital naevus. Although the naevus is largely confined to the papillary dermis, naevus cell aggregates surround adnexae and vessels also in the deep reticular dermis (HE, × 35).

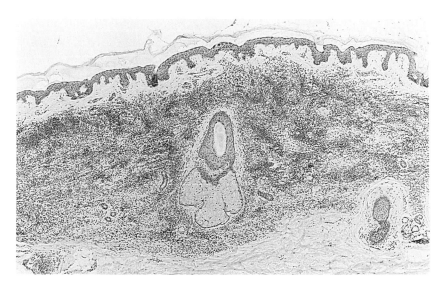

Figure 6.7 Congenital naevus confined to the reticular dermis. Such lack of papillary and adventitial dermal involvement strongly suggests a congenital naevus (HE, × 35).

appendageal and perivascular extension into the lower dermis marking the congenital nature of these naevi. In others, the papillary dermis and perifollicular adventitial dermis are totally uninvolved, the naevus being confined wholly to the reticular dermis (Figure 6.7). However, most commonly, the naevus involves the full thickness of the dermis (Figure 6.8) including the lower two-thirds of the reticular dermis. Growth is often preferentially along skin appendages and blood vessels (Figure 6.9(a)), resulting in a characteristic low-power appearance of a scatter of islands of naevus cells in the deep portions of the dermis. Other cases exhibit a diffuse pattern of growth, so that adnexae and vessels are engulfed in a sea of melanocytes.

At higher power, extension into the reticular dermis often exhibits a characteristic single cell- or Indian file-type of growth between pre-existent collagen bundles (Mark *et al.*, 1973). Cell nests sometimes bulge into vascular lumina, but are covered by an intact layer of endo-thelium (Mark *et al.*, 1973; Figure 6.10). In contrast to common acquired naevi, growth into sebaceous glands, arrector pili muscles (Figure 6.9(b)) and nerves is commonly seen. There is often an increase in number and size of dermal elastic fibres, closely packed around naevus cells (Massi, 1989).

The melanocytes may extend into the subcutis, usually along inter-lobular fibrous septa. Extension into the subcutis is usually taken as proof that the naevus is congenital; however, the recently described 'deep penetrating naevus' (p. 93; Seab *et al.*, 1989) may be an exception to this generalization. The subcutis may also be involved by blue naevi, especially the cellular variant.

Subcutaneous striated muscle tissue of the facial musculature and platysma may become involved by a congenital naevus; this should not be interpreted as a sign of malignancy.

Often, there is some degree of neuroid change and neurotropism, i.e. location of naevus cells within and adjacent to nerves. Fusiform or elongated naevus cells, arranged in ill-defined bundles or sometimes 'lames foliacées' (foliate laminae) resembling Wagner–Meissner cor-puscles, are not infrequently seen (Figure 6.10). Neuroid change in congenital naevi is often more extensive than in acquired naevi, and may be present superficially as well as deep within the naevus (Figure 6.10). Extensive neuroid change in a giant congenital naevus should not be confused with cutaneous neurofibroma; giant congenital naevus and neurofibromatosis are not related (Solomon *et al.*, 1980). Many mast cells may be present in naevi with extensive neuroid change; a mastocytoma arising in a congenital naevus was reported by Silverman and Zaim (1988).

Growth around nerves in the dermis and subcutis may be seen in

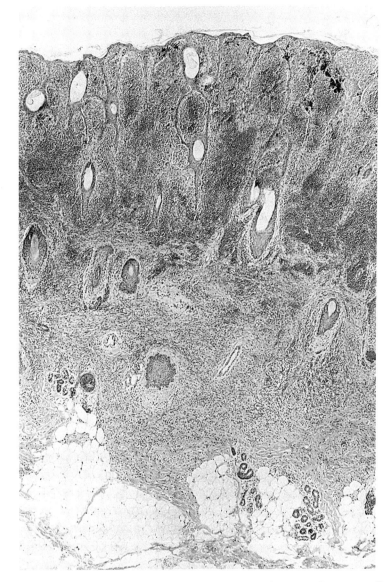

Figure 6.8 Congenital compound naevus. The proliferation of naevus cells extends throughout the papillary and reticular dermis and reaches the fibrous septa of the subcutis (HE, × 45).

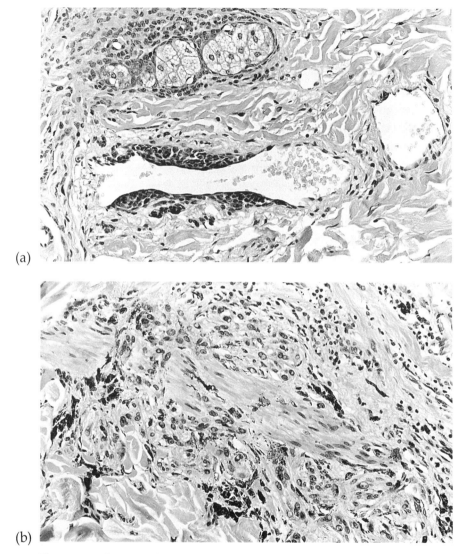

(a)

(b)

Figure 6.9 Congenital naevus. (a) Melanocytes closely surround sebaceous gland (top) and bulge into the lumen of a thin-walled vessel (bottom) (HE, × 185). (b) Melanocytes infiltrate an arrector pili muscle (HE, × 185).

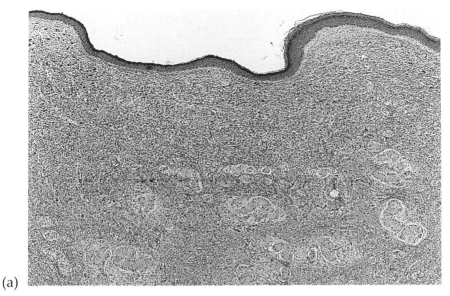

(a)

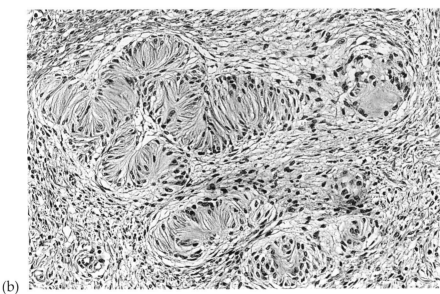

(b)

Figure 6.10   Neuroid change in a congenital naevus. (a) Scattered 'pseudotactile corpuscles' are seen (HE, × 35). (b) These pseudotactile corpuscles show a transversely fibrillary structure; nuclei are arranged at the periphery (HE, × 185).

some congenital naevi and by itself should not be interpreted as a sign of malignancy.

Some congenital naevi show areas with the histological features of common or cellular blue naevi (Reed *et al.*, 1965): such lesions can be considered *congenital combined naevi* (Figure 6.11). Other cases show features of Spitz naevus. Fibrosis and *'degenerative cytological atypia'* (p. 81) may also be encountered (Figure 6.12). In some giant congenital naevi, lipomas, fibromas or vascular proliferations are found, and occasionally, cartilage is formed (Ainsworth *et al.*, 1979).

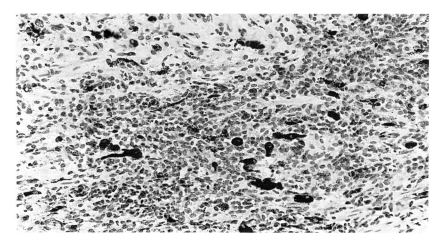

Figure 6.11   Congenital combined naevus. Scattered heavily pigmented unipolar and bipolar melanocytes are seen between conventional naevus cells (HE, × 185).

6.3   The distinction between congenital and acquired naevi

Walsh and MacKie (1988) compared the histology of 43 congenital and 64 acquired naevi and were able to separate the two groups in all but five cases. The main discriminating features were: the presence of melanocytes within arrector pili muscles and around eccrine sweat glands, sebaceous glands and blood vessel walls, and papillary dermal sparing.

However, some acquired naevi are said to show features similar to congenital naevi (Clemmensen and Kroon, 1988), and the opposite also holds. Everett (1989) found that most of 39 small congenital naevi did not show the classical features of congenital naevi; he concluded that it is the size rather than the congenital nature of the naevus that determines the histological features: accordingly, the histological diagnosis

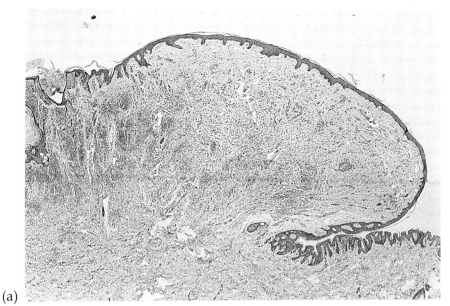

(a)

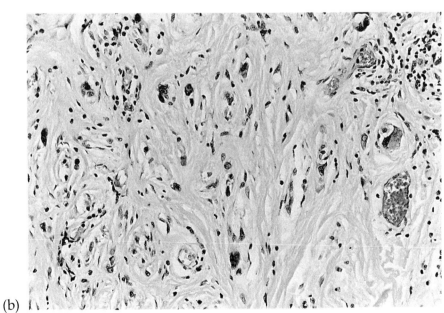

(b)

Figure 6.12 (a) A focus of regressive fibrosis in a congenital naevus leads to an asymmetrical shape (HE, × 20). (b) At higher power, cellular degenerative atypia (p. 81) is seen; mitoses are absent (HE, × 185).

of medium-sized and large congenital naevi is easier, but of course, the congenital nature of such naevi is also obvious clinically.

An estimate of the predictive value of histological criteria is hampered by the fact that exact figures concerning the relative prevalence of congenital naevi in the total of excised naevi is insufficiently known (Rhodes *et al.*, 1985). When assessing the possible congenital nature of a naevus, it is important to bear in mind that acquired naevi are much more common, so that the many features seen commonly in congenital naevi and only rarely in acquired naevi may in practice still carry only limited predictive value (p. 28).

6.4   Malignant transformation of congenital naevi

It has been well established that there is a significant risk of malignant transformation in large congenital naevi. The risk is partly dependent on the histological growth pattern, the presence of deep dermal and subcutaneous penetration being associated with a higher risk, which has been estimated at up to 8%, and also with earlier development of melanoma, often in childhood or adolescence (Quaba and Wallace, 1986). Early surgical removal of large congenital naevi is therefore advocated. The histological type of melanoma differs depending on the type of pre-existing congenital naevus: in the report by Illig and co-workers (1985), all 47 melanomas contiguous with a pre-existing congenital naevus limited to the upper two-thirds of the skin were of epidermal origin and mainly of superficial spreading type (p. 275). None of these tumours arose before puberty. In contrast, the malignancies developing in congenital naevi with deep dermal penetration and subcutaneous involvement are often located deep within the naevus (Hundeiker, 1987). The histological appearance of these deeply-located malignant tumours varies considerably and includes malignant schwannoma (Weidner *et al.*, 1985), round-cell or spindle-cell undifferentiated patterns, rhabdomyosarcoma and liposarcoma (Hendrickson and Ross, 1981); these tumours are discussed further in Chapter 9 (p. 276).

The degree of melanoma risk in small congenital naevi remains unclear. Whether it is wise to excise small congenital naevi prophylactically has not yet been settled. If the location allows for easy removal with good cosmetic results, many dermatologists and surgeons prefer to do so.

6.5   Subtypes of congenital naevus

Several clinical subtypes of congenital naevus have been described and will be discussed briefly.

6.5.1   Congenital acral melanocytic naevus

Three cases of benign congenital naevi, located at acral sites in young white adults presenting with an alarming clinical picture strongly suggestive of acral lentiginous melanoma, were reported by Botet and colleagues (1981). The lesions exhibited recent growth, large size (several centimetres), crusting, and irregular contours and colour; however, the histology revealed the features of a benign congenital compound naevus.

6.5.2   Speckled lentiginous naevus

This lesion consists of many small, darkly pigmented macules super-imposed on a homogeneous light-brown background (Stewart et al., 1978). It is usually congenital or appears shortly after birth, in females and males alike, and is most commonly localized on the trunk, lower limbs, or head and neck region. Its prevalence in a Caucasian popula-tion is estimated at about 2% (Kopf et al., 1985b). Occasionally, con-genital speckled lentiginous naevus exhibits a dermotomal distribution ('zosteriform lentiginous naevus'; Ruth et al., 1980).

Histologically, the lightly pigmented background shows the features of lentigo simplex, whereas the darker spots usually correspond to junctional or compound naevi. These may show an intimate asso-ciation with eccrine sweat ducts ('eccrine-centred naevus') or with hair follicles (Mishima, 1973; Morishima et al., 1976).

The term 'naevus spilus' has been used by some as a synonym of speckled lentiginous naevus; however, others have adhered to the original definition of naevus spilus, i.e. a uniform macular spot of hyperpigmentation, without superimposed dark speckles (p. 39; Stewart et al., 1978). Because the term 'naevus spilus' is used differently by different authors, it is best avoided.

6.5.3   Cerebriform congenital intradermal naevus

Congenital melanocytic naevus is sometimes the cause of cutis verticis gyrata, a clinical term with various histological substrates, and which consists of an area of convoluted folds of greatly thickened skin, usually occurring on the scalp, which may reach a size of more than 20 cm. Cutis verticis gyrata caused by a congenital naevus is known as cerebriform intradermal naevus. Females are affected somewhat more commonly. The lesion is present at birth or arises early in life as a skin-coloured or pigmented spot, enlarging in size especially between 5 and 10 years of age and gradually becoming cerebriform in appearance. It is sharply demarcated and is often associated with hair loss.

The histology is that of a congenital naevus; there may be extensive neuroid differentiation, resulting in a close resemblance to neurofibroma. Complete excision is advocated, in view of the severe cosmetic and psychological problems, and the risk of development of melanoma, which occurred in two out of 50 cases reviewed in the literature (Orkin *et al.*, 1974).

6.6 Meningeal melanocytic lesions associated with congenital naevi (neurocutaneous melanosis)

Congenital naevi located in the region of the head and neck may be associated with melanocytic proliferations of the meninges covering the brain and spinal cord (*meningeal melanocytosis*; Reed *et al.*, 1965). The base of the brain is usually most heavily involved; extensive involvement of the brain stem may lead to hydrocephalus, seizures, mental retardation and motor deficits. Such cases carry a poor prognosis.

Histologically, scattered dendritic melanocytes are present, or actual tumours may be formed; some of these show little cytological atypia, are associated with a relatively indolent biological behaviour and are designated *meningeal melanocytomas*. In contrast, *meningeal melanomas* show marked cytological atypia, mitotic activity and necrosis, and are associated with aggressive growth as well as metastasis. These meningeal tumours are discussed more extensively in Chapter 11 (p. 369).

6.7 Placental naevus cell aggregates

Rarely, a giant congenital naevus is associated with the presence of clusters of melanocytes within the placenta, located within the stroma of stem villi as well as within some secondary and tertiary villi (Demian *et al.*, 1974; Sotelo-Avila *et al.*, 1988). This may be visible macroscopically as dark spots in the placental tissue. Histologically, there are no signs of malignancy. It is unclear whether this phenomenon is due to aberrant migration of melanoblasts from the neural crest or to 'benign metastasis' from the cutaneous lesion.

References

Ainsworth, A. M., Folberg, R., Reed, R. J. and Clark, W. H. (1979) Melanocytic nevi, melanocytomas, melanocytic dysplasias, and uncommon forms of melanoma. In *Human Malignant Melanoma* (eds W. H. Clark, L. I. Goldman and M. J. Mastrangelo). New York: Grune & Stratton, pp. 167–208.

Botet, M. V., Caro, F. R. and Sánchez, J. L. (1981) Congenital acral melanocytic nevi clinically simulating acral lentiginous melanoma. *J. Am. Acad. Dermatol.*, 5, 406–10.

Castilla, E. E., De Graca, D. M. and Orioli-Parreiras, J. M. (1981) Epidemiology of congenital pigmented nevi, incidence rates and relative frequencies. *Br. J. Dermatol.*, **104**, 307–15.

Clemmensen, O. J. and Kroon, S. (1988) The histology of 'congenital features' in early acquired melanocytic nevi. *J. Am. Acad. Dermatol.*, **19**, 742–6.

Consensus Conference (1984) Precursors to malignant melanoma. *J. Am. Med. Assoc.*, **251**, 1864–6.

Demian, S. D. E., Donnelly, W. H., Frias, J. L. and Monif, G. R. G. (1974) Placental lesions in congenital giant pigmented nevi. *Am. J. Clin. Pathol.*, **61**, 438–42.

Enhamre, A. (1986) Relative area index in congenital nevi. *Arch. Dermatol.*, **122**, 501–2.

Enhamre, A. (1987) Congenital nevi: accuracy of relative area index measurements. *Arch. Dermatol.*, **123**, 709–10.

Everett, M. A. (1989) Histopathology of congenital pigmented nevi. *Am. J. Dermatopathol.*, **11**, 11–12.

Hasegawa, J. I., Maeda, N., Kanzaki, T. and Mizuno, N. (1987) Spontaneous regression of congenital giant cell pigmented nevus with malignant melanoma. In *Clinical Dermatology. The CMD Case Collection* (eds D. S. Wilkinson, J. M. Mascaró and C. E. Orfanos) Stuttgart: Schattauer, pp. 46–47.

Hendrickson, M. R. and Ross, J. C. (1981) Neoplasms arising in congenital giant nevi. *Am. J. Surg. Pathol.*, **5**, 109–35.

Hundeiker, M. (1987) Diagnose und Therapie der kongenitalen Pigmentzellnaevi. *Dtsch. Med. Wocherschr.*, **112**, 807–9.

Illig, L., Weidner, F., Hundeiker, M. *et al.* (1985) Congenital nevi ≤10 cm as precursors to melanoma. 52 cases, a review, and a new conception. *Arch. Dermatol.*, **121**, 1274–81.

Kerl, H., Smolle, J., Hödl, S. and Soyer, H. P. (1989) Kongenitales Pseudomelanom. *Zeitschr. Hautkrankh.*, **64**, 564–8.

Kikuchi, I., Inoue, S., Ogata, K. and Idemoni, M (1984) Disappearance of a nevocellular nevus with depigmentation. *Arch. Dermatol.*, **120**, 678–9.

Kopf, A. W., Levine, L. J., Rigel, D. S., Friedmann, R. J. and Levenstein, M. (1985a) Congenital nevus-like nevi, nevi spili, and café au lait spots in patients with malignant melanoma. *J. Derm. Surg. Oncol.*, **11**, 275.

Kopf, A. W., Levine, L. J., Rigel, D. S., Friedmann, R. J. and Levenstein, M. (1985b) Prevalence of congenital nevus-like nevi, nevi spili, and café au lait spots. *Arch. Dermatol.*, **121**, 766–9.

Kuchnl-Petzoldt, C., Kunze, J., Mueller, R., Volk, B. and Petres, J. (1984) Histology of congenital nevi during the first year of life. *Am. J. Dermatopathol.*, **6**, 1S-8S.

Langer, K. and Konrad, K. (1990) Congenital melanocytic nevi with halo phenomenon: report of two cases and a review of the literature. *J. Dermatol. Surg. Oncol.*, **16**, 377–80.

Mancianti, M.-L., Clark, W. H., Hayes, F. A. and Herlyn, M. (1990) Malignant melanoma simulants arising in congenital melanocytic nevi do not show experimental evidence for a malignant phenotype. *Am. J. Pathol.*, **136**, 817–29.

Mark, G. J., Mihm, M. C., Liteplo, M. G., Reed, R. J. and Clark, W. H. (1973) Congenital melanocytic nevi of the small and garment type. Clinical, histologic, and ultrastructural studies. *Hum. Pathol.*, **4**, 395–418.

Massi, G. (1989) Elastic fibers in congenital melanocytic nevus. *Arch. Dermatol.*, **125**, 299–300.

Mishima, Y. (1973) Eccrine-centered nevus. *Arch. Dermatol.*, **107**, 59–61.

Morishima, T., Endo, M., Imagawa, I. and Morioka, S. (1976) Clinical and histopathological studies on spotted grouped pigmented nevi with special reference to eccrine-centered nevus. *Acta Derm. Venereol. (Stockh.)*, **56**, 345–51.

Nickoloff, B. J., Walton, R., Pregerson-Rodan, K., Jacobs, A. H. and Cox, A. J. (1986) Immunohistologic patterns of congenital nevocellular nevi. *Arch. Dermatol.*, **122**, 1263–8.

Orkin, M., Frichot III, B. C. and Zelickson, A. S. (1974) Cerebriform intradermal nevus. Cause of cutis verticis gyrata. *Arch. Dermatol.*, **110**, 575–82.

Quaba, A. A. and Wallace, A. F. (1986) The incidence of malignant melanoma (to 15 years of age) arising in 'large' congenital nevocellular nevi. *Plast. Reconstr. Surg.*, **78**, 174–9.

Reed, W. B., Becker, S. W., Becker, S. W. Jr. and Nickel, W. R. (1965) Giant pigmented naevi, melanoma, and leptomeningeal melanocytosis. *Arch. Dermatol.*, **91**, 100–19.

Rhodes, A. R. (1986) Congenital nevomelanocytic nevi. Histologic patterns in the first year of life and evolution during childhood. *Arch. Dermatol.*, **122**, 1257–62.

Rhodes, A. R., Silverman, R. A., Harrist, T. J. and Melski, J. W. (1985) A histologic comparison of congenital and acquired nevomelanocytic nevi. *Arch. Dermatol.*, **121**, 1266–73.

Ruth, W. K., Shelburne, J. D. and Jegasothy, B. V. (1980) Zosteriform lentiginous nevus. *Arch. Dermatol.*, **116**, 1980.

Seab, J. A., Graham, J. H. and Helwig, E. B. (1989) Deep penetrating nevus. *Am. J. Surg. Pathol.*, **13**, 39–44.

Silverman, R. A. and Zaim, M. T. (1988) Mastocytoma arising within a congenital nevocellular nevus. *Arch. Dermatol.*, **124**, 1016–8.

Silvers, D. N. and Helwig, E. B. (1981) Melanocytic nevi in neonates. *J. Am. Acad, Dermatol.*, **4**, 166–75.

Solomon, L., Eng, A. M., Bené, M. and Loeffel, D. (1980) Giant congenital neuroid melanocytic nevus. *Arch. Dermatol.*, **116**, 318–20.

Sotelo-Avila, C., Graham, M., Hanby, D. E. and Rudolph, A. J. (1988) Nevus cell aggregates in the placenta. A histochemical and electron microscopic study. *Am. J. Clin. Pathol.*, **89**, 395–400.

Stenn, K. S., Arons, M. and Hurwitz, S. (1983) Patterns of congenital nevocellular nevi. A histologic study of thirty-eight cases. *J. Am. Acad. Dermatol.*, **9**, 388–93.

Stewart, D. M., Altman, J. and Mehregan, A. H. (1978) Speckled lentiginous nevus. *Arch. Dermatol.*, **114**, 895–6.

Walsh, M. Y. and MacKie, R. M. (1988) Histological features of value in differentiating small congenital melanocytic naevi from acquired naevi. *Histopathology*, **12**, 145–54.

Walton, R. G., Jacobs, A. H. and Cox, A. J. (1976) Pigmented lesions in newborn infants. *Br. J. Dermatol.*, **95**, 389–96.

Weidner, N., Flanders, D. J., Jochimsen, P. R. and Stamler, F. W. (1985) Neurosarcomatous malignant melanoma arising in a neuroid giant congenital melanocytic nevus. *Arch. Dermatol.*, **121**, 1302–6.

Zitelli, J. A., Grant, M. G., Abell, E. and Boyd, J. B. (1984) Histologic patterns of congenital nevocytic nevi and implications for treatment. *J. Am. Acad. Dermatol.*, **11**, 402–9.

7 Spitz naevus, desmoplastic Spitz naevus and pigmented spindle cell naevus

Several decades ago it was believed that the prognosis of melanoma was markedly better in childhood (Pack *et al.*, 1947). At that time there was speculation about possible hormonal influences to account for this. However, Spitz (1948) demonstrated that there were major histological differences between these childhood lesions, previously erroneously diagnosed as melanomas, and true metastasizing melanomas. Subsequently it became apparent that similar 'Spitz naevi' occurred also in adults, albeit less commonly (Allen and Spitz, 1953; Kernen and Ackerman, 1960).

The difficulty of distinguishing this type of naevus from melanoma was stressed by a series of reports of melanocytic lesions closely resembling these naevi histologically, but leading to metastases and death (p. 264; Brunck, 1953; Yagawa and Nakamura, 1954; Okun, 1979; Peters and Goellner, 1986). Indeed, the large number of diagnostic criteria put forward in the literature is an indication of the difficulty of making the diagnosis, and emphasizes that no single criterion or small set of criteria can consistently separate Spitz naevi from melanomas. Moreover, when reviewing the literature, a critical evaluation of some of these criteria is not always possible, since the follow-up data are often incomplete and the periods of follow-up too short. Reported disease-free survival periods of two years or even six months do not prove benignity, and cannot be accepted as conclusive evidence that in such cases a diagnosis of Spitz naevus was correct, and that the validity of the diagnostic criteria has been corroborated.

Since the early descriptions of Spitz naevus, it has become apparent that the spectrum of histological appearances is quite varied, and some variants have now been recognized. Of these, desmoplastic Spitz naevus and pigmented spindle cell naevus will be included in this chapter.

7.1 Terminology

The original term used by Spitz was 'juvenile melanoma', a term which, although unsatisfactory and now abandoned, highlights two important aspects: a tendency to occur in the young and a resemblance to melanoma. However, since the same lesion also occurs in adulthood and especially since the term 'melanoma' indicates malignancy, the term juvenile melanoma has since been discarded (Kernen and Ackerman, 1960). A variety of other terms has been proposed: 'benign juvenile melanoma' is a contradiction in terms, and does not take into account that the lesion may occur in adults. The term 'spindle and epithelioid cell naevus' proposed by Helwig (1955), which does not have these disadvantages, has gained considerable popularity especially in the United States. However, it is long and a little cumbersome, tempting pathologists to use the cryptic abbreviation 'SEN'. More importantly, the naevus may consist solely of spindle cells or epithelioid cells. The use of the separate terms 'spindle cell naevus' and 'epithelioid cell naevus' (Kernen and Ackerman, 1960) makes two diagnoses out of the ends of what is a continuous spectrum. 'Naevus of large spindle and/or epithelioid cells' (Paniago-Pereira et al., 1978) is probably the most accurate term, but it is also the most cumbersome!

The term Spitz naevus has retained considerable popularity: it has the advantage of being short and, even if it is not intrinsically informative, it does not carry misleading connotations. Eponyms not uncommonly pay tribute to the wrong person, but in this instance it is wholly justified.

7.2   Clinical features

As is the case with many benign and harmless lesions, epidemiological data concerning the incidence, age distribution and sex preference of Spitz naevi in the general population are difficult to ascertain with any precision. Spitz naevus occurs mainly in Caucasians; it is rare in blacks and orientals. Most cases are diagnosed in childhood and adolescence. In an early series of 262 cases, 85% of patients were infants and children (Allen, 1960). However, in later series, over 25% were adults (Coskey and Mehregan, 1973; Weedon and Little, 1977; Paniago-Pereira et al., 1978). Because Spitz naevus was initially described as a lesion of childhood, there is probably referral bias resulting in over-representation of adult patients in later series, based at least partly on consultation cases: the adult age of the patient may have caused concern and led to referral of the case for a second opinion (Weedon and Little, 1977). Rarely, Spitz naevus occurs at the extremes of age: it may be congenital (McWhorter and Woolner, 1954; Palazzo and Duray, 1988), whereas probably the oldest patient on record was 81 years of age (Coskey and Mehregan, 1973).

There is no obvious sex preponderance; Spitz naevi are perhaps slightly more common in females; in one series, this difference was most marked in the 15–44 years age group, when cosmetic considerations may have been especially important (Paniago-Pereira *et al.*, 1978).

Spitz naevus occurs anywhere on the body, but there appears to be a preference for the face, especially the cheeks, and the lower extremities (Kernen and Ackerman, 1960; Allen, 1960; Peters and Goellner, 1986); however, the trunk was a common site in one series (Weedon and Little, 1977).

Spitz naevus often presents as a nonpigmented and hairless nodule, usually measuring less than 1 cm, although sizes up to 3 cm have been recorded (Allen, 1960). Moderate or even marked pigmentation occurs in a minority of cases, most often in adolescence and adulthood (Echevarria and Ackerman, 1967; Peters and Goellner, 1986). In young children, especially, it often has a pink or reddish hue, because of associated dilatation of superficial capillaries, and there may be a close resemblance to pyogenic granuloma. In adults the naevus tends to present as a firm, skin-coloured or evenly pigmented nodule (Paniago-Pereira *et al.*, 1978). Some Spitz naevi are tender or pruritic (Weedon, 1984); ulceration and bleeding are uncommon and, when present, are probably due to trauma (Weedon and Little, 1977). At the time of diagnosis many Spitz naevi have been noted only a few months, but some have been known to be present for several years.

The clinical features of Spitz naevus are usually insufficiently distinctive to warrant a positive diagnosis: a correct clinical diagnosis was reported in about 20% of childhood cases and less than 10% of adult cases (Weedon, 1984). However, *in conjunction with the histological appearances, clinical data are very important*: for instance, a lesion composed exclusively of large epithelioid melanocytes in an adult is more likely to be a melanoma than in a child, since the large majority of Spitz naevi in adults are of the spindle cell or mixed variety.

Multiple Spitz naevi have been repeatedly observed, either clustered together (agminate) or disseminated on the skin, but sparing palms, soles and mucous membranes. Hamm and co-workers (1987) reviewed 33 cases from the literature: females were somewhat more often affected and, in half of the cases, the naevi were located on the face, most often on the cheeks, the others being divided between the trunk and extremities. Three-quarters of cases occurred before the age of six, and some were congenital (Palazzo and Duray, 1988) or developed on the basis of a congenital naevus. *Agminate Spitz naevi* have been reported after sun exposure, sunburn, radiotherapy or a variety of traumata including previous excision of a solitary Spitz naevus. The latter situation may closely mimic the development of multiple satellites and *in transit* metastases of malignant melanoma (Paties *et al.*, 1987).

Histologically, such cases show the usual features of Spitz naevus, but occasionally there may be a marked increase in junctional proliferation together with some irregularity of rete ridges, together with sub-epidermal fibrosis (Hamm *et al.*, 1987).

7.3   Histological features

Spitz naevus consists of a proliferation of large epithelioid or spindle-shaped melanocytes, or an admixture of both. It is symmetrical and shows a sharp demarcation of the junctional component.

Spitz naevi differ in several respects from common acquired naevi. They differ cytologically in being composed of large plump spindle cells and/or epithelioid cells, with or without epithelioid giant cells. There is penetration of the reticular dermis to an extent not seen in common acquired naevi. There is often telangiectasia and oedema of the superficial stroma. Lymphocyte infiltration is often a feature.

Spitz naevi share with common acquired naevi certain important features. There is symmetry from side to side, with sharp margination. There is usually some 'maturation' from above downwards. Epithelioid giant cells, if present, and any stromal changes found superficially,

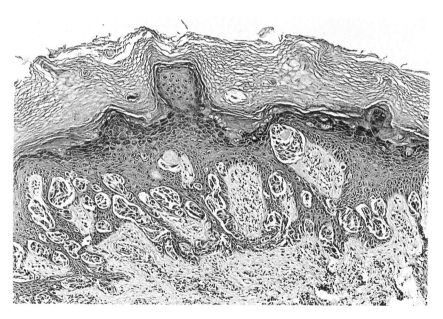

Figure 7.1   Junctional Spitz naevus. Small nests of large melanocytes are seen at the dermoepidermal junction; note also epidermal hyperplasia and hyperkeratosis (HE, × 90).

together with maturation of the deeper component, contribute to the zoned structure of Spitz naevi: this zoning is a feature of most types of benign naevi, with the obvious exception of blue naevi.

Spitz naevi may be junctional (Figure 7.1), compound, or intradermal; the compound type is most common, encompassing about two-thirds of cases; wholly junctional lesions account for only 5–10% of cases (Paniago-Pereira *et al.*, 1978). Intradermal Spitz naevi are mainly seen in adulthood (Mérot and Frenk, 1989).

Architecturally as well as cytologically there is a wide spectrum of appearances. As indicated above, there are two main cell types, epithelioid cells and spindle cells, which may be seen either exclusively, or together. In all age groups, spindle cell Spitz naevi are the most common type. Spitz naevi composed wholly or largely of epithelioid cells are seen mainly in childhood. Spitz naevi of adulthood are usually composed largely of spindle cells, and tend to be more often pigmented and sometimes sclerosed. Mostly, pigmentation is slight and shows a symmetrical and regular distribution, and is most prominent in superficial parts of the lesion. Importantly, the cells of all types of Spitz naevus are larger than the melanocytes of which congenital and common acquired naevi are composed.

The melanocytes in *epithelioid-type Spitz naevus* are round, oval or polygonal, large, and sometimes strikingly pleomorphic (Figures 7.2 and 7.3). The nuclei are round, oval or somewhat irregularly shaped, and often contain one, centrally placed, large nucleolus; a minority of cells may possess a greatly enlarged nucleus with an irregularly shaped nucleolus. The nuclei show a finely stippled or moderately coarse chromatin distribution, or are vesicular. Multinucleated cells are often seen and are numerous in some lesions. There is usually a generous amount of acidophilic or amphophilic cytoplasm, often with a homogeneous, 'ground-glass' appearance. Melanin is usually absent. Cellular borders are often sharp and distinct. In general, cells with large nuclei have much cytoplasm, so that the N/C ratio is not high. The cells are usually weakly to moderately positive for S-100 and NSE (Rode *et al.*, 1990).

Mitoses may be absent, rare, or fairly common, and are mostly located in superficial parts of the lesion. An occasional atypical mitosis is sometimes seen and does not in itself indicate malignancy, although we view such lesions with more suspicion than other Spitz naevi. Mitoses located at the base of the naevus are very uncommon.

Epithelioid-type Spitz naevus is usually of the compound type; the junctional nests are often small, consisting of only a few cells. This contrasts with the spindle cell variant of Spitz naevus, which often contains large, vertically orientated junctional nests. The epidermis is

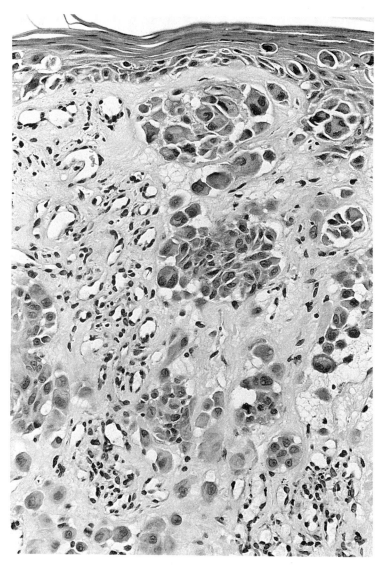

Figure 7.2 Epithelioid-type Spitz naevus. Loosely grouped, large, round or polygonal, sometimes binucleated melanocytes are present in a slightly oedematous dermis containing increased numbers of capillaries. A few melanocytes ascend into suprabasal layers of the epidermis (HE, × 225).

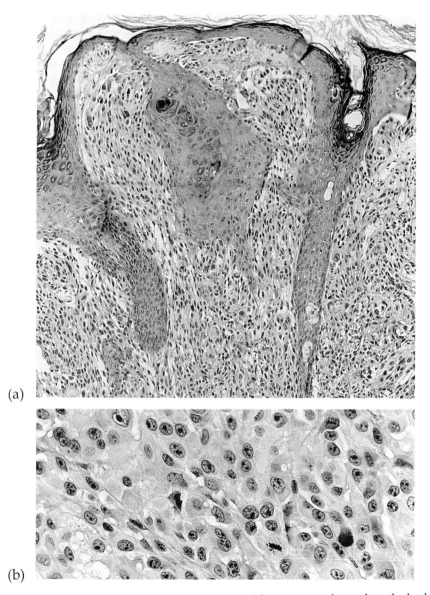

(a)

(b)

Figure 7.3 Mixed spindle cell and epithelioid Spitz naevus, located on the back of a 7-month-old infant. (a) Preferential vertical orientation of spindle cells arranged in large nests; epidermal hyperplasia. (b) At high power, compact groups of large and polymorphic melanocytes with large nuclei containing prominent nucleoli are seen. The cellular features closely resemble those of some melanomas (Figure 9.30, p. 262). In such cases, the architecture of the lesion and the clinical context are of paramount importance to avoid a misdiagnosis of melanoma (HE, × 370).

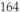

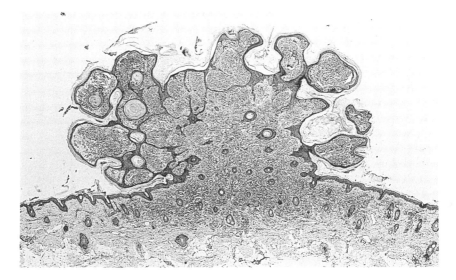

Figure 7.4   Papillomatous Spitz naevus on the face of a 6-year-old girl. Note symmetry and marked papillomatosis. The epidermis is thin but intact (HE, × 20).

usually intact, unless it has been traumatized, which may occur especially in papillomatous Spitz naevi (Figure 7.4), which often exhibit marked dermal oedema, telangiectasia, proliferation of dermal capillaries and thinning of epidermal suprapapillary plates. Epidermal rete ridges are often hyperplastic, showing irregular elongation and sometimes thickening (Figure 7.5). Frank pseudoepitheliomatous hyperplasia is, however, uncommon in epithelioid-type Spitz naevus.

At the dermoepidermal junction, collections of amorphous, diastase-resistant PAS-positive, eosinophilic globules, so-called *Kamino bodies*, are found in about 60% of Spitz naevi, but commonly several sections have to be searched in order to find them (Figure 7.6). These Kamino bodies often coalesce to form irregular structures (Arbuckle and Weedon, 1982). They constitute an important histological diagnostic clue, since they are rare in melanoma (Kamino *et al.*, 1979), where they are usually smaller, with less tendency to coalesce (Weedon, 1984). Rarely, Kamino bodies are seen in common acquired naevi (p. 74). Ultrastructurally, Kamino bodies consist of amorphous masses and bundles of filaments; immunohistochemically, basement membrane components, including collagen types IV and VII and laminin, can be demonstrated (Havenith *et al.*, 1989; Schmoeckel *et al.*, 1990); degenerate melanocytes and keratinocytes probably also contribute to these structures (Kamino *et al.*, 1979).

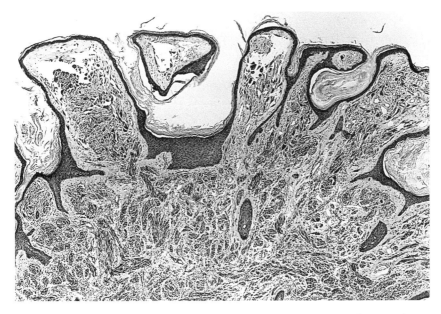

Figure 7.5 Papillomatous Spitz naevus. In the upper dermis, oedema and dissociation of melanocytic nests is seen, whereas in deeper parts more compact strands are formed (HE, × 35).

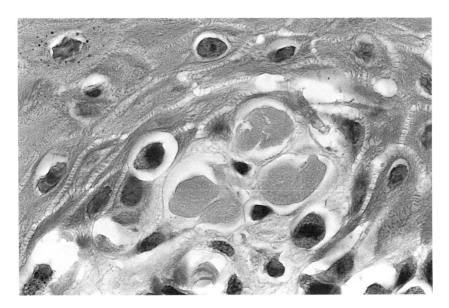

Figure 7.6 Kamino bodies, consisting of round or slightly irregular, densely eosinophilic amorphous masses at the dermoepidermal junction (HE, × 920).

Upward spread and transepidermal elimination of nests of mel-anocytes is seen in a minority of cases (Mérot, 1988). In childhood especially, but also occasionally in adolescence and rarely in early adult life, it may be associated with upward spread of single mel-anocytes (Mérot and Frenk, 1989). However, intraepidermal pagetoid spread in a lateral direction is absent in Spitz naevus and, when present in a lesion, is likely to be indicative of melanoma. The lateral border of the intraepidermal component of a Spitz naevus is sharp, consisting of a nest rather than of a gradual petering-out of solitary melanocytes.

In epithelioid-type Spitz naevi, the presence of distinctly atypical melanocytes lying scattered in the oedomatous dermis and forming compact nests in the upper dermis, may cause some alarm, especially in case of an inappropriate, incomplete biopsy, which precludes a proper evaluation of the architecture of the lateral and deep borders of the lesion.

Lymphatic invasion has been documented convincingly in 7 out of a series of 49 Spitz naevi in children, and did not lead to evidence of metastasis during the follow-up period ranging from 2 to 14 years (Howat and Variend, 1985). Recently, Smith and colleagues (1989)

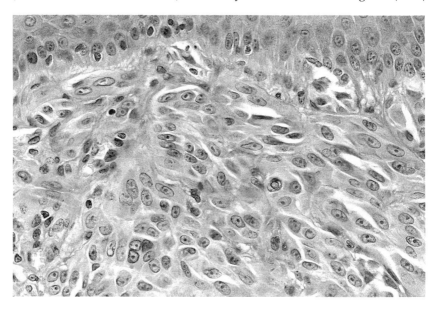

Figure 7.7   Spindle cell Spitz naevus. The oval or elongated melanocytes possess slightly pleomorphic nuclei with a prominent central nucleolus and a well-defined nuclear membrane. There is a moderate amount of cytoplasm; cell borders are ill-defined (HE, × 370).

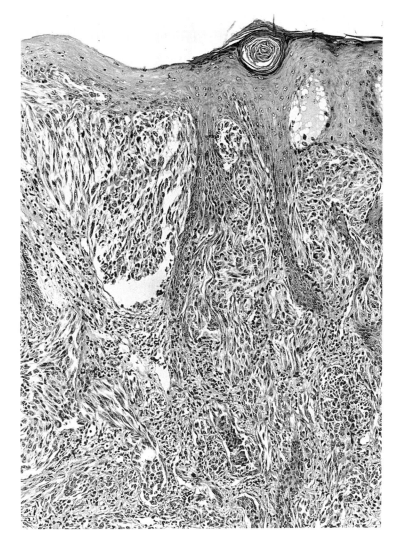

Figure 7.8   Spindle cell Spitz naevus (upper lip, 2-year-old boy). Note
epidermal hyperplasia and vertical arrangement of nests and strands of
fusiform melanocytes (HE, × 115).

raised the possibility that 'benign metastasis' similar to that seen with
some cellular blue naevi (p. 124) may occur in a subgroup of Spitz naevi
which are exceptional in their large size and deep, pushing penetration
of the dermis and subcutis; however, the alternative approach, i.e. to
consider these tumours as melanomas resembling Spitz naevus, poss-

ibly with a less aggressive course of disease than ordinary melanomas, is also applicable to the presently available data. This matter is therefore discussed further in Chapter 9 (p. 264).

A perivascular *lymphocytic infiltrate* is often seen, but a basal band-like infiltrate is rare. Occasionally Spitz naevi regress: in the first stage of the process, a dense infiltrate of lymphocytes and histiocytes disrupts and breaks down dermal naevus cell aggregates. Plasma cells are usually scarce or absent, except in some ulcerated lesions. At a later phase, fibrosis ensues, with disappearance of the infiltrate and the naevus cells. Such regressive changes involve the whole lesion in a symmetrical fashion: partial, asymmetrical regression is highly suggestive of malignancy.

In a *spindle cell Spitz naevus*, the melanocytes are oval or elongated (Figure 7.7). They possess a moderately large, centrally located oval nucleus with usually a dispersed or finely stippled chromatin pattern and a single centrally located round or slightly irregular nucleolus. The well-developed cytoplasm is amphophilic or eosinophilic and usually well demarcated. At the dermoepidermal junction, these cells form elongated, vertically orientated nests (Figure 7.8), which are often separated from the adjacent, irregularly elongated epidermal rete ridges by a cleft-like retraction space, a result of tissue shrinkage during processing. Small nests and solitary cells are usually present also, but large nests predominate over solitary cells (Ackerman, 1989). Nests may be so large that they reach from the dermoepidermal junction upward into the stratum corneum or even to the surface. Transepithelial elimination of nests may be present (Kantor and Wheeland, 1987) and is occasionally accompanied by ascent of a small number of solitary cells, especially in the centre of the lesion, most commonly in cases occurring in childhood. Kamino bodies, described above, are also commonly present in spindle cell Spitz naevus. The epidermis is often hyperplastic and may even exhibit pseudoepitheliomatous hyperplasia (Figure 7.9).

The dermal melanocytes of a spindle cell Spitz naevus are arranged in fascicles and loose aggregates, which gradually diminish in size and merge with a diffuse pattern of growth at the base, where melanocytes lie singly between collagen fibres of the reticular dermis (Figure 7.10). Spitz naevi usually show considerable *infiltration of the reticular dermis*; not uncommonly, arrector pili muscles are invaded by the naevus cells (Ainsworth *et al.*, 1979). Deep parts of the naevus merge gradually with the normal dermal architecture at the borders of the lesion. The basal border is often very indistinct, small collections or solitary spindled melanocytes being present at a considerable distance from the main mass of the lesion (Figure 7.11; Weedon, 1984). *The growth pattern at*

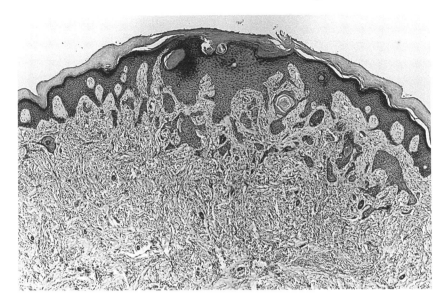

Figure 7.9   Pseudoepitheliomatous hyperplasia in Spitz naevus. This feature may be conspicuous in Spitz naevi, but it is also seen in some melanomas (HE, × 35).

the base of the naevus is infiltrating rather than 'pushing': compact nodules with pushing margins in deeper parts should raise suspicion of melanoma. It should be noted, however, that this is in sharp contrast to the pigmented spindle cell naevus described later in this chapter (p. 178). In deep parts of the naevus, the cells usually diminish gradually in size ('maturation').

Some lesions show an abrupt change to a smaller cell type, conforming to common intradermal naevus cells (Weedon and Little, 1977). Such a common acquired naevus component is usually present lateral to the Spitz naevus. In our experience, the Spitz naevus component of such lesions is often more strongly pigmented than most pure Spitz naevi (Figure 7.12). The presence of a focus with a larger cell type and increased pigmentation may raise a suspicion of malignant transformation. However, the large-cell type exhibits a regular, infiltrating type of growth rather than forming compact nodules, and other features suggestive of malignancy are also lacking.

Recurrent Spitz naevus may result from incomplete excision or curettage of a Spitz naevus, after a period of several months or years (Stern, 1982). These recurrences may show more architectural irregularity than the original lesions, and obviously the index of suspicion is

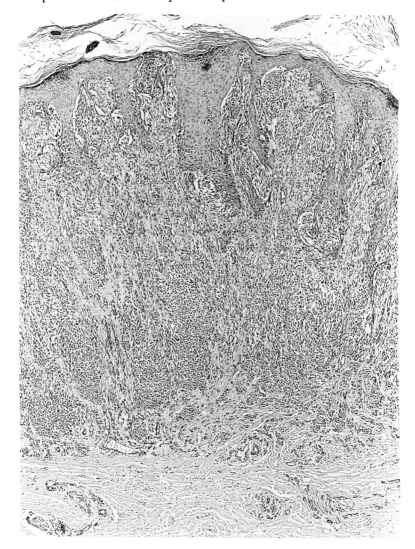

Figure 7.10   Spindle cell Spitz naevus. Epidermal hyperplasia, large vertically oriented nests at the dermoepidermal junction, regular architecture of the dermal component, infiltrating rather than pushing growth at the base (HE, × 45).

raised because the lesion is a recurrent one. Rarely, the recurrence may take the form of a large number of agminate Spitz naevi (p. 159).

The main characteristics of Spitz naevus are summarized in Table 7.1.

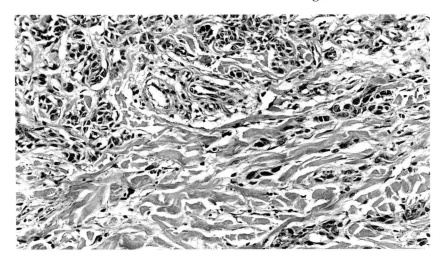

Figure 7.11   Spitz naevus; penetration of reticular dermis. The dermal component of Spitz naevi exhibits an infiltrating rather than a pushing type of growth (HE, × 185).

Table 7.1 Spitz naevus

Clinical features
Nodule, most often nonpigmented, usually less than 1 cm
Moderate or marked pigmentation in some, especially in adolescence and
    adulthood
Majority diagnosed before adulthood
Slight preference for face and lower extremities

Histological features
Spindle-cell, epithelioid-cell or mixed type
Symmetry
Sharp lateral demarcation of junctional component
Epidermal hyperplasia
Retraction spaces between intraepidermal nests of melanocytes and adjacent
    epidermis
Ascending melanocytes usually absent or rare except in young children
Colloid bodies (Kamino bodies) at dermoepidermal interface
Oedema and telangiectases of superficial dermis in some
Regular architecture of dermal component, infiltrating margins
Maturation with increasing depth
Mitoses in superficial parts, but absent or very rare in deep parts; atypical
    mitoses very rare
Perivascular or diffuse inflammatory infiltrate
Lymphangio-invasive growth sometimes present

Remarks
Multiple (agminate or disseminated) Spitz naevi occur, the agminate type
    most often on the face of young children

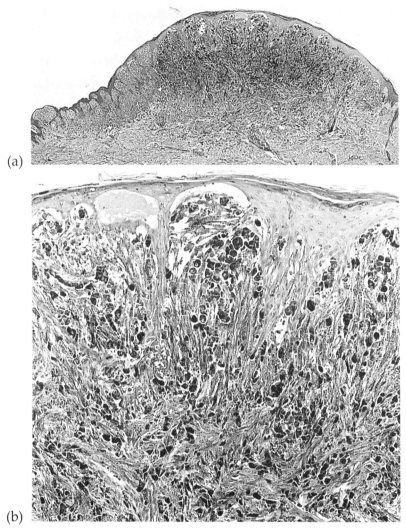

Figure 7.12 Common acquired and Spitz naevus. (a) To the left, a common compound naevus component is present; to the right, a heavily pigmented spindle cell component is seen (HE, × 25). (b) At higher power, a predominantly vertical arrangement of cells, superficial dermal oedema and an infiltrating rather than pushing growth pattern; this argues in favour of a benign lesion. Mitoses, ascent of melanocytes and necrosis are absent (HE, × 115).

7.4 Differential diagnosis

Numerous criteria have been proposed for the diagnosis of Spitz naevus, and there is no doubt that on the basis of these one can confidently distinguish between a typical Spitz naevus and a typical melanoma. However, as outlined above, difficult cases are not uncommon and require a very careful assessment of the clinical and histological features in conjunction with a detailed knowledge of diagnostic criteria and their relative value. The usefulness of criteria based on series of indubitable cases may be limited to the diagnosis of only such indubitable cases. In our experience, the difficulties encountered in the differential diagnosis of Spitz naevus *vs* 'Spitz-like' melanoma (p. 264) are considerable. In Table 7.2, the most important differential diagnostic features are listed.

We think it is wise to be cautious with the diagnosis of Spitz naevus, and not to be tempted into diagnostic heroism in those cases in which the clinical and histological data are not typical. In these circumstances, we prefer to explain the diagnostic difficulty to the clinician, and to make a guarded diagnosis, stating specifically that the possibility of melanoma cannot be totally excluded. Similarly, one should not make a positive diagnosis of melanoma unless one is certain of malignancy: this could lead to overtreatment, with all its possible sequelae, as well as undue psychological stress for the patient, and it could also influence the follow-up data of clinical trials. The optimal treatment for such patients should be discussed on an individual basis, weighing the degree of suspicion of malignancy against the various therapeutic options.

Apart from melanoma, some nonmelanocytic lesions have to be considered in the differential diagnosis. In *juvenile xanthogranuloma*, a junctional component is lacking, Touton-type giant cells and eosinophils are present and the lesional cells are S-100 negative. *Cellular neurothekeoma* (Barnhill and Mihm, 1990) also lacks junctional nests, individual cells infiltrating the dermis, maturation or melanin pigment, whereas there is usually a myxoid stroma. *Epithelioid cell histiocytoma* (Wilson Jones *et al.*, 1989) is also wholly intradermal, occurs in adulthood, mostly on the lower limbs, exhibits an epidermal collarette and consists of a proliferation of epithelioid, often triangular, large cells which do not diminish in size towards the base. *Reticulohistiocytoma of the skin*, which shows giant cells with a large amount of cytoplasm and greatly enlarged and hyperchromatic nuclei, occurs in adults, in whom purely epithelioid-type Spitz naevus is rare.

The diagnosis of Spitz naevus currently rests on light microscopical morphological features; additional techniques thus far appear to be of limited value in the differential diagnosis between Spitz naevus and melanoma. Differences in lectin-binding patterns (Kohchiyama *et al.*, 1987) and image analysis cytometry (LeBoit and Fletcher, 1987) may possibly be of some use. Recently, Rode and co-workers (1990) reported that Spitz naevi showed a less strong immunoreactivity for S-100 protein

Table 7.2 Differential diagnosis Spitz naevus *vs* melanoma

Feature	Spitz naevus	Melanoma
Size	mostly <1 cm	any size
Shape	symmetrical	often asymmetrical
Lateral demarcation	sharp	sharp or ill-defined
Epidermal thinning of suprapapillary plates	often +	+ or −
Epidermal hyperplasia	often +	+ or −
Retraction spaces between intraepidermal nests of melanocytes and surrounding epidermis	often +	+ or −
Ascending melanocytes	usually absent except in young children	often present
Colloid bodies at dermoepidermal interface	often present	rare
Oedema and teleangiectases of superficial dermis	often +	+ or −
Architecture of dermal component	regular, pre-existent dermal collagen pattern	abrupt changes sometimes
'Maturation'	may be evident	usually absent (beware 'pseudo-maturation')
Deep border	indistinct, individual cells	nodules, more compact
Mitoses in deep parts of dermal component	very rare	often
Atypical mitoses	very rare	not uncommon
Dermal inflammatory infiltrate	perivascular, diffuse (in epithelioid variant), rarely band-like	band-like or perivascular
Irregular regression	absent	sometimes

and NSE, when compared to melanoma, a finding that could be expressed objectively by computerized image analysis. Ploidy assessment was also said to be of help in the distinction between Spitz naevus and melanoma. A difference in numbers of AgNORs (p. 25) between Spitz naevi and melanomas has been reported (Howat *et al.*, 1989) but there was overlap in the numbers, so that there appears to be no immediate diagnostic applicability to this finding. Ultrastructurally, Spitz naevus has been reported to contain a distinctive type of cell with a large number of premelanosomes, orientated around the Golgi complex, without melanin synthesis; these cells were considered diagnostic of Spitz naevus and therefore of potential practical use in the differential diagnosis (Ainsworth *et al.*, 1979).

7.5   Desmoplastic Spitz naevus

This variant of Spitz naevus is characterized by prominent collagen production within the intradermal component (Reed *et al.*, 1975; Paniago-Pereira *et al.*, 1978; Barr *et al.*, 1980). It is usually wholly intradermal or shows only a minor junctional component.

Clinically, desmoplastic Spitz naevus presents as a dome-shaped nodule, most often located on the extremities. A minority of cases occurs on the head and neck, which is the most common site of desmoplastic melanoma. Generally, desmoplastic Spitz naevus occurs in adulthood with a peak incidence in the third decade, but some are encountered in children and adolescents. Usually it has been noted several months to many years prior to treatment. The desmoplastic response does not seem to be related to trauma as has been suggested previously.

Histologically the desmoplastic naevus consists of an intradermal, poorly circumscribed proliferation of large elongated melanocytes, associated with an increase in collagen (Figure 7.13). Compact nests and aggregates are often present in superficial parts, whereas in deeper parts the cells lie singly between the collagen bundles. The melanocytes possess hyperchromatic nuclei with finely dispersed or sometimes clumped chromatin. Small nucleoli may be present. Intradermal multinucleated cells are sometimes seen. In contrast to blue naevi, the cells possess a moderate to large amount of eosinophilic or amphophilic cytoplasm, especially in the upper parts of the lesion, and only scanty melanin pigment or none at all. Mitoses are scarce, usually <1 per 20HPF. Importantly, the size of the melanocytes and their nuclei gradually diminishes towards the base of the lesion (Figure 7.14). Some lymphohistiocytic inflammatory infiltrate may be present.

The main features of desmoplastic Spitz naevus are listed in Table 7.3.

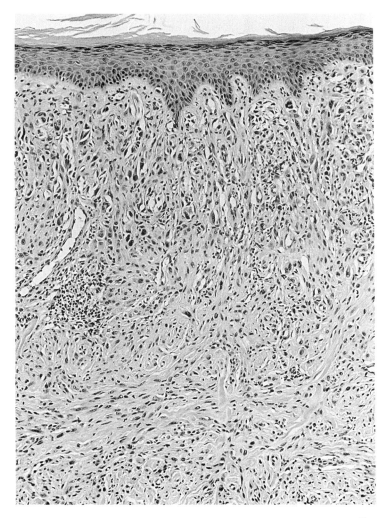

Figure 7.13 Desmoplastic naevus. This variant of Spitz naevus is usually wholly intradermal and is characterized by a fibrotic reaction. Note the gradual diminution in size of the melanocytes towards the base of the naevus (HE, × 115).

Desmoplastic Spitz naevus may cause differential diagnostic difficulties with desmoplastic melanoma (p. 253), combined naevus, blue naevus and deep penetrating naevus, as well as with a variety of nonmelanocytic dermal spindle cell lesions, such as dermatofibroma, reticulohistiocytoma (Barr *et al.*, 1980) and the recently described epithelioid cell histiocytoma (Wilson Jones *et al.*, 1989).

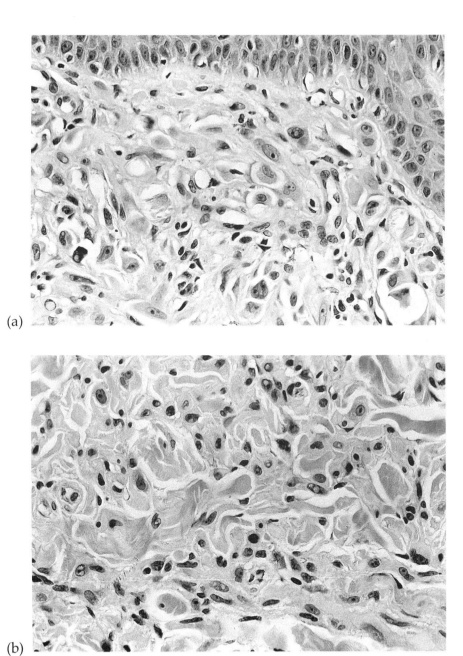

Figure 7.14 Desmoplastic naevus, same case as Figure 7.13. (a) In upper parts of the lesion, the melanocytes are large and there is distinct cellular pleomorphism (HE, × 370). (b) At the base, the cells are smaller and less pleomorphic (HE, × 370).

Table 7.3 Desmoplastic Spitz naevus

Clinical features
  Dome-shaped nodule
  Most common on extremities
  Peak incidence in 3rd decade

Histological features
  Intradermal proliferation of elongated cells
  Increase in dermal collagen
  Multinucleate cells sometimes present
  Small amount of melanin sometimes present
  Scarce mitoses
  Sometimes junctional component, without atypia
  'Maturation'

Remarks
  Differential diagnosis desmoplastic melanoma (p. 253)
  Differential diagnosis other spindle cell lesions: presence of melanin,
    intranuclear cytoplasmic invaginations, immunostaining

As indicated above, there is usually no intraepidermal component; when it is present, it shows a regular architecture and lacks cytological atypia. In contrast, most *desmoplastic melanomas* show melanoma *in situ* or at least hyperplasia of atypical melanocytes within the overlying epidermis. Table 9.2 provides criteria for the differential diagnosis between desmoplastic naevus and desmoplastic melanoma (p. 259).

The presence of intranuclear cytoplasmic invaginations is of help in identifying the melanocytic nature of the lesion. The distinction between desmoplastic naevus and *nonmelanocytic spindle cell lesions* is facilitated by melanin stains and immunostains (p. 22).

7.6   Pigmented spindle cell naevus ('Reed's pigmented spindle cell tumour')

This lesion is usually regarded as a variant of Spitz naevus, but it shows a number of distinctive features so that a good case can be made for regarding it as a separate entity. It often gives rise to differential diagnostic difficulties with melanoma, since it occurs more often in adults; it is generally heavily pigmented and it is less common than the classical Spitz naevus so that its features are less well-known (Reed *et al.*, 1975; Gartmann, 1981; Smith, 1987).

Pigmented spindle cell naevus is a symmetrical, sharply confined, often darkly pigmented papule or small nodule, usually less than

0.6 cm in diameter; it is occasionally surrounded by a hypopigmented halo (Gartmann, 1981). Most are of recent onset, and there is a preference for the extremities, especially the upper leg, more rarely trunk and arm; pigmented spindle cell naevus is distinctly uncommon in the head and neck region. It may occur in childhood as well as in late adult life, but the peak incidence is around the age of 30. It appears to be somewhat more common in females (Reed *et al.*, 1975; Smith, 1987).

Histologically, the lesion is a small, symmetrical, compound or junctional naevus with an expansile growth pattern (Figure 7.15). The pushing margin contrasts with the infiltrative growth pattern of Spitz naevus; however, occasionally, some degree of infiltration by melanocytes away from the main part of the lesion can be present (Sagebiel *et al.*, 1984; Smith, 1987). Generally fusiform, pigmented melanocytes are arranged in nests of varying size, which are characteristically closely positioned and often fused, occupying a large portion of the dermoepidermal junction and sometimes involving skin appendages in the upper dermis. Increased numbers of single melanocytes can also be present, but nests predominate. Because of cellular shrinkage during tissue processing, clefts are often formed around and within these nests, resulting in a 'torn apart' appearance of the tissue. The lesion

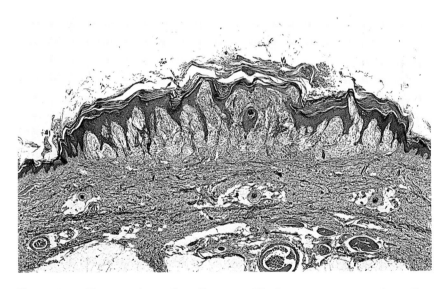

Figure 7.15 Pigmented spindle cell naevus. The lesion is symmetrical, small, flat, highly cellular and exhibits confluence of large and irregular nests, with a predominantly vertical orientation. In this instance, there is only little pigment production (HE, × 20).

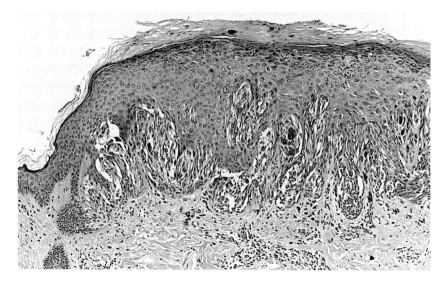

Figure 7.16   Pigmented spindle cell naevus. Confluent vertically orientated nests. Note sharp lateral demarcation (left) (HE, × 90).

occupies an expanded papillary dermis and has a sharply delineated deep margin due to the expansile nature of the proliferation abutting the reticular dermis. In contrast to Spitz naevi, extension into the reticular dermis is rare.

Pigmented spindle cell naevi are generally thin: in one series, mean thickness was 0.65 mm, with a range 0.2–2.4 mm (Smith, 1987).

A moderate degree of epidermal hyperplasia is common, but elongation of rete ridges is usually less striking than in Spitz naevus; Kamino bodies are less frequent but, when searched for in step sections, can be found in the majority of cases (Wistuba and Gonzalez, 1990). Usually, the naevus has a sharp, nested lateral border (Figure 7.16); in a small proportion of cases, however, a lentiginous proliferation of single melanocytes is present at the edge (Barnhill and Mihm, 1989).

Nests of melanocytes may reach upward into the stratum corneum and transepidermal elimination of nests is not uncommon (Sau *et al.*, 1984). In addition, upward migration of a few single melanocytes is occasionally seen (Barnhill and Mihm, 1989; Wistuba and Gonzalez, 1990). Pigmentation of suprabasal keratinocytes and the horn layer is common, resulting in a very dark colour of some of these lesions.

An inflammatory infiltrate composed of lymphocytes and melanophages is usually present at the deep margin of the tumour, a feature accentuating the resemblance to melanoma. However as in other benign melanocytic lesions, plasma cells are usually absent or rare (Sagebiel *et al.*, 1984). In contrast to Spitz naevus, oedema and vascular ectasia in the papillary dermis are absent. Subepidermal lamellar fibrosis, as found in dysplastic naevi, is seen only in a minority of cases and, when present, is inconspicuous.

As its name implies, the pigmented spindle cell naevus consists predominantly of pigmented spindle-shaped melanocytes (Figure 7.17). A minor component of epithelioid cells is present in a few cases

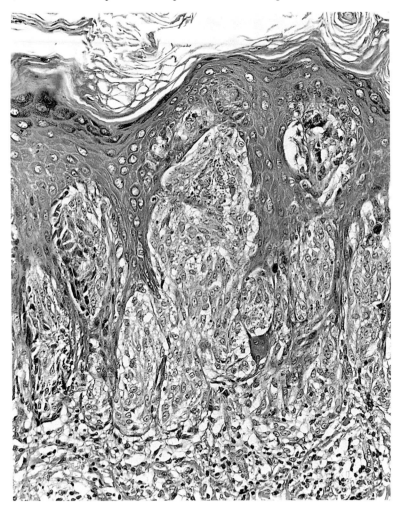

Figure 7.17 Pigmented spindle cell naevus. Confluence of closely apposed, irregular nests of fusiform, variably pigmented melanocytes is seen. There is some lymphocytic response in the papillary dermis (HE, × 225).

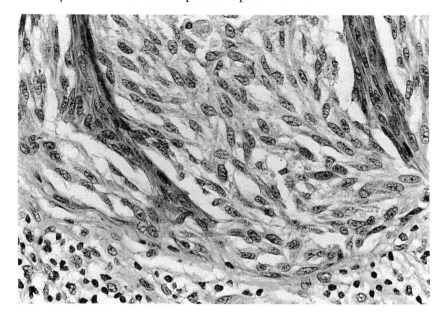

Figure 7.18   Pigmented spindle cell naevus, cytological features. The melanocytes are elongated and possess monomorphic oval nuclei, sometimes containing a small nucleolus (HE, × 370).

Table 7.4   Pigmented spindle cell naevus (Reed)

Clinical features
Symmetrical evenly pigmented macule or nodule
Usually smaller than 0.6 cm
Most often in early adulthood (range: childhood–middle age)
Most often extremities (especially upper leg)

Histological features
Symmetrical, sharply demarcated junctional or compound naevus
Large, fusiform, pigmented naevus cells
Confluence of adjacent nests results in irregular shapes
Epidermal hyperplasia
Nests predominate over solitary melanocytes
Sometimes transepidermal elimination of nests
Occasionally upward spread of a few solitary cells
Pushing, expansile growth pattern in dermis; superficial growth rather than
    the deeper dermal penetration commonly seen in Spitz naevus and spindle
    cell melanoma
Little cellular pleomorphism
Usually few mitoses, but may be present even at the base of the lesion
Kamino bodies sparse

(Smith, 1987). Importantly, there is uniformity of cell size and nuclei in the junctional component. Usually, the melanocytes are equal in size to, or smaller than, adjacent keratinocytes (Sagebiel *et al.*, 1984). Nuclei are oval and contain finely stippled chromatin. Decrease in cellular and nuclear size towards the base may be inconspicuous or absent, but the lesion is thin. Significant nuclear pleomorphism and anisochromasia are absent, which is important diagnostically (Figure 7.18). However, some lesions otherwise typical of pigmented spindle cell naevus exhibit some degree of nuclear pleomorphism (Sagebiel *et al.*, 1984). Prominent nucleoli are seen in up to 50% of cases (Smith, 1987). Abrupt changes in architecture or cell type, so-called intralesional transformation, is a feature of melanoma, and effectively excludes a diagnosis of pigmented spindle cell tumour.

A few mitoses are found in about one-third of cases (Sagebiel *et al.*, 1984; Smith, 1987). Mitoses at the deep border of this tumour are more often detected than in Spitz naevus, but it should be borne in mind that these lesions are generally thin. Smith (1987) stressed that mitotic figures are not atypical: a solitary illustrated example is the exception proving the rule.

The melanin pigmentation is moderate to marked in over 80% of cases, the remaining ones being lightly pigmented. In some lesions most of the melanin is present in melanophages.

The main features of pigmented spindle cell naevus are provided in Table 7.4.

References

Ackerman, A. B. (1989) Differentiation of benign from malignant neoplasms by silhouette. *Am. J. Dermatopathol.*, **11**, 297–300.

Ainsworth, A. M., Folberg, R., Reed, R. J. and Clark, W. H. (1979) Melanocytic nevi, melanocytomas, melanocytic dysplasias, and uncommon forms of melanoma. In *Human Malignant Melanoma* (eds W. H. Clark, L. I. Goldman and M. J. Mastrangelo). New York: Grune & Stratton, pp. 167–208.

Allen, A. C. (1960) Juvenile melanomas of children and adults and melanocarcinomas of children. *Arch. Dermatol.*, **82**, 325–35.

Allen, A. C. and Spitz, S. (1953) Malignant melanoma: a clinico-pathological analysis of the criteria for diagnosis and prognosis. *Cancer*, **6**, 1–45.

Arbuckle, S. and Weedon, D. (1982) Eosinophilic globules in the Spitz nevus. *J. Am. Acad. Dermatol.*, **7**, 324–7.

Barnhill, R. L. and Mihm, M. C. (1989) Pigmented spindle cell naevus and its variants: distinction from melanoma. *Br. J. Dermatol.*, **121**, 717–26.

Barnhill, R. L. and Mihm, M. C. (1990) Cellular neurothekeoma. A distinctive variant of neurothekeoma mimicking nevomelanocytic tumors. *Am. J. Surg. Pathol.*, **14**, 113–20.

Barr, R. J., Morales, R. V. and Graham, J. H. (1980) Desmoplastic nevus. A distinct histologic variant of mixed spindle cell and epithelioid cell nevus. *Cancer*, **46**, 557–64.

Brunck, J. (1953) Über einen metastasierenden, aber klinisch gutartig verlaufenden Naevus mit blasig entarteten Naevuszellen und über deren Genese. *Arch. Dermatol. Syph.*, **196**, 170–5.

Coskey, R. J. and Mehregan, A. (1973) Spindle cell nevi in adults and children. *Arch. Dermatol.*, **108**, 535–6.

Echevarria, R. and Ackerman, L. V. (1967) Spindle and epithelioid cell nevi in the adult. Clinicopathologic report of 26 cases. *Cancer*, **20**, 175–89.

Gartmann, H. (1981) Der pigmentierte Spindelzellentumor. *Z. Hautkrankh.*, **56**, 862–76.

Hamm, H., Happle, R. and Bröcker, E. (1987) Multiple agminate Spitz naevi: review of the literature and report of a case with distinctive immunohistological features. *Br. J. Dermatol.*, **117**, 511–22.

Havenith, M. G., van Zandvoort, E. H. M., Cleutjens, J. P. M. and Bosman, F. T. (1989) Basement membrane deposition in benign and malignant naevo-melanocytic lesions: an immunohistochemical study with antibodies to type IV collagen and laminin. *Histopathology*, **15**, 137–46.

Helwig, E. B. (1955) Seminar on skin neoplasms and dermatoses. In *Proceedings of the Twentieth Seminar of the American Society of Clinical Pathologists*, Sept. 11, 1954. Am. Soc. Clin. Pathol., pp. 63–7.

Howat, A. J. and Variend, S. (1985) Lymphatic invasion in Spitz nevi. *Am J. Surg. Pathol.*, **9**, 125–8.

Howat, A. J., Giri, D. D., Cotton, D. W. K. and Slater, D. N. (1989) Nucleolar organizer regions in Spitz nevi and malignant melanomas. *Cancer*, **63**, 474–8.

Kamino, H., Misheloff, E., Ackerman, A. B., Flotte, T. J. and Greco, M. A. (1979). Eosinophilic globules in Spitz's nevi. New findings and a diagnostic sign. *Am. J. Surg. Pathol.*, **1**, 319–24.

Kantor, G. R. and Wheeland, R. G. (1987) Transepidermal elimination of nevus cells. A possible mechanism of nevus involution. *Arch. Dermatol.*, **123**, 1371–4.

Kernen, J. A. and Ackerman, L. V. (1960) Spindle cell nevi and epithelioid cell nevi (so-called juvenile melanomas) in children and adults: a clinico-pathological study of 27 cases. *Cancer*, **13**, 612–25.

Kohchiyama, A., Oka, D. and Ueki, H. (1987) Differing lectin-binding patterns of malignant melanoma and nevocellular and Spitz nevi. *Arch. Dermatol.*, **279**, 226–31.

LeBoit, P. E. and Fletcher, H. V. (1987) A comparative study of Spitz nevus and nodular malignant melanoma using image analysis cytometry. *J. Invest. Dermatol.*, **88**, 753–7.

McWhorter, H. E. and Woolner, L. B. (1954) Pigmented nevi, juvenile melanomas, and malignant melanomas in children. *Cancer*, **7**, 564–85.

Mérot, Y. (1988) Transepidermal elimination of nevus cells in spindle and epithelioid cell (Spitz) nevi. *Arch. Dermatol.*, **124**, 1441–2.

Mérot, Y. and Frenk, E. (1989) Spitz nevus (large spindle and/or epithelioid cell nevus). Age-related involvement of the suprabasal epidermis. *Virchows Arch. A (Pathol. Anat).*, **415**, 97–101.

Okun, M. R. (1979) Melanoma resembling spindle and epithelioid cell nevus. *Arch. Dermatol.*, **115**, 1416–20.

Pack, G. T., Persik, S. L. and Scharnagel, I. M. (1947) Treatment of malignant melanoma: report of 862 cases. *Calif. Med.*, **66**, 283–7.

Palazzo, J. P. and Duray, P. H. (1988) Congenital agminated Spitz nevi: immunoreactivity with a melanoma-associated monoclonal antibody.

J. Cutan. Pathol., **15**, 166–70.

Paniago-Pereira, C., Maize, J. C. and Ackerman, A. B. (1978) Nevus of large spindle and/or epithelioid cells (Spitz's nevus). *Arch. Dermatol.*, **114**, 1811–23.

Paties, C. T., Borroni, G., Rosso, R. and Vassallo, G. (1987) Relapsing eruptive multiple Spitz nevi or metastatic Spitzoid malignant melanoma? *Am. J. Dermatopathol.*, **9**, 520–7.

Peters, M. S. and Goellner, J. R. (1986) Spitz naevi and malignant melanomas of childhood and adolescence. *Histopathology.*, **10**, 1289–1302.

Reed, R. J., Ichinose, H., Clark, W. H. and Mihm, M. C. (1975) Common and uncommon melanocytic nevi and borderline melanomas. *Sem. Oncol.*, **2**, 119–47.

Rode, J., Williams, R. A., Jarvis, L. R., Dhillon, A. P. and Jamal, O. (1990) S100 protein, neurone specific enolase, and nuclear DNA content in Spitz naevus. *J. Pathol.*, **161**, 41–5.

Sagebiel, R. W., Chinn, E. K. and Egbert, B. M. (1984) Pigmented spindle cell nevus. Clinical and histologic review of 90 cases. *Am. J. Surg. Pathol.*, **8**, 645–53.

Sau, P., Graham, J. H. and Helwig, E. B. (1984) Pigmented spindle cell nevus. *Arch. Dermatol.*, **120**, 1615.

Schmoeckel, C., Stolz, W., Burgeson, R. and Krieg, T. (1990) Identification of basement membrane components in eosinophilic globules in a case of Spitz's nevus. *Am. J. Dermatopathol.*, **12**, 272–4.

Smith, N. P. (1987) The pigmented spindle cell tumor of Reed: an underdiagnosed lesion. *Sem. Diagn. Pathol.*, **4**, 75–87.

Smith, K. J., Skelton, H. G., Lupton G. P. and Graham, J. H. (1989) Spindle cell and epithelioid cell nevi with atypia and metastatis (malignant Spitz nevus). *Am. J. Surg. Pathol.*, **13**, 931–39.

Spitz, S. (1948) Melanomas of childhood. *Am. J. Pathol.*, **24**, 591–609.

Stern, J. (1982) Recurrent spindle and epithelioid cell nevi. *Abstr. Am. Soc. Dermatopathol., 20th Ann. Meeting*, New Orleans, p. 19.

Weedon, D. (1984) The Spitz naevus. *Clin. Oncol.*, **3**, 493–507.

Weedon, D. and Little, J. H. (1977) Spindle and epithelioid cell nevi in children and adults. A review of 211 cases of the Spitz nevus. *Cancer*, **40**, 217–25.

Wilson Jones, E., Cerio, R. and Smith, N. P. (1989) Epithelioid cell histiocytoma: a new entity. *Br. J. Dermatol.*, **120**, 185–95.

Wistuba, I. and Gonzalez, S. (1990) Eosinophilic globules in pigmented spindle cell nevus. *Am. J. Dermatopathol.*, **12**, 268–71.

Yagawa, K. and Nakamura, K. (1954) Autopsy case of widely metastasized juvenile malignant melanoma arised from 'naevus pigmentosus'. *Gann*, **45**, 278–80.

8 Dysplastic naevus

Malignant change at the site of an acquired naevus is a well-recognized phenomenon. Some melanoma patients give a history of the presence of a pigmented lesion at the site of the tumour many years or even decades before it suddenly changed and the clinical features of melanoma became apparent; also, and more definitively, remnants of benign melanocytic naevi can be recognized histologically within or immediately adjacent to about 10–20% of melanomas in Caucasians (Cochran, 1969; Crucioli and Stilwell, 1982; Ackerman, 1988). Since a pre-existing naevus may be destroyed by the growing melanoma, Stolz and colleagues (1989) investigated a series of early, thin melanomas, and arrived at the even higher figure of 27%. Thus, it is clear that the chance of developing a melanoma in a naevus is several orders of magnitude greater than in a corresponding area of normal skin. This is in accordance with the increased incidence of melanoma in individuals with large numbers of naevi (reviewed by Greene *et al.*, 1987a). The increased risk is at least partially explained by the fact that so many more melanocytes are present in a naevus than in normal skin.

Since in most countries the annual incidence of melanoma is less than 30 per 100 000, the association between naevus and melanoma is obviously very weak and has no concrete clinical application, since removal of all naevi in the general population is clearly impractical; furthermore, it would not prevent the development of melanoma in clinically normal skin.

However, the fact that a significant number of melanomas develop in naevi, poses the question whether one can recognize a specific subtype of naevus which is associated more closely with the development of melanoma. In other words: is there a distinct type of naevus, identifiable clinically and histologically, which carries a *clinically significant* risk of malignant transformation?

In the past 10–15 years, the dysplastic naevus, first described in the context of familial melanoma (Frichot *et al.*, 1977; Clark *et al.*, 1978), and subsequently also as a sporadic lesion (Elder *et al.*, 1980), has emerged as a possible candidate; it has become the subject of intense debate regarding terminology, clinical and pathological diagnosis, epidemiology and premalignant potential.

No consensus of definition. Before discussing the features of these lesions and their putative relation to melanoma, some general comments on epidemiological and clinicopathological studies of dysplastic naevi merit attention. It is important to emphasize that at present a general consensus concerning the criteria for the diagnosis of dysplastic naevus has not been achieved and that individual clinicians and pathologists diagnose these lesions very differently. Therefore, published data concerning their prevalence are not easily compared and it is no surprise that there are large discrepancies between different series, resulting in different conclusions and recommendations.

Insufficient follow-up. Estimates of the premalignant potential of these lesions is hampered by the fact that, when a definitive histological diagnosis has been obtained, this means that the lesion has been completely removed so that its natural course can no longer be investigated. There are few follow-up data of incompletely removed dysplastic naevi. In one report, it was mentioned that no melanoma developed after partial removal (shave biopsy) of 21 naevi said to be dysplastic (Ackerman and Mihara, 1985); however, in contrast to many others, these authors did not require cytological atypia for the diagnosis of dysplastic naevus (p. 203).

Relationship of dysplastic naevus to melanoma. A further caveat should be entered about the putative relationship of dysplastic naevus to melanoma: morphological similarities between melanoma and dysplastic naevus might suggest that such a naevus has a greater likelihood of developing into melanoma. However, in itself, it does not provide firm evidence: for instance, Spitz naevus may also show considerable resemblance to melanoma, but this does not make it a premalignant lesion. One needs to find evidence of transition from dysplastic naevus to melanoma and, since follow-up studies cannot supply this, it has to be looked for by studying established melanomas.

Spurious lumping together of different entities. Unless the 'dysplastic naevus' can be defined with reasonable precision histologically, there is a serious danger that a heterogeneous group of lesions is assembled, consisting of essentially benign lesions which for various reasons appear worrisome, on the one hand, and of underdiagnosed malignancies, on the other. *Such lumping together of different lesions can easily create a spurious concept of an entity with a high premalignant potential.*

Terminology. Another problem concerns the use of the term 'dysplasia'. Ackerman (1988) has repeatedly emphasized that in pathology the term 'dysplasia' has been used in totally different ways and that a uniform definition is lacking. Partly because of this, some authors have abandoned the term 'dysplastic naevus' altogether (Seywright *et al.*, 1986; Ackerman, 1988). However, it should be pointed out that the exact meaning of many pathological terms has historically been subject to change. As long as a precise definition of dysplasia is provided in the context of melanocytic lesions of the skin, the fact that the same word carries a different meaning in, say, developmental pathology, does not pose an insuperable obstacle.

Here the term 'dysplasia', in the context of the 'dysplastic naevus', is used to indicate the constellation of architectural and cytological features described and discussed in Sections 8.4 and 8.5. We do not think that anything is gained by trading the term dysplastic naevus for any of the alternative or related terms proposed, such as 'atypical mole', 'intraepidermal melanocytic neoplasia' (Frankel, 1987) or 'intra-epidermal proliferation of atypical melanocytes' (Urso *et al.*, 1990).

Clinical implications. One further point to be made at the outset is that the clinical implications of the diagnosis of dysplastic naevus depend more on the clinical context than on the histological features: sporadic dysplastic naevi carry only a very small risk of melanoma, whereas in the familial dysplastic naevus syndrome, the risk to the patient is very high.

8.1   Familial melanoma and the dysplastic naevus syndrome

The association of familial melanoma with the presence of large numbers of clinically atypical moles was first described by Frichot and colleagues (1977); however, it is the more extensive report by Clark and colleagues appearing one year later that is often taken as the landmark description of what is now known as the familial dysplastic naevus syndrome.

Clark and associates (1978) described two families in whom about half of the members had large numbers of clinically and histologically atypical naevi and who had a very high incidence of melanoma (Clark *et al.*, 1978; Reimer *et al.*, 1978). In a prospective study of dysplastic naevus-bearing *vs* clinically normal members of such melanoma-prone families, age-adjusted incidence rates of melanoma were 14.3 and 0 per 1000, respectively, indicating the very close relation between the presence of dysplastic naevi and melanoma risk in these families (Greene *et al.*, 1985a). In the same study, a pre-existent naevus was found at the margin of 85% of melanomas; in 70% of cases, these naevi showed histological evidence of dysplasia, suggesting strongly that the dysplastic naevi found in this setting are actually the precursor lesions of the melanomas developing in the familial dysplastic naevus syndrome.

In some dysplastic naevus syndrome kindreds, an increase in internal neoplasms has been reported (Lynch *et al.*, 1983; Bergman *et al.*, 1986), but this was not found in other families (Greene *et al.*, 1985b; 1987b).

Segregation studies suggested that in these families the dysplastic naevus and melanoma traits are both effects of a single gene with an autosomal dominant mode of inheritance (Greene *et al.*, 1983; Bale *et al.*, 1986). A patient with a large number of dysplastic naevi confined to the left upper quadrant of the body was reported by Sterry and Christophers (1988): such a distribution is thought to be due to a somatic mutation during early embryonic development, and supports the concept of a single autosomal trait. A segregation study of a panel of polymorphic DNA markers in affected families in the United States pointed to a probable location of the putative gene distally on the short arm of chromosome 1 (Bale *et al.*, 1989). However, this finding could not be confirmed in Dutch and Australian dysplastic naevus syndrome families (Salomon *et al.*, 1989; Gruis *et al.*, 1990). Linkage analyses may be influenced markedly by nonpenetrance of the trait under study or by a high prevalence of sporadic cases in the general community; both these factors may be of importance in the case of the dysplastic naevus syndrome (Kefford, 1990) and may perhaps have brought about these apparently conflicting results; alternatively, it is possible that different genes are involved. There are some indications that abnormal sensitivity to UV-induced cellular damage caused by a defect in early excision repair of DNA plays a role in the pathogenesis of the disease (Howell *et al.*, 1984; Roth *et al.*, 1988).

The syndrome was initially designated *B–K mole syndrome* (Clark *et al.*, 1978), after the initials of the families' surnames, or the *FAMMM syndrome* (familial atypical multiple mole melanoma syndrome; Lynch *et al.*, 1978, 1981). Later, the term *dysplastic naevus syndrome* was introduced (Greene *et al.*, 1980). On the basis of the clinical and histopathological appearances, several names were proposed for the naevi encountered in these patients: epithelioid melanocytic dysplasia (Clark *et al.*, 1978), large atypical mole, melanocytic dysplasia (Elder *et al.*, 1980), atypical melanocytic hyperplasia (Sagebiel, 1979), and *dysplastic naevus* (Greene *et al.*, 1980; Elder *et al.*, 1981). The latter term has gained popularity, despite attempts to discourage its use (Cook and Robertson, 1985; Ackerman and Mihara, 1985; Ackerman, 1988).

In the past decade, many more melanoma-prone families have been identified and the occurrence of dysplastic naevi in the context of many such families, as well as their association with greatly increased risk for development of melanoma, has now become generally acknowledged.

Close follow-up, aiming at early clinical detection of melanoma in affected family members is the basis of clinical management. The patient's skin is examined thoroughly, including the scalp, ears, external genitalia, intergluteal fold and feet; photographs are an important aid in detecting subsequent changes in naevi, especially when these are very numerous (Rivers *et al.*, 1990). One or a few lesions are excised to confirm the diagnosis; it is wise to remove prophylactically lesions located on the scalp, because changes here are less easily noticed; all changing or otherwise suspicious lesions are also removed; follow-up is carried out at least once a year, and patients are advised as to self-examination, observation of family members, and sun-avoidance. Screening should include all first degree relatives older than 10 years (Greene *et al.*, 1987a). Excision of all naevi is a futile exercise: new dysplastic naevi continue to develop, as was illustrated by a case in which total removal of all pigmented lesions was undertaken (Barnes and Nordlund, 1987).

The efficacy of early detection of melanoma during follow-up of dysplastic naevus syndrome patients is shown in a recent study, published twice (Rigel *et al.*, 1989; Rivers *et al.*, 1990), in which 452 such patients were followed for a period averaging 27 months. Melanoma developed in 18 patients: 12 of these were *in situ* melanomas, while the remaining six were all under 0.89 mm in thickness and therefore also had an excellent prognosis.

8.2   Sporadic dysplastic naevus syndrome and solitary dysplastic naevus

In 15 out of a series of 79 nonfamilial melanoma patients studied prospectively, Elder and colleagues (1980) found moles on the covered buttock area, where moles are normally rare; seven of these 15 patients had large and abnormal naevi with the histological features of dysplastic naevi (section 8.3). In the melanomas of five of these patients, there were remnants of a pre-existing dysplastic naevus in contiguity with the melanoma. The authors concluded that, phenotypically, these sporadic cases were very similar to the affected members of dysplastic naevus syndrome families. Such an apparently sporadic case may of course be the first member of a dysplastic naevus syndrome family to come to clinical attention; alternatively, it may represent a germinal mutation (Greene *et al.*, 1987a).

Interestingly, seven cases of eruptive dysplastic naevi in HIV-positive patients occurring at the transition to AIDS or AIDS-related complex were described by Duvic and associates (1989).

English and colleagues (1986) reported clinical evidence of the dysplastic naevus syndrome in 27% of a series of melanoma patients with either a positive family history of melanoma, or multiple melanomas, or a histologically proved dysplastic naevus, as opposed to 6% in other melanoma patients; melanoma patients in the context of dysplastic naevus syndrome tended to be younger, with a male predominance.

Simultaneously with the recognition of the sporadic form of the dysplastic naevus syndrome, characterized by the presence of a large number of irregular and abnormally large naevi, also at unusual sites, reports began to indicate that *solitary dysplastic naevi are not uncommon in the general population*: indeed, depending on the diagnostic criteria used, their overall prevalence has been estimated at about 2–9% (Rhodes *et al.*, 1980; Sheiber *et al.*, 1981; Crutcher and Sagebiel, 1984; Greene *et al.*, 1987a; Cook *et al.*, 1989). They are found most frequently in persons with many naevi; indeed, Nordlund and colleagues (1985) reported clinically dysplastic naevi (defined as naevi larger than 5 mm, and with irregular borders and irregular pigmentation) in as many as 19% of persons with more than 30 naevi. In the same study, clinically dysplastic naevi were found in no less than 34% of nonfamilial melanoma patients, as opposed to 7% in control subjects without melanoma.

In order to categorize the various clinical situations in which dysplastic naevi are diagnosed, and to assign specific risk factors for each, Kraemer and co-workers (1983) proposed the categories summarized in Table 8.1. Type D2 patients have a life-time risk of melanoma approaching 100%; for the other subgroups, especially for the large group of type A patients with a solitary dysplastic naevus and a negative personal and family history for melanoma, precise figures are not available for the reasons discussed; the relative risk appears to be

Table 8.1 Summary of clinical categories of dysplastic naevi (after Kraemer *et al.*, 1983)

Type A: true sporadic type (no family history of melanoma or dysplastic naevi)

Type B: no melanoma, but dysplastic naevi in two or more family members

Type C: patient has dysplastic naevi and melanoma, but no family history of dysplastic naevi or melanoma

Type D1: one family member with dysplastic naevi and melanoma, other family members with dysplastic naevi

Type D2: two or more family members with melanoma as well as dysplastic naevi in the order of three-fold when only a few dysplastic naevi are present; this risk is similar to that of red-haired individuals with easily sun-burned skin (Elder and MacKie, 1990).

When a histological diagnosis of a dysplastic naevus is made, it is wise to investigate the entire skin for the presence of multiple abnormal pigmented lesions, and to assess whether there is a personal or family history of melanoma. The identification of new familial cases of dysplastic naevus syndrome is obviously of great importance. However, the familial dysplastic naevus syndrome is rare, and *the large majority of dysplastic naevi encountered are isolated cases*. The prevalence of solitary dysplastic naevi in the general population implies that the large majority never lead to melanoma. Therefore, when there are no other clinically abnormal naevi, the number of naevi is not clearly excessive, and the personal and family history of melanoma is negative, there appears to be no need for further action. When there is a history of melanoma, life-long surveillance has been advocated (Elder and MacKie, 1990).

8.3   Clinical features

Dysplastic naevi may occur singly or in large numbers; they are found on sun-exposed skin as well as on covered areas of the body such as the scalp, breast and buttocks. They appear in adolescence and early adulthood (Consensus Conference, 1984). They are often larger than usual naevi, which generally do not exceed 8 mm in diameter. It has been advocated to exclude lesions up to 5 mm in diameter, in order to avoid the inclusion of simple lentigines and junctional naevi into the group of dysplastic naevi (Elder and MacKie, 1990). Dysplastic naevi often show an irregular contour, a somewhat varied degree of pigmentation, and they may be surrounded by a reddish hue, which is no longer visible in the excision specimen. They are raised or flat, or may show a papular centre and macular periphery (Elder *et al.*, 1982). In adulthood, a completely macular pigmented lesion exceeding 4 mm is suspect of being a dysplastic naevus, except on palms, soles and external genitalia, where simple lentigines and common junctional naevi often exceed that size (Elder, 1985). Once they are fully developed, they remain stable clinically; subsequent change, after a period of stability, is suspect of malignant change, and such a lesion should be excised (Elder and MacKie, 1990).

8.4   Pathological features

Dysplastic naevi are junctional or compound naevi; the latter are more common and, in these, the junctional component usually extends

lateral to the intradermal component over a distance of at least three
rete ridges ('shoulder phenomenon'; Clark *et al.*, 1984; Elder, 1985).
This may be macroscopically evident as a flat extension of the pigmentation around a central raised portion. The lateral margins are often
poorly defined.

Sometimes, the histological features of dysplastic naevus are present
in a congenital naevus. As indicated above, they may be seen in
contiguity with melanoma, a finding with a possible bearing on the
nature of the lesion and its precancerous potential.

8.4.1   *Architecture of junctional component and reactive epidermal changes*

In dysplastic naevi, there is a very marked increase in number of
junctional melanocytes, which are arranged in a lentiginous and/or
nested pattern. Nests are irregular in size and shape and are irregularly
spaced over the naevus (Figures 8.1–8.4). Rete tip preference (p. 63) of
these nests is usually absent; however, it should be borne in mind that
in papillomatous compound naevi, rete tip preference may also be
absent (p. 65). In contrast to common acquired naevi, nests are com-

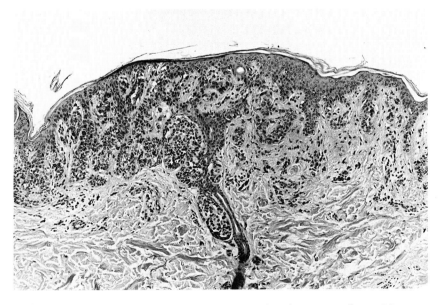

Figure 8.1   Dysplastic junctional naevus. Irregular elongation of rete ridges;
proliferation of melanocytes at the dermoepidermal junction, in a lentiginous
pattern as well as in the form of unevenly spaced nests, which also extend
along a sweat gland duct. There is mild subepidermal fibrosis (HE, × 90).

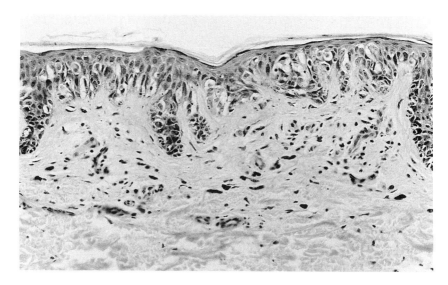

Figure 8.2 Dysplastic junctional naevus. Extensive lentiginous and irregularly nested proliferation of melanocytes; mild subepidermal fibrosis and inflammation; 47-year-old female with a history of melanoma (HE, × 185).

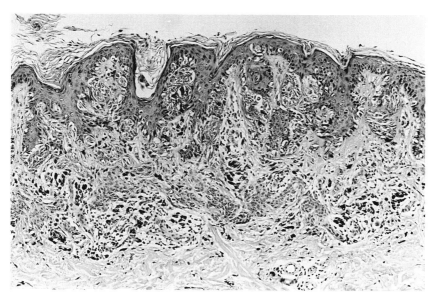

Figure 8.3 Dysplastic compound naevus. Irregular and extensive lentiginous and nested proliferation of melanocytes along the dermoepidermal junction; fibrosis and patchy inflammatory infiltrate in the upper dermis (HE, × 90).

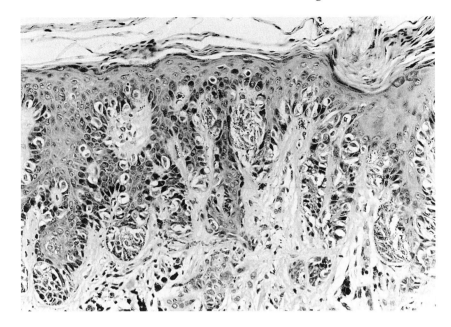

Figure 8.4   Dysplastic compound naevus. Marked increase in melanocytes at the dermoepidermal junction, in a lentiginous and nested pattern. Melanocytes vary in size, orientation and shape. (HE, × 185).

monly orientated horizontally and may form bridges between adjacent rete ridges. Retraction artefacts around nests and solitary melanocytes sometimes result in a moth-eaten appearance of the dermoepidermal junction.

There is usually some elongation of epidermal rete ridges which may be accompanied by mild thickening of the suprapapillary plates. However, prominent acanthosis and hyperkeratosis are absent; if present, they should raise a suspicion of melanoma. The elongated rete ridges often show an irregular shape and arrangement (Figure 8.5), with various oblique orientations and, as indicated above, they may be interconnected by horizontally orientated melanocytic nests.

In contrast to *in situ* melanoma, ascent of atypical melanocytes into the upper layers of the epidermis and pagetoid lateral spread are absent. Apart from the distinction from *in situ* melanoma discussed later (p. 204), the lesion should be distinguished from lentigo maligna (p. 240), which also exhibits a proliferation of atypical melanocytes, but in the context of an atrophic epidermis and signs of actinic damage in the dermis. Rhodes and co-workers (1983) considered lentigo maligna a separate and unrelated melanocytic dysplasia since, in their material, it

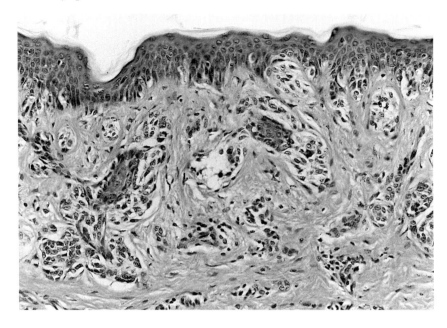

Figure 8.5 Dysplastic compound naevus. Subepidermal fibrosis with distortion of rete ridges and irregular melanocytic proliferation (HE, × 185).

was not associated with a dermal naevus component, did not occur in association with melanoma in relatives and showed a different topographical distribution. Dysplastic naevi do occur in sun-exposed skin, but these are associated with irregular elongation of epidermal rete ridges rather than epidermal atrophy, and are otherwise also identical with dysplastic naevi in other sites.

8.4.2 Cytological atypia of melanocytes

The melanocytes at the dermoepidermal junction show some degree of variation in size, shape and orientation. Some have a dark, irregular or crescent-shaped nucleus, while others show a slightly larger, vesicular nucleus containing a prominent nucleolus. Also, the cytoplasm varies in amount, stainability, and melanin content. There is often an admixture of dusty and finely granular melanin pigment in the cytoplasm. As a result of these variations, the dysplastic naevus exhibits an impression of cytological variability, even within individual nests of melanocytes, or within one stretch of melanocytes in lentiginous arrangement (Figure 8.6). Even if each individual cell could perhaps also be encountered in common acquired naevi, it is the variability

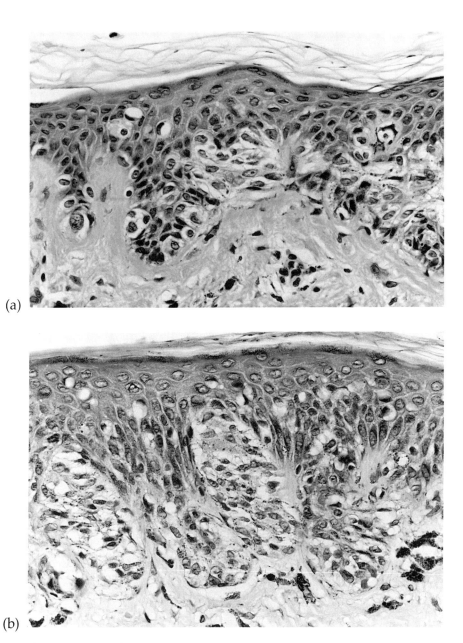

Figure 8.6 Dysplastic junctional naevus, cytological atypia. Melanocytes are increased in number and exhibit varying degrees of nuclear enlargement and increased cytoplasmic stainability (a, b) (HE, × 370).

between cells, enhancing the impression of irregularity caused by the architectural features described above, that is an important feature of the dysplastic naevus. In some dysplastic naevi the flat periphery of the lesion exhibits the most distinct cytological atypia (Elder, 1985).

There is some controversy as to whether this cytological atypia is present in *all* dysplastic naevi, i.e. whether cytological atypia is an obligatory criterion for the diagnosis of dysplastic naevus; this will be dealt with in section 8.5. Suffice it, to say here, that we agree with Clark and co-workers (1984) that the presence of cellular and nuclear pleomorphism as described above, and sometimes designated *'random cytological atypia', is an important diagnostic feature of the dysplastic naevus.*

A minor degree of cytological atypia is occasionally present in common junctional and compound naevi which we would not consider to be dysplastic naevi. Also, some architectural features of dysplastic naevi, such as markedly increased junctional activity and subepidermal fibrosis, are not uncommon in naevi which we would not consider dysplastic. Even a very mild irregularity of cytological features in addition to slight architectural irregularity is not uncommon: it is likely that such lesions probably cause the very marked differences in prevalence figures given for 'dysplastic naevi' in the general population. In our view, it is the combination of marked, irregular hyperplasia and cytological atypia that is necessary for the diagnosis of dysplastic naevus. Such lesions can be recognized clinically, and are certainly not common.

8.4.3   *Intradermal component, dermal reactive changes*

The dermal portion of a dysplastic compound naevus consists of strands, nests and aggregates; in some instances, these may show no or hardly any 'maturation' (p. 65), i.e. the cells do not gradually diminish in size towards the base of the lesion. This feature may be difficult to evaluate, since 'maturation' may also be absent in common compound naevi, especially in thin lesions. There is often a subtle degree of nuclear atypia in the dermal component. Mitoses, which are occasionally seen in the junctional component of the naevus, are absent or very rare in the dermal portion. Some melanin may be produced also at the base of the lesion, and pigmentation may be somewhat irregular in distribution.

Dysplastic naevi commonly show a fibrotic stromal response, which is especially prominent around rete ridges and vessels. This is manifested as an increase of strongly eosinophilic and slightly refractile collagen fibres (*'eosinophilic fibroplasia'*). To some extent, this change is

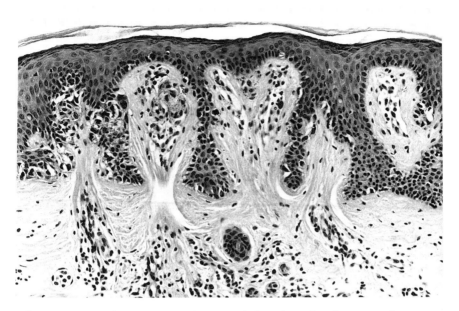

Figure 8.7 Dysplastic junctional naevus. Subepidermal and perivascular lamellar fibroplasia (HE, × 185).

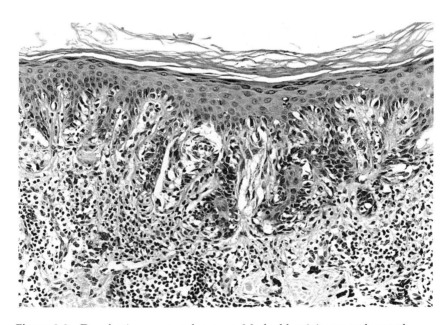

Figure 8.8 Dysplastic compound naevus. Marked lentiginous and nested proliferation of melanocytes, marked inflammatory infiltrate in upper dermis, some subepidermal fibrosis and irregularity of rete ridges (HE, × 185).

Table 8.2 Dysplastic naevus, clinical and histological features

Clinical features
>5 mm; often larger than other acquired naevi
Irregular outline
Predominantly macular, sometimes papular centre and macular periphery
Variations in degree of pigmentation
Surrounding red hue
Sometimes large numbers, most common on upper trunk and extremities, but also on covered sites (buttocks, groins, scalp, breasts)
Sporadic and familial cases, with or without association with melanoma in patient or family

Histological features
Architectural features
Marked proliferation of melanocytes at dermoepidermal junction in a lentiginous pattern with or without nests
Absence of 'rete tip preference' of nests
Irregular size and shape of nests
Nests bridging adjacent rete ridges
Irregular shape and orientation of rete ridges
Junctional component extending ≥3 rete ridges beyond margins of dermal component (when present)
Impairment of maturation of dermal component (when present)
Eosinophilic and lamellar fibroplasia
Lymphocytic infiltrate (focal, perivascular)
Capillary proliferation within superficial dermis

Cytological features
Enlargement of some melanocytes and their nuclei, 'random atypia'
Nuclear hyperchromasia
Prominent nucleoli
Dusty melanin pigment

Remarks
Familial dysplastic naevus syndrome is rare; solitary dysplastic naevi are not uncommon
Familial and sporadic cases show similar histology
In common acquired naevi, several of the features may be present ('active naevi')
Melanoma risk depends more on patient and family history and clinical appearance (number of atypical moles) than on histology

also seen in many lentigines and early junctional naevi. Stacks of dense collagen lamellae may be formed around rete ridges and vessels: this more distinctive change is referred to as *'lamellar fibroplasia'* (Figure 8.7). Fibroblasts within the papillary dermis are slightly increased in number and there is usually some increased vascularity. A mild or moderate *perivascular lymphocytic infiltrate* (Figure 8.8) is invariably present and is often associated with scattered *melanophages*. Importantly, a basal, band-like lymphocytic infiltrate is not seen and plasma cells are scarce. However, active regression may result in a diffuse inflammatory infiltrate disrupting dermal naevus cell nests; this may be difficult to distinguish from regressing melanoma. In the absence of previous trauma, focal and asymmetrical regression is very suggestive of malignancy.

The pathological features of dysplastic naevi are summarized in Table 8.2.

8.5   Histological criteria for the diagnosis

The criteria cited in the literature for the diagnosis of dysplastic naevus have varied considerably, necessitating discussion of some major publications in this field. Rather than attempting a complete review of the extensive literature on this subject, we have chosen a few key articles which illustrate important issues in the debate. It is important to appreciate at the outset that all authorities aim to base the diagnosis on concrete and evaluable criteria, and agree that *one should not use the diagnosis of dysplastic naevus as a 'ragbag for all histologically worrying but probably benign lesions'* (Cook and Fallowfield, 1990).

Clark and co-workers (1984) cited five diagnostic criteria: persistent lentiginous hyperplasia, melanocytic nuclear atypia, lamellar fibroplasia, concentric eosinophilic fibroplasia and sparse patchy lymphocytic infiltrates.

In Elder's view (1985), the histological diagnosis hinges on two major criteria: lentiginous or epithelioid 'immature' hyperplasia, and 'random cytological atypia'; in addition, five minor criteria are given: nests bridging or adjacent to rete ridges, lamellar fibroplasia, eosinophilic or nonspecific fibroplasia, patchy lymphocytic response, and psoriasiform elongation of rete ridges.

Ackerman and Mihara (1985) commented on the criteria for dysplastic naevus previously proposed by others. These authors criticized the use of the term dysplasia, and indicated that in their experience, naevi 'referred to as dysplastic naevi' are very common in the general population. They did not consider cytological atypia a prerequisite for the diagnosis. A further discussion of this and other important papers by Ackerman will be included in the following subsection which focuses further on the distinction between common acquired and dysplastic naevi.

Steijlen and colleagues (1988) performed a discriminant analysis of the diagnostic features of dysplastic naevi, comparing 36 dysplastic naevi (derived from 18 sporadic and 18 familial cases of clinically evident dysplastic naevus syndrome) with 326 naevi obtained from

routine autopsies. These authors concluded that the dysplastic naevi
were identified most accurately on the basis of the presence of a
lymphocytic infiltrate together with at least two of the following four
features: markedly increased junctional activity, irregular nests, large
melanocytic nuclei, and dust-like melanin. With these criteria, positive
and negative predictive values of 89 and 98% were reached. When all
four features were present, the lesion was considered to be a 'severely
dysplastic' naevus: such naevi were found exclusively in the dysplastic
naevus syndrome group.

In this study of Steijlen and colleagues (1988), there was a significant
age difference between test and control groups, and several features of
dysplastic naevus were seen more often in younger cases of the control
group, so that the histological differences between naevi in test and
control groups were greater than they would have been had perfectly
age-matched controls been available for study. Also, a histological
diagnosis of dysplastic naevus had apparently been taken into account
in the selection of cases for the test group, which introduced an element
of circular reasoning into the study. Furthermore, the positive predictive
value obtained does not reflect the value that would be obtained with
nonselected material, in view of the markedly different prevalences of
dysplastic and common acquired naevi (p. 28). However, the important contribution made by Steijlen and colleagues is that their study
provides quantitative data showing that the diagnosis of dysplastic
naevus, and consequently figures for its *prevalence* in the general
population, *depends to a large extent on the minimum diagnostic criteria
required to make this diagnosis.*

Barnhill and colleagues (1990) investigated the relation of nuclear
atypia of melanocytes and a variety of architectural features in a series
of 153 naevi removed from patients with nonfamilial melanoma. These
authors concluded that the diagnosis of dysplastic naevus should be
based on a combination of nuclear atypia and abnormal architecture,
especially abnormal patterns of intraepidermal melanocytic proliferation,
with or without confluence, and with variation in size, shape and
location of nests, as well as confluence of nests.

8.5.1 *Dysplastic naevus* vs *common acquired naevus*

The concept of the 'dysplastic naevus' has met with considerable
criticism, much of which concerns its distinction from common acquired naevi. In this respect, it is important to realize that common
naevi of the type described in Chapter 4 as 'active naevi' (Eng, 1983;
Holman *et al.*, 1983; Armstrong *et al.*, 1984; Rosai, 1989), exhibit a
spectrum of appearances which shows some overlap with the features

of dysplastic naevus. Such 'active' or 'hot' naevi show an association with sunlight exposure, pregnancy, previous incomplete excision, location on the genitalia, or the presence of a melanoma elsewhere. However, they may also occur in the absence of these factors, especially in young persons.

Probably the most outspoken critic of the concept of the dysplastic naevus is Ackerman (1985, 1988; Ackerman and Mihara, 1985). He considers dysplastic naevi to be 'extremely common'. Ackerman and Mihara (1985) stated that 'most compound nevi that are confined to the epidermis and the papillary dermis are dysplastic nevi'. Furthermore, according to Ackerman's experience, 'melanocytic naevi said to be dysplastic naevi are diagnosable easily under scanning magnification' (Ackerman, 1988). This, however, is in contrast with the experience of many others. Significantly, Ackerman considers evaluation of cytological atypia unnecessary for the diagnosis of dysplastic naevus (Ackerman and Mihara, 1985); the architecture of the lesion is considered the only useful histological parameter. In fact, in this Ackerman receives support from an earlier Consensus Conference (1984) where it was also stated that cytological atypia is not essential for the diagnosis of dysplastic naevus.

However, this contrasts with the viewpoint of many workers who have put forward criteria for the distinction of common acquired naevi and dysplastic naevi. One of the two main criteria for the diagnosis of dysplastic naevus put forward by Elder (1985) is 'random cytological atypia'. In the study by Steijlen and co-workers (1988), two of the four most discriminating features, i.e. the presence of large nuclei and dust-like melanin pigment, were also cytological rather than architectural. Greene and colleagues (1987a) emphasized that, in their opinion, 'the criterion of random cytologic atypia is necessary for the diagnosis'. In an attempted consensus meeting in 1987, cytological atypia scored highest (17 out of 22 participants) as a distinguishing feature of dysplastic naevi (Greene *et al.*, 1987a). Barnhill and colleagues (1990) also stressed the importance of nuclear atypia in the diagnosis of dysplastic naevus. This is in contrast to Ackerman and Mihara (1985) who maintain that atypia is not necessary for the diagnosis of a dysplastic naevus. Inevitably, the latter authors, in not accepting cytological atypia as a prerequisite for the diagnosis of dysplastic naevus, diagnose dysplastic naevus far more often than others and, indeed, so often that Ackerman (1988) proposes to rename the dysplastic naevus 'the common naevus'. Indeed, some of Ackerman's illustrations of 'dysplastic naevi' (1988, figures 2 and 3) would in our opinion not justify a diagnosis of dysplastic naevus; we agree that the naevi depicted in these illustrations are very common, but to us they are not dysplastic naevi! If the diagnosis of dysplastic naevus is restricted to lesions showing the combination of cytological and architectural abnormalities listed in Table 8.2, then dysplastic naevi are certainly not 'extremely common'. Recently, Murphy and Halpern (1990) discussed the criteria of the diagnosis of dysplastic naevus and arrived at the same conclusion, namely, that 'using architectural criteria alone, many acquired nevi will be erroneously judged to be dysplastic'.

The discrepancies between series are largely caused by the inclusion of common lesions showing only a few of the features of dysplastic naevus. We do not advocate making a diagnosis of dysplastic naevus in such cases.

We recommend that the diagnosis of dysplastic naevus is reserved for lesions exhibiting cytological atypia together with distinct architectural abnormalities as indicated in Table 8.3. Ascent of more than a very rare atypical melanocyte into the granular and cornified layers must be absent (see below). Cytological atypia as well as the characteristic architectural features are required for a diagnosis of dysplastic naevus. If this combination of features is not clearly present, we diagnose common acquired naevus rather than dysplastic naevus.

Table 8.3 Recommended criteria for histological diagnosis of dysplastic naevus

Cytological atypia of some melanocytes: nuclear pleomorphism, anisochromasia; increase in cytoplasm; dusty pigment

Distinct *architectural abnormalities*
  Marked increase in number of junctional melanocytes, arranged in
    irregularly distributed nests and/or lentiginous patterns
  Irregular size and shape of nests
  Horizontal orientation of nests with rete ridge-bridging, fusion of nests
  Irregularity of rete ridges
  Subepidermal 'lamellar' fibrosis
  Vascular proliferation and/or prominence
  Perivascular lymphocytic infiltrate

NB: ascent of more than a very occasional atypical melanocyte into the granular
  and cornified layers must be absent

8.6 Dysplastic naevus *vs in situ* melanoma

It is not always realized how difficult it is to arrive at a biologically correct histological diagnosis of *in situ* melanoma. The morphological arguments to consider a lesion an *in situ* melanoma are based on the resemblance of a lesion to the intraepidermal component of an invasive melanoma, *i.e.* a combination of irregular lateral spread (lentiginous and/or pagetoid), poor demarcation, asymmetry, ascent of solitary melanocytes and cytological atypia. However, each of these features may be absent or very inconspicuous in the intraepidermal part of some invasive melanomas, and it is therefore clear that not all these melanomas would have qualified as malignant if examined in their previous *in situ* phase. *In situ* melanoma, as it is currently recognized, resembles the intraepidermal component of only *some* invasive melanomas, and it is therefore probable that not all *in situ* melanomas are diagnosed as such.

These problems are reflected in the literature on the distinction between *in situ* melanoma and dysplastic naevus. Ackerman and Mihara (1985) stated that 'unlike malignant melanomas *in situ*, in both junctional and compound dysplastic nevi single melanocytes and nests of melanocytes are seated almost wholly at the dermoepidermal junction, and not above it. An occasional melanocyte, and even small nests of melanocytes, may be present above the junction in the lower portion of the spinous zone, but *extensive* scattering of melanocytes in the upper regions of the epidermis across an entire front of a dysplastic nevus is *almost* never seen. If such scattering is seen, the diagnosis is *likely to be* malignant melanoma' (our italics). We do not agree with this description: in the presence of extensive scattering of melanocytes across the entire front of a melanocytic lesion, a definitive diagnosis of melanoma is appropriate. Furthermore, in the same article it is stated that that 'at the earliest stages of malignant melanomas *in situ*, atypical melanocytes are arranged only as solitary units at the dermoepidermal junction'. With these statements side-by-side there is no way one could distinguish architecturally between dysplastic naevus and *in situ* melanoma, because the definitions have been so constructed as to allow for greater architectural alterations in dysplastic naevus than are required for a diagnosis of malignant melanoma. Apparently, the presence or absence of nuclear atypia is considered the key factor, but this is impossible to reconcile with the statement that atypia is present in some (even though not in all) dysplastic naevi (Ackerman and Mihara, 1985).

We consider an intraepidermal proliferation of atypical melanocytes, melanoma *in situ*, when there is distinct nuclear atypia of all these melanocytes, together with ascent of such atypical melanocytes, several of which reach the granular layer. When this is not present in a section of a markedly atypical melanocytic proliferation, we require additional sections; if ascending atypical melanocytes remain absent or extremely rare, a diagnosis of dysplastic naevus is made. This approach allows relatively consistent diagnosis but it is possible that some *in situ* melanomas will be underdiagnosed as dysplastic naevi, since ascent of single cells will occasionally also be absent in invasive melanoma.

An important problem in the definition of melanoma *in situ* lies in the interpretative element it entails, in addition to the morphological identification: the resemblance of an *in situ* melanoma to the intra-epidermal component of an invasive melanoma does not constitute definitive proof that the cells of which it consists are, in fact, fully malignant; the two key criteria of malignancy, i.e. invasion and metastasis, are absent by definition. Whether the intraepidermal proliferation preceding the invasive melanoma consists of fully malignant cells, as Ackerman implies, or whether a further change in these cells has to occur in order to attain a fully malignant potential, as is implied by the transition from radial to vertical growth phase (p. 235), and proposed by Clark and associates (1986), remains a moot point which can never be decided on morphological grounds.

Recently, Moore and colleagues (1990) briefly reported an epidemiological study in which they found significant discordance in the risk factors of *in situ* melanoma and invasive melanoma, which one would not expect if the former were merely an early phase of the latter. This study indicates that the transition from '*in situ* melanoma to invasive melanoma is associated with additional important events at the cellular level, rather than just the passage of time'.

It will be evident that follow-up data cannot be of much help in distinguishing between dysplastic naevus and *in situ* melanoma: both types of lesion should carry an increased risk of invasive melanoma. More cogently, as argued at the start of this chapter, those lesions which are available for histological investigation have been totally removed and are not available for follow-up.

8.7   Additional diagnostic techniques

In view of the difficulties in establishing dysplastic naevus as an entity distinct from common naevi and from melanoma, several groups have attempted to substantiate the morphological distinction by means of histochemistry, immunocytochemistry, electron microscopy and morphometry.

It is important to bear in mind the precise objectives and limitations of studies introducing new techniques in a classification in order to evaluate that classification. Either the study relies on initial correct identification of lesions, in which case the usefulness of the technique as a diagnostic adjunct is under study, or, alternatively, if pilot studies indicate that the new technique allows a more precise and possibly better distinction between cases, it could lead to a new classification, a validation of which needs follow up of cases. In that case, the validity of the older techniques, on which the old classification was based, is under question.

As discussed previously, it is clear that assessment of numbers of

AgNORs does not distinguish between dysplastic naevi and common naevi (p. 25). Abnormal *DNA histograms* have been reported in a large proportion of dysplastic naevi with marked architectural and cytological atypia (Bergman *et al.*, 1988), but only in a minority of naevi which were considered dysplastic naevi with slight atypia: it seems therefore unlikely that ploidy assessments can be used to distinguish dysplastic naevi as a group. *Immunoreactivity with HMB-45* has been reported in melanocytes of the dermal portion of dysplastic compound naevi but not in the dermal portion of common acquired naevi (Smoller *et al.*, 1989). However, Spitz naevi, blue naevi and some naevi, which in our view are not dysplastic, may show positivity so that there is no direct diagnostic applicability, and conclusions in terms of premalignant potential of dysplastic naevi drawn from such very circumstantial evidence should be viewed with caution.

Ultrastructural abnormalities of melanosomes in dysplastic naevi and melanomas have been described (Takahashi *et al.*, 1985, 1987; Rhodes *et al.*, 1988). In addition to melanosomes with normal morphological features, dysplastic naevi and melanomas contain abnormal melanosomes, with a spherical form and an irregular, often granular or vacuolated content. Such melanosomes were very rare in common acquired naevi and normal skin (Rhodes *et al.*, 1988).

8.8   Histological grading of dysplastic naevi to identify dysplastic naevi associated with high risk

Attempts to identify different grades of dysplasia in dysplastic naevi have been undertaken, in the hope of identifying subgroups of patients with different risks of melanoma. Bergman and colleagues (1988) reported that in dysplastic naevi with a high degree of cytological and architectural atypia, a higher number of positive histories of previous melanoma was found. The presence of a dysplastic naevus with mild atypia was considered to be insignificant clinically, unless there was a positive family history or the presence of many atypical moles. Dysplastic naevi with severe atypia more commonly showed abnormally high levels of expression of MHC Class I molecules, as well as an increase in the numbers of tetraploid and aneuploid melanocytes. It is probable that the 'dysplastic naevi with severe atypia' of the study of Bergman and co-workers (1988) are the lesions which we would diagnose as dysplastic naevi, whereas most of their cases with mild atypia would be diagnosed by us as common acquired naevi. Their study provides additional arguments for being restrictive with the diagnosis of dysplastic naevus.

Grading of dysplastic naevi is also implied in the study of Steijlen and co-workers (1988), who identified a subgroup of dysplastic naevi with 'severe atypia'. Black and Hunt (1990) used a scoring system to grade atypia in dysplastic naevi, taking into account the extent of melanocytic hyperplasia, cytological atypia, and lymphocytic infiltration. These authors also found that lesions with highest grades were most commonly encountered in subjects with a personal or family history of melanoma.

Jones (1989) collected the opinions of a number of leading authorities in this field: a clear majority opposed the use of a grading system of dysplastic naevi, most often because of the difficulties (interobserver variation) inherent in the diagnosis of dysplastic naevus. Some were confident that subtyping had no relevance, whereas others, more cautiously, felt that a possible relevance was not known.

In view of the difficulties of arriving at a consistent diagnosis of dysplastic naevus, we agree that it is premature to attempt a subdivision of dysplastic naevi, since this would require an even more refined histological differential diagnosis, with a further increase in interobserver variability. *It is not practical at present to attempt a formal grading system.*

8.9 Histological evidence of dysplastic naevi as precursors of melanoma

Following the detailed discussion of the histological features of dysplastic naevi and their distinction from common naevi and *in situ* melanoma, it is of interest to look again at the evidence for their premalignant potential.

Elder and colleagues (1982) found dysplastic naevi in contiguity with 36% of an unselected series of 261 superficial spreading melanomas, and in the majority of melanomas with a positive family history. Similar frequencies were reported by others: 22% in a series of 225 melanomas (Rhodes *et al.*, 1983), 6 out of 13 cases (Duray and Ernstoff, 1987) and 32% (Black, 1988). Cook and Robertson (1985) found 'melanocytic dysplasia' in 34% of a series of 226 primary cutaneous melanomas; in some of their cases a diffuse mottling or freckling of the skin, corresponding histologically to 'diffuse melanocytic dysplasia', surrounded the melanoma. These cases were associated with a high incidence of multiple primary melanomas (Robertson and Cook, 1987). In the series of Rhodes *et al.* (1983), 22 out of 49 dysplastic naevi ('atypical melanocytic hyperplasia in lentiginous pattern') associated with melanoma, showed an intradermal naevus component, strengthening the case for the existence of a pre-existing naevus at the site of the melanoma.

In contrast to these reports, Ackerman and Mihara (1985) stated that in their experience, the melanocytic lesion usually associated with a melanoma, when present at all, is the intradermal naevus. However, when a remnant of a pre-existing naevus is only seen in the dermis, this cannot be accepted as evidence that the pre-existent naevus was wholly intradermal.

When reviewing the figures for the prevalence of dysplastic naevi in contiguity with melanoma, it should be borne in mind that the histological differences between melanoma and dysplastic naevus are subtle and often quantitative rather than qualitative: for instance, an intra-epidermal proliferation of mildly atypical melanocytes without ascent into the granular layer would be diagnosed as a dysplastic naevus when viewed in isolation. However, in a melanoma, ascent of melanocytes may be present only focally and cytological atypia may be moderate. Therefore, if ascent is present on only one side of a superficial spreading melanoma, this could be interpreted as either a pre-existing dysplastic naevus or as part of the melanoma; there are no hard criteria to distinguish between the two. We agree with Ackerman and Mihara (1985) that, *if such cases are interpreted as remnants of a dysplastic naevus, this would lead to an overestimation of the frequency of such an association*.

Rhodes *et al.* (1983) also recognized this problem when they wrote: 'an important premise upon which we (and others) attribute the origin of some melanomas to DMN (dysplastic melanocytic naevi), is that AMHL (atypical melanocytic hyperplasia in a lentiginous epidermal pattern) can be distinguished histologically from intra-epidermal melanoma'. These authors further remarked that in their cases 'there was a spectrum of melanocytic hyperplasia and melanocytic cytologic atypism, usually progressing from slight to moderate atypism at the extreme lateral margin of the histologic section to more marked atypism as intra-epidermal (*in situ*) melanoma was approached'. Such a finding, however, which is in accordance with our own experience and that of others (Barnhill, 1990), does not necessarily indicate that the 'extreme lateral margin' represents a pre-existent, premalignant lesion: indeed, a sharp demarcation between the malignant tumour and an adjacent atypical melanocytic proliferation would make a stronger case that the latter represents a pre-existent naevus.

However, the fact that dysplastic naevi in contiguity with melanoma are present in 20–35% of invasive melanomas, that these are histologically identical to dysplastic naevi occurring in isolation, their presence at one side only of the melanoma, and their association with a dermal naevus component, provides strong arguments, albeit not quite conclusive ones, in favour of a pre-existing dysplastic naevus (Rhodes *et al.*, 1983).

8.10   Conclusion

From the above discussion, it will be apparent that several vital questions remain to be solved, before a consensus is possible regarding the concept of the dysplastic naevus as well as its diagnosis. Nonetheless, we feel that sufficiently corroborated data have become available to allow a reasonably accurate distinction between dysplastic naevus, common acquired naevus and melanoma. The diagnosis of dysplastic naevus should be reserved for those cases showing unequivocally the combination of cytological and architectural irregularities described above. In this way, the inclusion of large numbers of minor variations of common naevi can be avoided.

Since the spectrum of histological abnormalities ranges from very mild to very severe, problems of classifying borderline cases are unavoidable. In our opinion these difficulties do not justify a nihilistic approach to the whole concept of dysplastic naevus. At the very least, one could say that dysplastic naevus, as defined here, describes a relatively uncommon form of naevus which is sufficiently worrying for a diagnosis of melanoma *in situ* to be considered in the differential diagnosis. A few of these cases may in fact represent *in situ* melanoma, but none of them after thorough sectioning satisfies the minimum histological criteria accepted as necessary for this diagnosis. There is a reasonable body of evidence that such dysplastic lesions are significant precursors of melanoma. Patients with many dysplastic naevi defined in this way, and with a positive personal or family history of melanoma, have a high risk of developing melanoma. However, it is equally clear that sporadic dysplastic naevi have only a slightly increased risk of malignancy, the precise level of which will be ascertained more accurately when a better agreement about the optimal clinical and histological criteria for the diagnosis has been reached.

References

Ackerman, A. B. (1985) Primary acquired melanosis. *Hum. Pathol.*, **16**, 1077–8.

Ackerman, A. B. (1988) What naevus is dysplastic, a syndrome and the commonest precursor of malignant melanoma? A riddle and an answer. *Histopathology*, **13**, 241–56.

Ackerman, A. B. and Mihara, I. (1985) Dysplasia, dysplastic melanocytes, dysplastic nevi, the dysplastic nevus syndrome, and the relation between dysplastic nevi and malignant melanomas. *Hum. Pathol.*, **16**, 87–91.

Armstrong, B. K., Heenan, P. J., Caruso, V., Glancy, R. J. and Holman, C. D. J. (1984) Seasonal variation in the junctional component of pigmented naevi. Letter to the Editor. *Int. J. Cancer*, **34**, 441–2.

Bale, S. J., Chakravarti, A. and Greene, M. H. (1986) Cutaneous malignant melanoma and familial dysplastic nevi: evidence for autosomal dominance and pleiotropy. *Am. J. Hum. Genet.*, **38**, 188–96.

Bale, S. J., Dracopoli, N. C., Tucker, M. A. *et al.* (1989) Mapping the gene for hereditary cutaneous malignant melanoma-dysplastic nevus to chromosome 1p. *New Engl. J. Med.*, **320**, 1367–72.

Barnes, L. M. and Nordlund, J. J. (1987) The natural history of dysplastic nevi. *Arch. Dermatol.*, **123**, 1059–61.

Barnhill, R. L. (1990) Response. *J. Am. Acad. Dermatol.*, **23**, 139–40.

Barnhill, R. L., Roush, G. C. and Duray, P. H. (1990) Correlation of histologic architectural and cytoplasmic features with nuclear atypia in atypical (dysplastic) nevomelanocytic nevi. *Hum. Pathol.*, **21**, 51–58.

Bergman, W., Palani, A. and West, L. N. (1986) Clinical and genetic studies in six Dutch kindreds with the dysplastic nevus syndrome. *Ann. Hum. Genet.*, **50**, 249–58.

Bergman, W., Ruiter, D. J., Scheffer, E. and Van Vloten, W. A. (1988) Melanocytic atypia in dysplastic nevi. Immunohistochemical and cytophotometrical analysis. *Cancer*, **61**, 1660–6.

Black, W. C. (1988) Residual dysplastic and other nevi in superficial spreading melanoma. Clinical correlations and association with sun damage. *Cancer*, **62**, 163–73.

Black, W. C. and Hunt, W. C. (1990) Histologic correlations with the clinical diagnosis of dysplastic nevus. *Am. J. Surg. Pathol.*, **14**, 44–52.

Clark, W. H., Reimer, R. R., Greene, M., Ainsworth, A. M. and Mastrangelo, M. J. (1978) Origin of familial malignant melanomas from heritable melanocytic lesions. 'The B–K mole syndrome'. *Arch. Dermatol.*, **114**, 732–8.

Clark, W. H., Elder, D. E., Guerry D, Epstein, M. N., Greene, M. H. and Van Horn, M. (1984) A study of tumor progression: the precursor lesions of superficial spreading and nodular melanoma. *Hum. Pathol.*, **15**, 1147–65.

Clark, W. H., Elder, D. E. and Van Horn, M. (1986) The biologic forms of malignant melanoma. *Hum. Pathol.*, **17**, 443–50.

Cochran, A. J. (1969) Histology and prognosis in malignant melanoma. *J. Pathol.*, **97**, 459–68.

Consensus Conference (1984) Precursors to malignant melanoma. *J. Am. Med Assoc.*, **251**, 1864–6.

Cook, M. G. and Fallowfield, M. E. (1990) Dysplastic naevi — an alternative view. *Histopathology*, **16**, 29–35.

Cook, M. G. and Robertson, I. (1985) Melanocytic dysplasia and melanoma. *Histopathology*, **9**, 647–58.

Cook, K. R., Spears, G. F. S., Elder, D. E. and Greene, M. H. (1989) Dysplastic nevi in a population-based survey. *Cancer*, **63**, 1240–4.

Crucioli, V. and Stilwell, J. (1982) The histogenesis of malignant melanoma in relation to pre-existing pigmented lesions. *J. Cutan. Pathol.*, **9**, 396–404.

Crutcher, W. A. and Sagebiel, R. W. (1984) Prevalence of dysplastic naevi in a community practice. *Lancet*, **1**, 729.

Duray, P. D. and Ernstoff, M. S. (1987) Dysplastic nevus in histologic contiguity with acquired nonfamilial melanoma. Clinicopathologic experience in a 100-bed hospital. *Arch. Dermatol.*, **123**, 80–4.

Duvic, M., Lowe, L., Rapini, R. P., Rodriguez, S. and Levy, M. L. (1989) Eruptive dysplastic nevi associated with human immunodeficiency virus infection. *Arch. Dermatol.*, **125**, 397–401.

Elder, D. E. (1985) The dysplastic nevus. *Pathology*, **17**, 291–7.

Elder, D. E. and MacKie, R. M. (1990) Dysplastic melanocytic nevi. Their nature and significance. In *Cutaneous Melanoma, Biology and Management* (eds N. Cascinelli, M. Santinami and U. Veronesi). Milano: Masson, pp. 93–104.

Elder, D. E., Goldman, L. I., Goldman, S. C., Greene, M. H. and Clark, W. H. (1980) Dysplastic nevus syndrome: a phenotypic association of sporadic cutaneous melanoma. *Cancer*, **46**, 1787–94.

Elder, D. E., Greene, M. H., Bondi, E. E. and Clark, W. H. (1981) Acquired melanocytic nevi and melanoma: the dysplastic nevus syndrome. In *Pathology of Malignant Melanoma* (ed. A. B. Ackerman). New York: Masson, pp. 185–215.

Elder, D. E., Green, M. H., Guerry, D., Kraemer, K. H. and Clark, W. H. (1982) The dysplastic nevus syndrome. Our definition. *Am. J. Dermatopathol.*, **4**, 455–60.

Eng, A. M. (1983) Solitary small active junctional nevi in juvenile patients. *Arch. Dermatol.*, **119**, 35–8.

English, D. R., Menz, J., Heenan, P. J., Elder, D. E., Watt, J. D. and Armstrong, B. K. (1986) The dysplastic naevus syndrome in patients with cutaneous malignant melanoma in Western Australia. *Med. J. Austral.*, **145**, 194–8.

Frankel, K. A. (1987) Intraepithelial melanocytic neoplasia: a classification by pattern analysis of proliferations of atypical melanocytes. *Am. J. Dermatopathol.*, **9**, 80–81.

Frichot, B. C., Lynch, H. T., Guirgis, H. A., Harris, R. E. and Lynch, J. F. (1977) A new cutaneous phenotype in familial malignant melanoma. *Lancet*, **1**, 864–5.

Greene, M. H., Clark, W. H., Tucker, M. A. *et al.* (1980) Precursor naevi in cutaneous malignant melanoma: a proposed nomenclature. *Lancet*, **2**, 1024.

Greene, M. H., Goldin, L. R., Clark, W. H. *et al.* (1983) Familial cutaneous malignant melanoma — an autosomal dominant trait possibly linked to the *Rh* locus. *Proc. Natl. Acad. Sci. USA*, **80**, 6071–5.

Greene, M. H., Clark, W. H., Tucker, M. A., Kraemer, K. H., Elder, D. E. and Fraser, M. C. (1985a) The high risk of malignant melanoma in melanoma prone families with dysplastic nevi. *Ann. Int. Med.*, **102**, 458–69.

Greene, M. H., Clark, W. H., Tucker, M. A. *et al.* (1985b) Acquired precursors of cutaneous malignant melanoma. The familial dysplastic nevus syndrome. *New Engl. J. Med.*, **312**, 91–7.

Greene, M. H., Elder, D. E., Tucker, M. A. and Guerry D. (1987a) The dysplastic nevus syndrome. In *Cutaneous Melanoma. Status of Knowledge and Future Perspective* (eds U. Veronesi, N. Cascinelli and M. Santinami). London: Academic Press, pp. 279–318.

Greene, M. H., Tucker, M. A., Clark, W. H., Kraemer, K. H., Elder, D. E. and Fraser, M. C. (1987b) Hereditary melanoma and the dysplastic nevus syndrome: the risk of cancers other than melanoma. *J. Am. Acad. Dermatol.*, **16**, 792–7.

Gruis, N. A., Bergman, W. and Frants, R. R. (1990) Locus for susceptibility to melanoma on chromosome 1p. *New Engl. J. Med.*, **322**, 853–4.

Holman, C. D. J., Heenan, P. J., Caruso, R. J. and Armstrong, B. K. (1983) Seasonal variation in the junctional component of pigmented naevi. *Int. J. Cancer*, **31**, 213–5.

Howell, J. N., Greene, M. H., Corner, R. C. *et al.* (1984) Fibroblasts from patients with hereditary cutaneous melanoma are abnormally sensitive to the mutagenic effect of simulated sunlight and 4-nitroquinoline 1-oxide. *Proc. Natl. Acad. Sci. U.S.A.*, **81**, 1179–83.

Jones, R. E. (1989) Questions to the editorial board and other authorities. *Am. J. Dermatopathol.*, **11**, 276–84.

Kefford, R. F. (1990) Genetics of melanoma. In *Cutaneous Melanoma: Biology and Management* (eds N. Cascinelli, M. Santinami and U. Veronesi). Milan: Masson, pp. 39–44.

Kraemer, K. H., Greene, M. H., Tarone, R., Elder, D. E., Clark, W. H. and Guerry, D. (1983) Dysplastic naevi and cutaneous melanoma risk. *Lancet*, **2**, 1076–7.

Lynch, H. T., Frichot, B. C. and Lynch, J. F. (1978) Familial atypical multiple mole melanoma syndrome. *J. Med. Gen.*, **15**, 352–6.

Lynch, H. T., Fusaro, R. M., Pester, J. and Lynch, J. F. (1981) Naming the melanoma-prone syndrome. *Lancet*, **2**, 817.

Lynch, H. T., Fusaro, R. M., Kimberling, W. J., Lynch, J. F. and Danes, B. S. (1983) Familial atypical multiple mole-melanoma (FAMMM) syndrome: segregation analysis. *J. Med. Genet.*, **20**, 342–4.

Moore, D. H., Schneider, J. S. and Sagebiel, R. W. (1990) Discordance of risk factors for invasive and non-invasive melanoma. *Lancet*, **1**, 1523–4.

Murphy, G. F. and Halpern, A. (1990) Dysplastic melanocytic nevi. Normal variants or melanoma precursors? *Arch. Dermatol.*, **126**, 519–22.

Nordlund, J. J., Kirkwood, J., Forget, B. M. *et al.* (1985) Demographic study of clinically atypical (dysplastic) nevi in patients with melanoma and comparison subjects. *Cancer Res.*, **45**, 1855–61.

Reimer, R. R., Clark, W. H., Greene, M. H. *et al.* (1978) Precursor lesions in familial melanoma: a new genetic preneoplastic syndrome. *J. Am. Med. Assoc.*, **239**, 744–6.

Rhodes, A. R., Sober, A. J., Mihm, M. C. and Fitzpatrick, T. B. (1980) Possible risk factors for primary cutaneous melanoma. *Clin. Res.*, **28**, 252A.

Rhodes, A. R., Harrist, T. J., Day, C. L., Mihm, M. C., Fitzpatrick, T. B. and Sober, A. J. (1983) Dysplastic melanocytic nevi in histologic association with 234 primary cutaneous melanomas. *J. Am. Acad. Dermatol.*, **9**, 563–74.

Rhodes, A. R., Seki, Y., Fitzpatrick, T. B. and Stern, R. S. (1988) Melanosomal alterations in dysplastic melanocytic nevi. A quantitative, ultrastructural investigation. *Cancer*, **61**, 358–69.

Rigel, D. S., Rivers, J. K., Kopf, A. W. *et al.* (1989) Dysplastic nevi. Markers for increased risk for melanoma. *Cancer*, **63**, 386–9.

Rivers, J. K., Kopf, A. W., Vinokur, A. F. *et al.* (1990) Clinical characteristics of malignant melanomas developing in persons with dysplastic nevi. *Cancer*, **65**, 1232–6.

Robertson, I. and Cook, M. G. (1987) Multiple melanomas associated with diffuse melanocytic dysplasia. *Histopathology*, **11**, 395–402.

Rosai, J. (1989) *Ackerman's Surgical Pathology*, 7th edn. St Louis: C. V. Mosby, p. 123.

Roth, M., Boyle, J. M. and Muller, H. J. (1988) Thymidine dimer repair in fibroblasts with dysplastic nevus syndrome (DNS). *Experientia*, **44**, 169–71.

Sagebiel, R. W. (1979) Histopathology of borderline and early malignant melanoma. *Am. J. Surg. Pathol.*, **3**, 543–52.

Salomon, J., Donald, J., Shaw, H., McCarthy, W. and Kefford, R. (1989) Linkage analysis of Australian hereditary melanoma kindreds using RFLP loci on chromosome 1p. *Abs, 2nd Int. Conference on Melanoma*, Abs 152.

Seywright, M. M., Doherty, V. R. and MacKie, R. M. (1986) Proposed alternative terminology and subclassification of so called 'dysplastic naevi'. *J. Clin. Pathol.*, **39**, 189–94.

Sheiber, A., Milton, G. W., McCarthy, M. H. and Shaw, H. (1981) Clinical features, prognosis and incidence of multiple primary cutaneous malignant melanoma. *Austral. NZ. J. Surg.*, **51**, 386.

Smoller, B. R., McNutt, N. S. and Hsu, A. (1989) HMB-45 staining of dysplastic nevi: support for a spectrum of progression toward melanoma. *Am. J. Surg. Pathol.*, **13**, 680–4.

Steijlen, P. M., Bergman, W., Hermans, J., Scheffer, E., Van Vloten, W. A. and Ruiter, D. J. (1988) The efficacy of histopathological criteria required for diagnosing dysplastic naevi. *Histopathology*, **12**, 289–300.

Sterry, W. and Christophers, E. (1988) Quadrant distribution of dysplastic nevus syndrome. *Arch. Dermatol.*, **124**, 926–9.

Stolz, W., Schmoeckel, C., Landthaler, M. and Braun-Falco, O. (1989) Association of early malignant melanoma with nevocytic nevi. *Cancer*, **63**, 550–5.

Takahashi, H., Horikoshi, T. and Jimbow, K. (1985) Fine structural characterization of melanosomes in dysplastic nevi. *Cancer*, **56**, 111–23.

Takahashi, H., Yamana, K., Maeda, K., Akutsu, Y., Horikoshi, T. and Jimbow, K. (1987) Dysplastic melanocytic nevus. Electron-microscopic observation as a diagnostic tool. *Am. J. Dermatopathol.*, **9**, 189–97.

Urso, C., Giannini, A., Bartolini, M. and Bondi, R. (1990) Histological analysis of intraepidermal proliferations of atypical melanocytes. *Am. J. Dermatopathol.*, **12**, 150–5.

9 Cutaneous melanoma

Cutaneous melanoma causes about 1–2% of cancer deaths. In recent times its incidence has risen considerably (Lee, 1985), doubling every decade in several countries with a predominantly Caucasian population; yearly incidence figures in many countries are now about 10–30 per 100 000. At the same time, an increased awareness of the early signs and symptoms of melanoma has led to earlier detection (Drzewiecki et al., 1990) and substantial improvement in 5-year disease-free survival figures, which are now in the order of 80%.

Melanoma affects patients in a broad age range; however, melanoma is rare in childhood and uncommon in adolescence. In Europe, female patients outnumber males by a factor of approximately 1.6, but in the United States and Australia there is a more equal distribution between the sexes. In males, most melanomas occur on the trunk, especially the back, and the head and neck; in females, they are most common on the limbs, especially the lower legs.

There is an important association between *skin type* and melanoma risk: those with a fair skin, who burn easily and tan not at all or with difficulty (skin types I and II; Fitzpatrick, 1988), have the highest risk (Elwood et al., 1985). Melanoma is rare in skin types V and VI, i.e. oriental and negroid races, and is then usually located on palms, soles, nail beds (Krementz et al., 1976; Takematsu et al., 1985), or juxtacutaneous mucous membranes (Chapter 11).

Exposure to sunlight plays an important role in the aetiology of cutaneous melanoma. However, the distribution of melanoma includes regions seldom or never exposed to direct solar irradiation and, apart from lentigo maligna melanoma, there is no relation to chronic solar damage of the skin. Instead, acute, intermittent exposure to sunlight, causing sunburn, appears to be important, especially when occurring early in life (Cooke and Fraser, 1985; MacKie et al., 1987). However, many persons who have experienced sunburn never develop melanoma and *vice versa*. Moreover, the risk of sunburn is closely related to skin type so that it is not an independent variable in the assessment of melanoma risk. Further studies are needed to investigate more precisely the aetiological significance of sun exposure.

The presence of a *large number of naevi*, even in the absence of histological signs of dysplasia, constitutes an important risk factor (Swerdlow *et al.*, 1986; Holly *et al.*, 1987), and although the exact percentage of melanomas developing in naevi is unclear, there is certainly an important association between the two (p. 56).

Correlations between *socioeconomic status* and melanoma risk (Gallagher *et al.*, 1987) may be related to differences in occupational and recreational acute sun exposure.

A possible role of *chemical substances* in the aetiology of melanoma has been proposed (Rampen and Fleuren, 1987) but remains to be investigated further.

Positive *family history* for melanoma, with or without the additional stigmata of the dysplastic naevus syndrome, is an important risk factor. About 5 to 8% of melanoma cases show the typical features of hereditary cancer: autosomal dominant pattern of inheritance, high degree of multiple primary tumours and earlier mean age of onset (Kefford, 1990).

Melanoma is one of the cutaneous malignancies developing in *xeroderma pigmentosum*, an autosomal recessive disease caused by a defect in DNA repair (English and Swerdlow, 1987). A familial association with osteosarcoma, chondrosarcoma and adrenal carcinoma has been reported, pointing to possible common genetic defects (Hartley *et al.*, 1987). A few cases have been reported in patients with neurofibromatosis (Silverman *et al.*, 1988; Specht and Smith 1988) and we recently encountered a family in which the two occurred together in several family members; it seems likely that at least in some of these instances the two diseases are linked.

There are scattered reports of melanoma developing after various forms of *physical trauma*, such as frostbite, thermal burns and radiotherapy (Inbar *et al.*, 1988), or in skin affected by postmastectomy lymphoedema (Sarkany, 1972).

Tindall and colleagues (1989) reported three cases of melanoma in HIV-positive men, in whom the clinical severity of disease was inversely proportional to the absolute numbers of CD4+ cells. Possibly, this may be related to *impaired immunosurveillance*; in kidney transplant recipients, there is also an increased incidence of melanoma.

A variety of *chromosomal structural abnormalities* (deletions, translocations, isochromosomes) have been found in melanoma, most commonly involving chromosomes 1, 6, 7, 10 and 11; those located on chromosomes 7 and 11 have been associated with an unfavourable prognosis (Trent *et al.*, 1990). At the molecular level, the pathogenesis of melanoma is still largely unknown. Point mutations in N-*ras* (Albino *et al.*, 1989; Van 't Veer *et al.*, 1989; Shukla *et al.*, 1989) as well as K-*ras* and H-*ras* (Shukla *et al.*, 1989) have been demonstrated in a minority of melanomas; N-*ras* point mutations have been related to a location on body sites generally exposed to sunlight (Van 't Veer *et al.*, 1989). The latter finding points to a possible direct link between ultraviolet irradiation and mutational activation of this oncogene known to be involved in the development of a variety of malignant tumours. K-*ras* mutations were found occasionally in dysplastic naevi (Shukla *et al.*, 1989).

On the basis of genetic linkage studies of polymorphic marker genes in dysplastic naevus families in the United States of America, a 'melanoma susceptibility gene' has been postulated on the short arm of chromosome 1 (p. 189; Bale *et al.*, 1989). However, in Dutch and Australian dysplastic naevus families this location was effectively excluded as the site of such a putative gene (p. 189; Van Haeringen *et al.*, 1989; Salomon *et al.*, 1989).

9.1 Macroscopical appearance

Clinically, melanoma exhibits a large variety of appearances. In its most classical form, it appears as an asymmetrical, irregularly pigmented macule, papule or nodule, with irregular, notched and sometimes indistinct borders, varying in size from a few millimetres to, rarely, several centimetres. In individual tumours, colours may vary from white, pink, slate-grey or bluish, to different shades of brown, and black. The overlying epidermis is intact or ulcerated. Irregular pink or white, sometimes depressed areas point to foci of tumour regression (Figure 9.1; p. 227). The tumour may arise *de novo* on previously normal skin, or may originate in a pre-existent naevus, the malignant transformation of which has as its hallmark a sudden change in size, shape and colour, together with the features mentioned above. 'Satellites' consist of small usually pigmented macules or papules in the surrounding skin within a distance of a few centimetres (different authors suggesting a distance of 2, 3 and 5 cm), or in-transit metastases, situated at a greater distance, in the skin region drained by the same lymph node basin.

Many of these clinical features of melanoma do not develop until relatively late in its natural course; *early detection of melanoma* is based on the accurate recognition of suspicious pigmented lesions, arising in previously unblemished skin, showing some degree of irregularity and asymmetry, together with variations in pigmentation, and sometimes itching or, alternatively, suspicious changes in hitherto

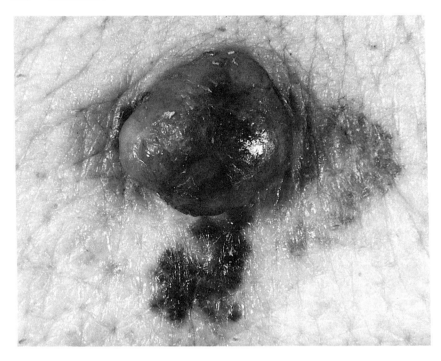

Figure 9.1 Cutaneous melanoma, showing many characteristic macroscopical features: large size, asymmetry, irregular contour, indistinct borders, variations in pigmentation, hypopigmented areas, eccentric ulcerating nodule (× 4).

quiescent moles. A large number of other melanocytic and non-melanocytic lesions may mimic melanoma clinically and sometimes also histologically: these include Spitz naevus, traumatized naevus, dysplastic naevus, basal cell carcinoma, pyogenic granuloma, sebor-rhoeic keratosis, pigmented solar keratosis, cutaneous histiocytoma and many others.

Clinical diagnosis is not sufficiently accurate to warrant definitive surgery. Recent improvements in clinical investigation, such as the application of surface microscopy of the lesion's pigment network, increase the accuracy of clinical diagnosis (Goldman, 1951; Soyer *et al.*, 1987, 1989), but some cases are still misdiagnosed on the basis of clinical appearance alone (Ledwig and Robinson, 1990). The conclusion of Kopf and colleagues (1975) that histological verification should precede the definitive treatment in all instances still holds.

As argued in Chapter 1 (p. 21), we do not advocate the use of frozen sections for quick diagnosis, because step sections are not available, morphology is suboptimal, much material is lost compared to paraffin sections and thickness measurements are unreliable. Tru-cut and fine needle aspiration biopsy of primary melanomas is also discouraged (p. 404). Thus, the diagnosis of melanoma should be based on histology of an excision, or rarely, incision (p. 17), of the lesion, performed with narrow margins, and followed by a re-excision with appropriate margins when the diagnosis has been established and tumour thickness has been measured.

9.2   Histological diagnosis

The histological diagnosis of melanoma is based on a constellation of cytological and architectural features, described in detail below, which must be evaluated together rather than in isolation, and considered in conjunction with clinical and macroscopical data. No single criterion or small set of criteria adequately distinguishes between melanoma and naevus in all instances.

It should be emphasized that *both cytological and architectural features are of importance in the diagnosis of melanoma*. Some melanomas consist of small and relatively monomorphic cells, so that the correct diagnosis rests mainly on architectural irregularities. However, others exhibit a quite regular architecture. Architectural signs of malignancy are often applicable only in one 'direction', e.g. asymmetry is usually a sign of malignancy but, especially in smaller lesions, symmetry does not prove benignity. Pagetoid spread usually indicates malignancy; however, some melanomas are well demarcated and pagetoid spread may be lacking. In such cases the diagnosis is largely based on cytological detail.

Several benign melanocytic tumours discussed in the previous chapters may be confused with melanoma. It is the specific context of a given case, including relevant clinical data such as age, localization and history of recent change, that determines what significance to attach to individual diagnostic features.

9.2.1   Architectural features

With the exception of the very rare intradermal melanoma arising in an intradermal naevus, the malignant blue naevus, and a minority of desmoplastic melanomas, cutaneous melanoma contains an intra-epidermal component which in all likelihood constitutes the site of origin of the tumour.

Several main architectural features that distinguish melanoma as a group from the various types of benign naevi will be discussed in this

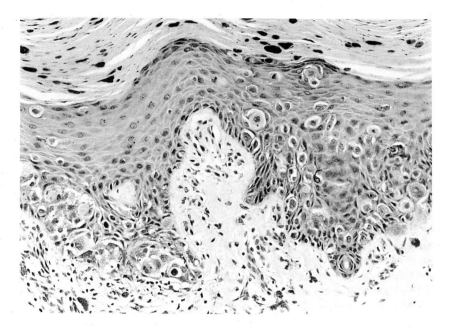

Figure 9.2 Ascent of melanoma cells. Single atypical melanocytes are seen throughout the thickness of the epidermis (HE, × 225).

section; the features characteristic of individual melanoma subtypes will be dealt with subsequently.

One of the most important features of malignancy is *asymmetry*. Benign lesions are more or less symmetrical, the plane of symmetry running vertically through the middle. Asymmetry in melanomas pertains to lateral extension, both intraepidermally and intradermally, extent of dermal involvement, architecture of epidermal and dermal component (nests, strands, nodules, sheets, fascicles), cell type, distribution and degree of pigmentation, and host response (inflammatory infiltrate, fibrosis).

Ascent (upward migration) of single atypical melanocytes (Figure 9.2), or small groups consisting of two or three such cells, into the granular layer and above, is a major histological hallmark of melanoma. However, in some benign melanocytic lesions such as Spitz naevus, pigmented spindle cell naevus, occasionally in volar junctional naevus and congenital naevus examined in early infancy, similar upward migration of solitary melanocytes may occur, albeit generally on a smaller scale, in the centre of the lesion rather than at its lateral borders, and in combination with upward migration of compact nests. In Spitz naevi, this is most common in children (Mérot and

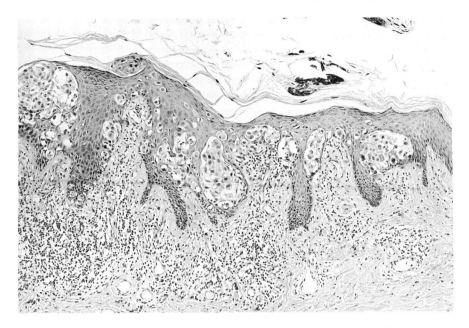

Figure 9.3 Melanoma. Irregular lateral pagetoid spread of nests and single atypical melanocytes along the dermoepidermal junction and also in suprabasal layers of the epidermis (HE, × 90).

Frenk, 1989). Importantly, such cells are devoid of distinct nuclear atypia. Thus, *before making a diagnosis of malignancy on the basis of melanocytic ascent, the presence of unequivocal cytological atypia is mandatory, and the above differential diagnostic possibilities should be considered.*

Characteristically, melanocytic ascent in melanoma is also present at the lateral margins of the tumour. This results in so-called *pagetoid spread* (Figure 9.3): polygonal or rounded tumour cells are scattered throughout the epidermal layers at the lateral borders of the lesions, and extend lateral to the main part of the tumour. This presumably represents an active infiltrative process, in a fashion strongly resembling mammary and extramammary Paget's disease. As the latter is also occasionally pigmented, the resemblance of the two lesions can be very close, the differences being dominantly cytological rather than architectural. The differential diagnosis is discussed in Chapter 3 (p. 49). Pagetoid spread of atypical melanocytes is an important sign of malignancy.

Apart from Paget's disease, ascent of melanocytes should be distinguished from Toker's clear cells of the nipple (Toker, 1970), and the very rare clear cell papulosis of the skin, consisting of a papular white eruption (Kuo *et al.*, 1987). These entities differ in clinical context, cytological features of the large pale intraepidermal cells, and the fact that these cells are EMA positive and S-100 negative.

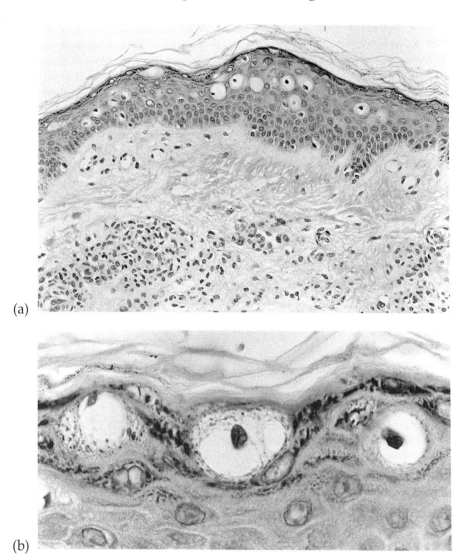

(a)

(b)

Figure 9.4 Vacuolization of keratinocytes, probably due to viral infection, overlying an intradermal naevus. (a) At low power, this may somewhat resemble ascent of melanocytes (HE, × 185). (b) At high power, it is readily apparent that the pale cells represent keratinocytes (HE, × 920).

A lesser degree of similarity with ascending melanoma cells may be seen in some cases of highly epidermotropic mycosis fungoides (Woringer-Kolopp disease), histiocytosis X, pigmented Bowen's disease, and by vacuolation of keratinocytes (Figure 9.4) as occurs in some viral diseases or as an artifact of tissue freezing (Mehregan and Pinkus, 1966) or poor fixation. Tangential sectioning through the basal layer of rete ridges may also rarely lead to problems. With good quality histological sections these mistakes are not likely to occur.

Melanocytic ascent should not be confused with transepidermal elimination of melanocytic nests, which travel as large clumps through the epidermis to reach the surface. This is seen not only in melanomas but also in Spitz naevi and occasional junctional and compound naevi. In Spitz naevi and pigmented spindle cell naevi, melanocytic nests may be so large that they reach from the dermoepidermal junction to the stratum corneum.

There is also some degree of *epidermal hyperplasia*, and this is occasionally so marked as to qualify as pseudoepitheliomatous hyperplasia (Figure 9.5; Levene, 1980; Kamino *et al.*, 1990).

When the atypical melanocytes spread into the underlying dermis, one speaks of invasion. Only at this stage can the tumour metastasize; the chance of metastasis is closely related to the maximal depth of this dermal invasion (Chapter 10).

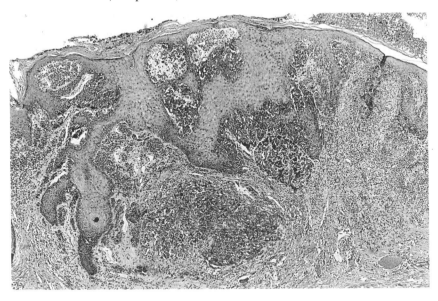

Figure 9.5 Melanoma. Pseudoepitheliomatous hyperplasia of the epidermis (HE, × 35).

When epidermal rete ridges are irregular and the dermoepidermal border is blurred because of subepidermal inflammatory infiltrate and oedema, microinvasion may be difficult to identify. Reticulin stains (Briggs, 1980) and immunostaining for collagen type IV are of help in outlining the dermoepidermal junction. However, when dermal invasion is so minimal that it is difficult to detect, it does not have an appreciable prognostic significance: it is only when there is obvious intradermal spread that there is a definite risk of metastasis. The only exception to this is melanoma with regressive changes (p. 316), in which intradermal tumour cells may be scarce or absent.

The dermal component consists of nests, strands, diffuse aggregates, trabeculae and fascicles. More rarely alveolar and pseudoglandular

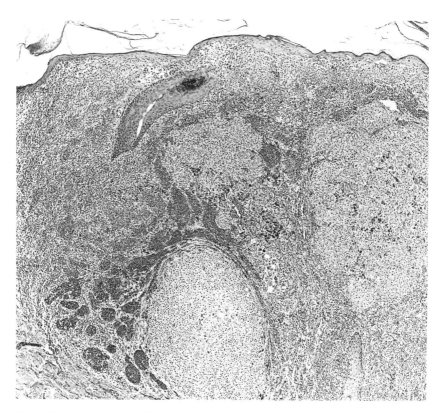

Figure 9.6   Melanoma. Abrupt changes in growth pattern and cell type, resulting in an irregular architecture (HE, × 35).

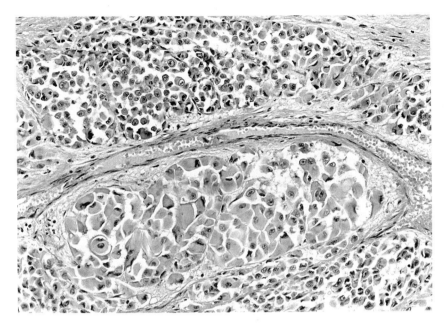

Figure 9.7   Melanoma. Abrupt changes in cell size. Within individual tumour cell nests and nodules, melanoma cells often resemble one another, while there is a clear difference in cytological features between different nests (HE, × 185).

structures are seen (Levene, 1980). Importantly, *the architectural pattern and cell type often vary from area to area* (Figures 9.6 and 9.7), *whereas benign melanocytic lesions generally show a similar architecture throughout*, for any given level. In many melanomas one can see groups or nodules of cells with identical nuclear and cytoplasmic features, but contrasting with different cytology in other areas of the invasive tumour (Clemente *et al.*, 1980). Compact nodules of melanocytes at the base are not uncommon in melanomas (Figure 9.8) but are absent in naevi. These features will be discussed more fully in the section 9.3.2.

There is often an *inflammatory infiltrate*, composed mainly of T-lymphocytes, Langerhans cells, histiocytes and plasmä cells (Ralfkiaer *et al.*, 1987). This infiltrate is often *band-like and located at the base of the melanoma*, but in other instances it is patchy and irregular in distribution, or diffusely involves the entire dermal component of the tumour, breaking up strands and nests of tumour cells in much the

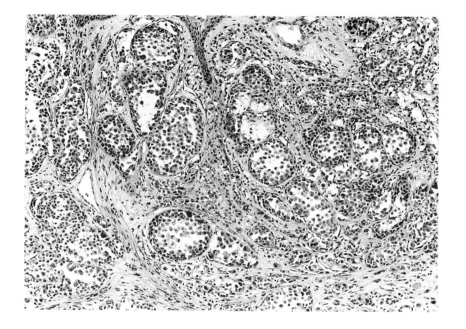

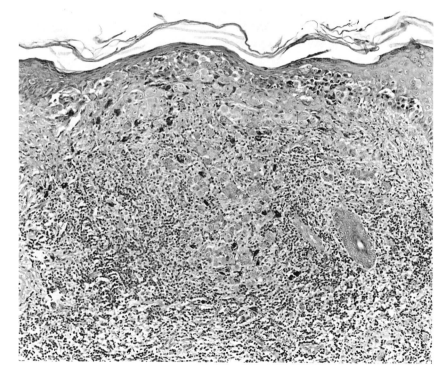

same way as in halo naevi (Figure 9.9). This is a sign of early, active *regression* and, in contrast to halo naevi, *it is often present in only part of the tumour.* In the later stages of regression the tumour cells disappear, and fibrosis of the dermis with scattered melanophages and sometimes an increased number of blood vessels is all that remains (Figure 9.10). When this happens throughout the melanoma, an absolute diagnosis of malignancy may eventually become impossible, although, in conjunction with a history of a previous melanotic lesion, the presence of a large area of superficial dermal scarring and melanin deposition is strongly suggestive of a regressed melanoma.

Sometimes, aggregates of much smaller melanocytes are present deep within the tumour; these must be differentiated from a pre-existent naevus component. In contrast to deeper parts of naevi, these aggregates of malignant small melanocytes are often compact and highly cellular, abnormally large, and irregular in size and contour, or form compact nests, and may contain melanin pigment. At high power the cells still show distinct nuclear atypia, especially hyperchromasia and coarse chromatin pattern, and mitoses are sometimes also found (Figure 9.11).

Lymphangioinvasive and haemangioinvasive growth is sometimes seen, but is usually difficult to detect with confidence unless special techniques are used (Fallowfield and Cook, 1989). Care should be taken not to mistake retraction artifacts or dissociation of tumour cell nests for vascular invasion.

9.2.2 Cytological features

There is an extraordinary variation in cytological morphology of melanoma cells. Since the architecture of melanoma also varies considerably between cases, as outlined in the previous section, it is no surprise that the diagnosis may cause substantial difficulties, especially when metastases are concerned. Here, we shall discuss the most common types of melanoma cells: these are descriptions of prototypes, but in practice, intermediate forms are also seen and different types occur together.

◀ **Figure 9.8** Melanoma, showing discrete, well-demarcated nests at all levels of the tumour (HE, × 90).

◀ **Figure 9.9** Melanoma, early regression. A dense predominantly lymphocytic infiltrate disrupts the dermal tumour component (HE, × 115).

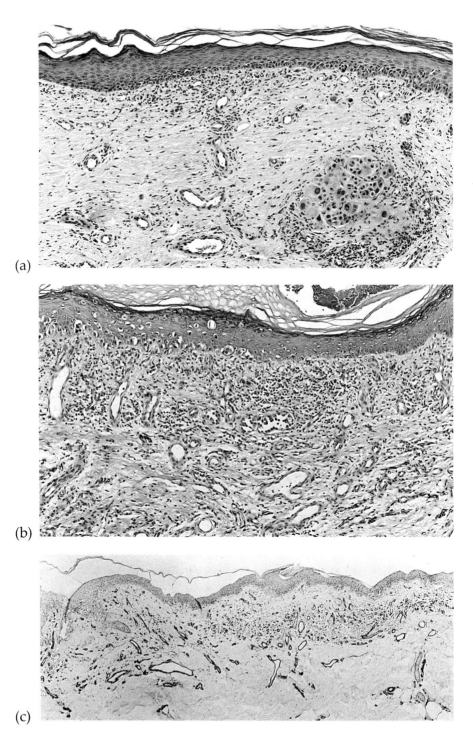

(a)

(b)

(c)

Melanoma cells may be polygonal, round, oval, spindled, bipolar, dendritic or irregular in shape, and vary in size from slightly larger than a lymphocyte to gigantic sizes. Multinucleate tumour cells may be present (Figures 9.11–9.13).

The *cytoplasm* is often eosinophilic or amphophilic and may be slightly granular, ground glass-like, or very pale and microvacuolar. Melanin pigment is granular, varying from very fine to very coarse, or dust-like, yielding a faint brownish, mauve or greyish tinge to the cytoplasm. In some primary tumours and' more commonly in metastases, melanin is completely absent (*amelanotic melanoma*). Large round poorly defined granular eosinophilic structures adjacent to the nucleus, staining strongly for vimentin, are seen in many melanomas with large or giant cell types. The periphery of such cells may be studded with small vacuoles. Rarely, large vacuoles or a central round area of cytoplasmic pallor may result in a strong resemblance to signet-ring cell adenocarcinoma (p. 282). Cytoplasmic borders are often indistinct and fuzzy.

In most melanomas some cells can be identified in which the cytoplasm invaginates into the nucleus, resulting in a horseshoe shape of the latter (Figure 9.14) or an apparent intranuclear 'pseudoinclusion', depending on the plane of section. Although this feature is not restricted to melanomas, it is sufficiently distinctive to be of help in differential diagnosis. Obviously these cytoplasmic pseudoinclusions should not be confused with nonspecific intranuclear vacuoles commonly seen after freezing and suboptimal tissue processing. Sometimes a small amount of melanin in such cytoplasmic pseudoinclusions is the only melanin encountered.

The *nucleus* is round, oval, irregular in shape, or elongated; the latter often shows a longitudinal groove or several irregular, mainly longitudinally oriented folds. The chromatin pattern is usually irregular and may be very coarse; in most melanomas, there is some degree of hyperchromasia and distinct anisochromasia. The nuclear membrane may be irregular in thickness. Sometimes nuclei are vesicular. There is often an eosinophilic nucleolus, most commonly located centrally

---

◀ **Figure 9.10** Regression of melanoma. (a) To the right, a small group of viable melanoma cells is present; elsewhere, the tumour is replaced by scar tissue with ectatic vessels and a sparse lymphocytic infiltrate (HE, × 90). (b) The dermal component of the tumour is almost totally replaced by scar tissue with many ectatic blood vessels. The overlying epidermis contains scattered tumour cells (HE, × 90). (c) The increased vascularity of the scar tissue is highlighted by collagen type IV immunostaining, which can be of help in outlining the area affected by regression (Immunoperoxidase, × 35).

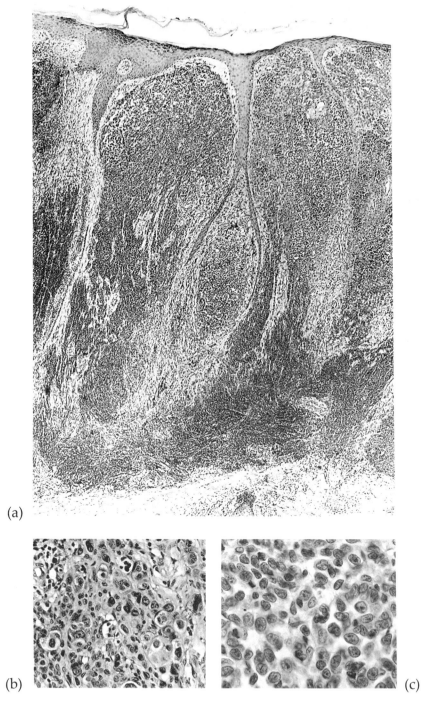

(a)

(b)

(c)

Figure 9.11 Melanoma, small cell type. (a) At low power, there is some resemblance to congenital naevus, but the proliferation is more compact (HE, × 35). Varying degrees of cellular atypia are found (b) HE, × 185; (c) HE, × 370.

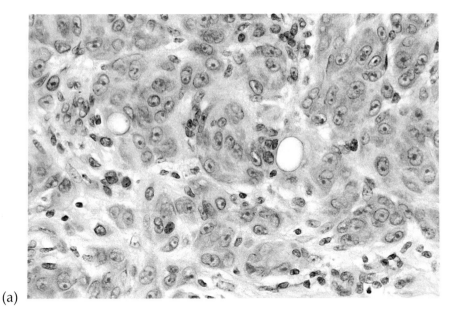

(a)

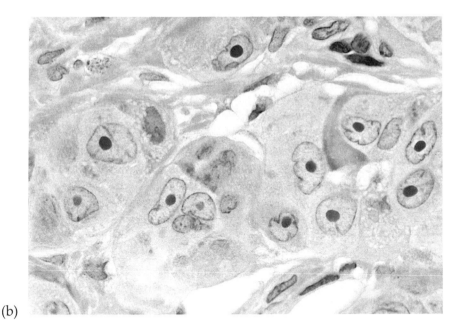

(b)

Figure 9.12 Epithelioid melanoma cells with relatively mild nuclear atypia. (a) paraffin section. Nuclei are slightly irregular and possess a prominent nucleolus; there is a moderate to large amount of cytoplasm. Two nuclei are greatly enlarged by a spherical, clear vacuole within them. Such vacuoles may be related to the cytoplasmic intranuclear herniations illustrated in Figure 9.14 (HE, × 370). (b) Plastic section (HE, × 920).

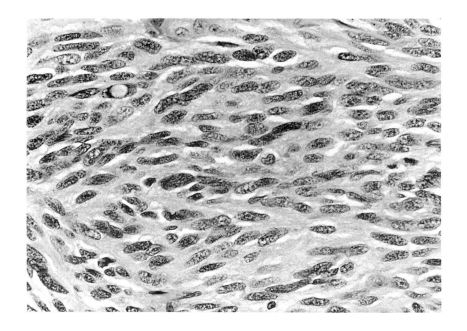

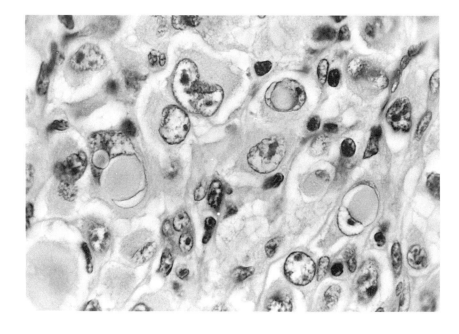

and sometimes irregular in shape. It is often prominent, especially in vesicular nuclei. Nucleoli are sometimes multiple. Irregularly shaped macronucleoli are found in some cases. Mitoses are usually present at the base of the tumour also, but they vary greatly in number; abnormal mitotic figures are not uncommonly present.

There is some *association of specific growth patterns and cell types* (Elder *et al.*, 1979; Reed, 1984, 1985). When the intraepidermal component shows a predominantly lentiginous type of growth, the intraepidermal tumour cells are often dendritic. When there is a pagetoid type of intraepidermal spread, the intraepidermal cells are generally rounded or polygonal and the invasive component often consists of rounded or polygonal epithelioid cells. In nodular melanoma, where intraepidermal lateral growth is absent, the invasive tumour may consist of either epithelioid or fusiform cells. However, the association between cell type and architecture is not very close and there are many combinations of different cell types.

9.3   Clinicopathological subtyping of melanoma

Cutaneous melanoma could be regarded as a single entity. However, since there is a considerable diversity in clinical and histological appearances, a number of macroscopical and histological subtypes have been recognized and proposed as distinct subtypes (Clark *et al.*, 1969, 1972, 1986; McGovern, 1982, 1983; McGovern and Murad, 1985; McGovern *et al.*, 1980, 1986; Reed, 1976). Some of these, notably superficial spreading, nodular, lentigo maligna- and acral lentiginous melanoma, have become widely accepted. Clinically, these subtypes relate to location, race, age distribution and, possibly, natural history.

9.3.1   *Problems of melanoma subtyping*

The subclassification of cutaneous melanoma is not free of serious conceptual and practical problems. Several of these relate to the fact

---

◀ **Figure 9.13**   Spindle-cell melanoma, cytological features. Nuclear pleomorphism is mild; there is a moderately coarse, speckled chromatin pattern, with a moderate degree of anisochromasia. Note intranuclear pseudoinclusion (upper left) (HE, × 370).

◀ **Figure 9.14**   Intranuclear cytoplasmic pseudoinclusions. Left of centre it is apparent that the intranuclear pseudoinclusion is part of the cytoplasm surrounded almost totally by a crescent-shaped nucleus. Melanin is occasionally found in these pseudoinclusions (HE, × 920).

that the current classification of cutaneous melanoma is not based on one single and logical system of histological criteria. Instead, it is partly based on growth pattern, especially of the *in situ* component, partly on cytological features, and partly on features of the surrounding skin and the tumour localization. It would clearly be preferable if the classification could be based on a system of criteria pertaining strictly to histopathological features of the invasive tumour.

As discussed above, different cell types occur with different architectural types and *vice versa*, so that the number of possible combinations of histological features is much larger than a simple subdivision of melanoma into a small number of subtypes would suggest. As a result, one may experience considerable difficulties in assigning an individual melanoma to a specific subtype. Even though classification of many individual melanomas is straightforward, about 10 to 20% do not fit easily into one of the subtypes: some do not fit any of the categories, whereas others fit more than one, e.g. the invasive portion of a lentigo maligna melanoma may qualify as a neurotropic melanoma, or a nodular melanoma may be compatible with the criteria proposed for 'minimal deviation' melanoma. Furthermore, the histological subtype may change during the course of the disease: the intraepidermal lateral spread which is the hallmark of superficial spreading melanoma may be obscured by subsequent nodular growth, leading to a change in histological subtype; a 'minimal deviation melanoma' may reach the subcutis and thus no longer qualify as minimal deviation melanoma purely because of this, again leading to a change in histological subtype. This is obviously not very satisfactory.

These and other points of criticism have been forcibly stressed by Ackerman (1980; 1982; Ackerman and David, 1986). It should, however, be admitted that these problems in the current classification of melanomas have their analogies in the classification of tumours in many other organs; they are not unique to melanomas. Indeed, the histological and biological variability of tumours of any organ is such that distinction of subtypes practically always results in a minority of problem cases which do not easily fit any of the subtypes. There are two lines of approach to this problem: either to use it as an argument to do away with the subtyping (the lumpers' approach) or to establish new subtypes based on these problem cases (the splitters' approach). To our mind, extreme rigidity in adhering to either of these approaches is not very helpful.

Partly because melanoma subtyping is widely practised, we prefer to include a discussion of the currently used subtypes, even though it is obvious that the system is less than perfect. A practical justification for it is given towards the end of this section.

9.3.2   Radial and vertical growth phases

An important concept in the current classification of melanoma is that of the radial and vertical growth phase: in superfical spreading, lentigo maligna- and acral lentiginous melanoma, a radial growth phase, confined to the epidermis and superficial papillary dermis (Elder *et al.*, 1979; Reed, 1984, 1985) precedes the downward growth into the deep dermis and underlying tissues.

According to Clark and colleagues (1972; 1986), the intradermal tumour cells in the *radial growth phase* resemble the intraepidermal ones, and lie as single cells or small clusters, numbering up to 15 cells, these nests being usually smaller than or equal in size to the intra-epidermal nests, while none of the dermal clusters has an apparent growth preference over the other clusters. There is usually a marked inflammatory response. The *vertical growth phase*, by contrast, consists of one or more larger aggregates composed of tumour cells which are often amelanotic and which may resemble each other closely but differ from the tumour cells of the radial growth phase; an inflammatory response is usually absent at the base of the vertical phase. Extension into the lower reticular dermis qualifies as vertical growth phase by definition (Clark *et al.*, 1986).

In a substantial number of cutaneous melanomas, one can indeed recognize such a focus of *'intralesional tumour progression'*, a term which is favoured by us, since it avoids too much emphasis on the direction of growth, which is not the key factor, but highlights what we consider the central issue, namely, the emergence of a clone of altered tumour cells which has a growth advantage over the others. However, there are many melanomas in which this phenomenon is absent or incon-spicuous, and, as Clark and colleagues (1986) admit, such tumours may extend into the lower dermis (this, according to these authors is vertical growth phase by definition, even when the other features of vertical growth phase are absent!). In our experience, based on a review of many hundreds of stage II and III melanomas, such tumours do occasionally metastasize to regional nodes and distant sites, occasion-ally even in the absence of lower dermal involvement.

'Intralesional progression' is commonly a feature at some stage of the development of a primary melanoma. It may occur early, leading to the development of a nodular melanoma, or late, resulting in the other three main histological types. Its recognition is an aid in the diagnosis of malignancy, but, as indicated above, in some metastasizing mel-anomas it may not occur or at least may be unrecognizable histologic-ally. Conversely, some benign naevi may show a focus of melanocytes with a different morphology, which may erroneously be interpreted as intralesional transformation and therefore as a sign of malignancy: these include balloon cell naevus (p. 90) and a combination of common acquired and Spitz naevus (p. 172).

There is no clear indication that intralesional tumour progression has a direct impact on prognosis, after stratification for the well-corroborated histological prognostic parameters described in the next chapter.

9.3.3   A pragmatic argument for melanoma subtyping

The problems inherent in the currently used melanoma classification cannot be lightly dismissed, nor are they easily amenable to solution. However, it remains obvious that there is a great macrosocopical diversity in melanomas and that this can, in part, be related to the diversity in histological features, and used in the subdivision of melanomas. These differences would not be reflected by diagnosing melanoma without further specification as to subtype. About 80–90% of melanomas can be classified into the four main subtypes, which does not compare unfavourably with classifications of other tumour types. For practical purposes, the main issue remains the distinction between benign and malignant lesions; the separate description of different types of melanoma is very helpful in this distinction, and for this reason alone the subtyping is of practical value.

9.3.4   The four classical subtypes of melanoma

The four major melanoma subtypes classically recognized are: *superficial spreading melanoma, nodular melanoma, lentigo maligna melanoma*, and *acral lentiginous melanoma*. The differences between these four types consist of a mixture of architectural, cytological and clinical features.

Lentigo maligna melanoma occurs on sun-damaged skin, especially on the face and distal upper limbs. Acral lentiginous melanoma is located on the palm, sole, and nail bed; melanomas with similar morphology occur in juxtacutaneous mucous membranes of the upper aerodigestive tract, anus and genitalia. Superficial spreading and nodular melanomas occur practically anywhere on the skin. All types except for nodular melanoma show intraepidermal lateral spread of tumour cells, which is predominantly pagetoid (cells scattered irregularly at all levels of the epidermis) in superficial spreading melanoma, and lentiginous (cells proliferating along the dermoepidermal junction) in lentigo maligna and acral lentiginous melanoma. The latter two types generally exhibit dendritic intraepidermal tumour cells, with or without an admixture of nondendritic polygonal or rounded cells. The intraepidermal part of superficial spreading and nodular melanoma

Table 9.1 Four main melanoma subtypes

	SSM	*NM*	*LMM*	*ALM*
Peak incidence	middle adult life	middle adult life	late adult life	late adult life
Race	usually whites	usually whites	only whites	all races
Localization	all skin	all skin	sun-damaged skin	palms, soles, subungual
Main cell type in epidermis	epithelioid	epithelioid	dendritic	dendritic
Pagetoid lateral spread	usual	absent or minimal	rare	rare
Lentiginous lateral spread	uncommon	absent	usual	usual
Epidermal hyperplasia	often	sometimes	absent	present
Epidermal atrophy	sometimes	sometimes	present	absent
Actinic damage of skin	sometimes	sometimes	present	absent
Relative frequencies (Clark *et al.*, 1986) Unclassifiable: 10%	67%	10%	9%	4%

SSM = superficial spreading melanoma
NM   = nodular melanoma
LMM = lentigo maligna melanoma
ALM = acral lentiginous melanoma

does not usually contain dendritic cells. A 'variant' growth pattern of superficial spreading melanoma with similarities to acral lentiginous melanoma has been described (Elder *et al.*, 1979), blurring the border between these two types.

The distinctive features are summarized in Table 9.1.

9.4   Superficial spreading melanoma

This most common melanoma subtype is characterized by significant intraepidermal lateral extension of malignant melanocytes, usually of the epithelioid type, with a pagetoid pattern of growth (Figure 9.3).

9.4.1   Clinical features

About two-thirds of cutaneous melanomas are of the superficial spreading type. The tumour has a wide age range which peaks in the fourth decade (Clark *et al.*, 1975). In its earliest phase, the lesion is flat; it may, however, arise in a pre-existing naevus which may be raised. Irregular pigmentation, with notched, irregular and sometimes indistinct borders are early signs. In addition there may be areas of depigmentation. Some lesions itch or give a burning sensation even at an early phase of their development. Later, sometimes only after many years, a nodule may develop as a sign of dermal invasive growth and expansion. Still later, the tumour may ulcerate and bleed, and satellites may develop.

9.4.2   Histological features

Many of the features of superficial spreading melanoma have been discussed already in the preceding paragraphs, since they pertain to all types of melanoma. The distinguishing feature of superficial spreading melanoma is the presence of *pagetoid spread of tumour cells within the epidermis over a distance of at least three rete ridges lateral to the lateral border of the dermal tumour component* (Clark *et al.*, 1969).

The intraepidermal tumour cells are irregularly scattered as unevenly spaced nests of various sizes and shapes, as well as single cells, both at the dermoepidermal junction and above it.

The epidermis is often irregularly thickened, with distortion of the rete ridges. Some superficial spreading melanomas, mostly occurring on the lower legs of elderly patients, show a verrucous surface and prominent hyperkeratosis: these have been designated *'verrucous-keratotic melanoma'* (Kuehnl-Petzold *et al.*, 1982). They should not be confused with verrucous naevoid melanoma, discussed below (p. 264): the similarity is one of name only.

The dermal component most commonly consists of atypical epithelioid melanocytes, lying together in irregular strands, clumps and nodules, or singly within a fibrotic or sometimes oedematous papillary dermis, and later extending into the reticular dermis and subcutis. Uncommonly, a spindle-shaped tumour cell type predominates.

Pagetoid spread of tumour cells has been discussed before, together with its differential diagnosis (p. 221), the most important one being extramammary Paget's disease, which may be pigmented, especially in negroid patients (p. 48).

Dermal invasion and tumour progression may result in a tumour nodule, but as long as the intraepidermal component extends laterally as mentioned above, the melanoma is designated superficial spreading melanoma, and not nodular melanoma. It will be apparent that the distinction between superficial spreading and nodular melanoma may at times be arbitrary, and that transition from superficial spreading to nodular melanoma can occur if the invasive dermal component outgrows the epidermal component (Ackerman, 1982; 1984).

Some superficial spreading melanomas occurring on hair-bearing skin, exhibit lentiginous intraepidermal spread and dendritic intraepidermal melanocytes, similar to acral lentiginous melanoma (Elder *et al.*, 1979).

9.5   Nodular melanoma

Nodular melanoma differs from superficial spreading melanoma by the *absence of significant intraepidermal lateral spread* characteristic of the latter.

9.5.1   Clinical features

Nodular melanoma comprises about 10% of cutaneous melanomas (Clark *et al.*, 1986). It occurs in a wide age range, and appears to be about twice as common in men as in women; in men they are located preferentially on the back and the head and neck region (Clark *et al.*, 1975). Often the tumour grows rapidly so that the history is short.

It has been argued that many, if not all, nodular melanomas may have started out as intraepidermal, radially spreading lesions, but that overgrowth of the nodular component subsequently obliterates the horizontal component, resulting in a transition from a superficial spreading to a nodular subtype. It seems likely that this indeed occurs in some instances; however, not uncommonly, nodular melanomas start out clinically as nodules rather than as flat lesions.

9.5.2   Histological features

Nodular melanoma resembles superficial spreading melanoma, but lacks the intraepidermal lateral spread that characterizes the latter. The tumour cells are usually of an epithelioid type, but some cases exhibit only a spindled or fusiform tumour cell population, which in general is more characteristic of the lentigo maligna and acral lentiginous variants of melanoma.

In some nodular melanomas there is only very little epidermal involvement, so that the lesion has to be distinguished from a cutaneous melanoma metastasis (for distinguishing features, see p. 277).

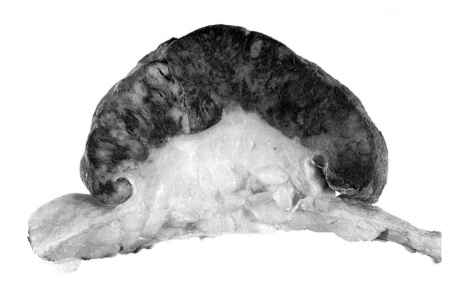

Figure 9.15   Polypoid nodular melanoma. The whole tumour is raised above the original surface of the skin. Such tumours are often thick and ulcerated (Magnification: × 4).

Several nonmelanocytic tumours also enter the differential diagnosis, especially atypical fibroxanthoma, spindle cell squamous carcinoma and angiosarcoma, especially when the tumour cells have a spindle shape; this is discussed in a separate section (p. 253). Merkel cell carcinoma (p. 45) has occasionally been confused with nodular melanoma.

'*Polypoid melanoma*' is a term sometimes used for a nodular (or, more rarely, superficial spreading or acral lentiginous) melanoma in which the whole of the tumour is raised above the original level of the epidermis (Figure 9.15). Such exophytic lesions, which frequently ulcerate, usually carry a poor prognosis, in keeping with their often considerable thickness and the presence of ulceration. They should not be confused with verrucous naevoid melanoma (p. 264).

9.6   Lentigo maligna and lentigo maligna melanoma

Lentigo maligna melanoma is the only melanoma type regularly *associated with chronic solar damage of the skin*, and it is often preceded for many years by lentigo maligna, an irregular hyper-pigmentation of the skin corresponding histologically to a proliferation of atypical melanocytes within an atrophic epidermis, in the presence

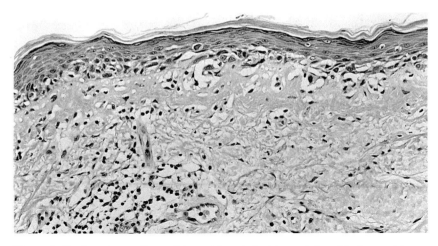

Figure 9.16   Lentigo maligna. The epidermis is thin and devoid of rete ridges; there is an almost continuous proliferation of atypical melanocytes at the dermoepidermal junction and focally ascending into suprabasal layers; the dermis shows fibrosis and a patchy lymphocytic infiltrate (HE, × 185).

of actinic damage to the dermis. Not unexpectedly, lentigo maligna may occur together with actinic keratosis.

9.6.1   Lentigo maligna

Lentigo maligna, synonyms of which are Hutchinson's freckle and *morbus* Dubreuilh (Hutchinson, 1890, 1894; Dubreuilh, 1894), is an irregularly shaped, flat, impalpable pigmented lesion, emerging in sun-damaged skin, most commonly on the face, usually in mid- or late adult life in white persons; it may attain a size of several centimetres. Various shades of brown are seen and there may be irregular depigmentation; however, some cases are uniformly light brown.

Histologically, the epidermis is atrophic and the dermis shows signs of actinic damage (dyselastosis, basophilic degeneration of collagen, telangiectasia, some perivascular round cell infiltrate), often with scattered melanophages. Early stages of the process consist of irregular epidermal hyperpigmentation together with a mild increase in number of melanocytes, located in the basal layer of the epidermis, and often extending along skin appendages, and which are arranged as solitary units rather than as nests (Figure 9.16). Usually these melanocytes possess dendrites which may be inconspicuous but which stand out more clearly when the cells are heavily pigmented or when melanin stains are used. Nuclear enlargement, pleomorphism and

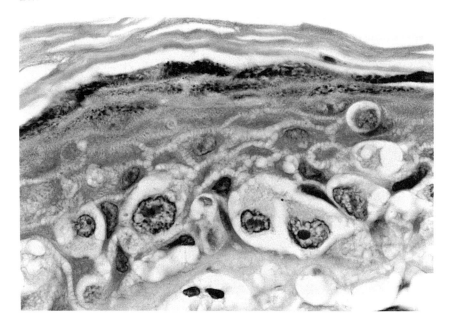

Figure 9.17 Prominent cytological atypia of melanocytes in lentigo maligna. In lentigo maligna, the degree of atypia varies greatly between cases, and sometimes also between sites in the same lesion (HE, × 920).

hyperchromasia are often inconspicuous at this stage. A biopsy of a clinically evident case may occasionally fall short of being diagnostic of lentigo maligna. In such cases, there is atrophy of the epidermis and actinic damage of the dermis, but the increase in number of basally located melanocytes is small, cytological atypia is mild, and ascending melanocytes are absent. The pathologist then reports that the histological features are compatible with, but not diagnostic of, lentigo maligna.

Later, a more pronounced melanocytic hyperplasia develops, together with an often marked increase in cellular atypia (Figure 9.17), and retraction of the cytoplasm, which may result in a moth-eaten appearance of the dermoepidermal junction. Irregular small nests of melanocytes may appear, but are less common than in superficial spreading melanoma. Atypical melanocytes ascend into the upper layers of the epidermis and usually extend along hair follicles and ducts of sweat glands.

Lentigo maligna should be differentiated from *lentigo simplex*, which exhibits elongation of rete ridges instead of epidermal atrophy, lacks melanocytic atypia, and does not involve skin appendages.

Clinically, lentigo maligna may resemble *pigmented solar keratosis*, which is a keratinocytic dysplasia with reactive hyperpigmentation. The histological distinction is usually not difficult: in the latter, the epidermis is usually thickened rather than thinned, and exhibits atypia of keratinocytes, especially the basally located ones, and parakeratosis. *Dysplastic naevi* on sun-damaged skin show basically the same features as those on covered skin. Instead of epidermal atrophy there is usually irregular elongation of rete ridges and subepidermal fibrosis including lamellar fibroplasia; also, many dysplastic naevi possess an intradermal component.

Excision of lentigo maligna offers the best chance of cure (Coleman et al., 1980); histological verification of the completeness of resection is very important. Radiotherapy, cryosurgery, curettage, electrodesiccation and topical application of toxic agents have also been used, but recurrence is more common with these treatments. When definitive ablative treatment of lentigo maligna is decided against, because of local extent of the lesion or advanced age and poor condition of the patient, follow-up intervals of 3 or at most 6 months are advocated. Even after definitive treatment, careful follow-up remains important since not all of the lesion may be pigmented, and there is a risk of recurrence since the lesion may extend irregularly beyond clinically detectable margins and, even histologically, its borders may be indistinct and difficult to assess.

9.6.2   Lentigo maligna melanoma

As indicated above, lentigo maligna is flat and impalpable; a palpable lesion arising in it is suspect. Invasive melanoma develops in only a small percentage of cases, usually after many years. Consequently, lentigo maligna melanoma is a melanoma of sun-damaged skin, occurring mainly in elderly white patients, with a peak incidence after the age of 60. There is no obvious sex preference, males predominating in some series and females in others.

Previously, the risk of melanoma development in lentigo maligna was considered to be of the order of 30% (Davis et al., 1967); however, this figure is too high and reflects patient populations diagnosed and treated clinically rather than the general population. Indeed, on the basis of age-specific prevalence figures of lentigo maligna and calculated figures of the age-specific incidence of lentigo maligna melanoma, Weinstock and Sober (1987) arrived at much lower figures: for lentigo maligna patients at ages 45 and 65, they estimated life-time risks of clinically diagnosed lentigo maligna melanoma of only 4.7 and 2.2%, respectively.

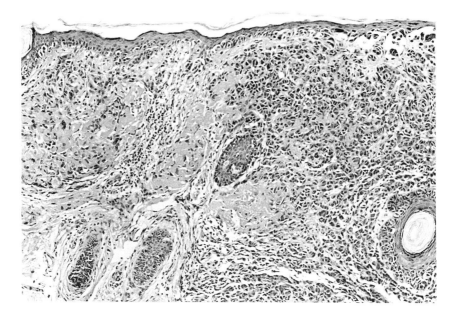

Figure 9.18 Lentigo maligna melanoma. Characteristics of lentigo maligna in the epidermis; invasion of the dermis. In this instance, the invasive cell type is predominantly epithelioid (HE, × 90).

Histologically, lentigo maligna melanoma may consist of rounded, epithelioid cells (Figure 9.18) but commonly shows an admixture of oval or spindle-shaped tumour cells (Figure 9.19), with or without the features of desmoplastic melanoma (Figure 9.27; p. 257). The spindle shape of tumour cells may occasionally cause some difficulty in the identification of microinvasion since the tumour cells may resemble reactive fibroblasts. Immunostaining with S-100 facilitates the detection of such invading tumour cells which, in one series, were encountered in as many as 14 out of 91 biopsy specimens in which invasion was difficult or impossible to identify on HE-stained sections; in 13 of these, there were multiple foci of invasion (Penneys, 1987). Invasive melanocytes can be distinguished from S-100-positive dendritic reticulum cells by their nuclear atypia and/or organization in small groups and bundles rather than as solitary cells.

Lentigo maligna melanoma usually has a protracted preinvasive phase, but once invasion develops and the main prognostic parameters such as thickness and ulceration are taken into account, the prognosis is similar to that of other melanoma types (Gussack *et al.*, 1983; Koh

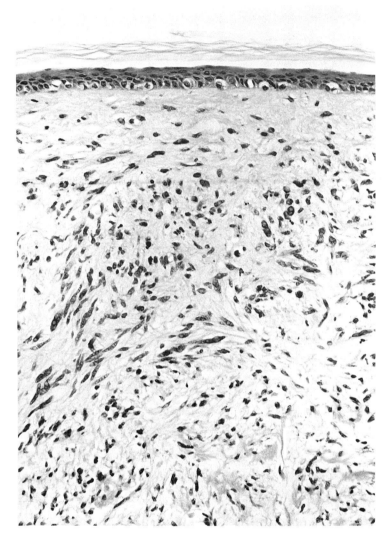

Figure 9.19   Lentigo maligna melanoma. In this instance the tumour cells are spindled and exhibit distinct nuclear enlargement and hyperchromasia (HE, × 225).

et al., 1984), despite early claims to the contrary (Wayte and Helwig, 1968; McGovern *et al.*, 1980). In a few instances the tumour becomes deeply invasive within a relatively short period of time (Michalik *et al.*, 1983).

9.7   Acral lentiginous melanoma

A lentiginous pattern of intraepidermal spread was noted in melanomas of acral sites by Seiji and Takahashi (1974), but the first detailed decriptions of acral lentiginous melanoma as a distinct clinicopathological subtype were presented a few years later (Reed, 1976; Arrington et al., 1977). These authors pointed out that many melanomas of palms, soles and nailbeds exhibited similar histological features, notably lentiginous intraepidermal spread of dendritic melanocytes, associated with reactive epithelial hyperplasia. Occasional melanomas of hair-bearing skin and many melanomas of mucous membranes (upper aerodigestive tract, genital tract, anus) share a similar histology (p. 333).

It should be noted that some melanomas of palms, soles and nailbeds show the histological features of superficial spreading or nodular melanoma (Feibleman et al., 1980; Arrington et al., 1977).

9.7.1   Clinical features

Acral lentiginous melanoma constitutes about 4% of melanomas in Caucasians (Clark et al., 1986), but is *the main cutaneous melanoma type occurring in other races* (Krementz et al., 1976; Takematsu et al., 1985). The tumour occurs throughout adulthood, with a mean age of approximately 60 years; it is exceedingly rare in childhood (Chapman et al., 1987). Acral lentiginous melanoma is found on volar (palmar and plantar) skin, and subungually; on palms and soles, it may appear as an irregular, sometimes linear pigmented macule, papule or nodule, or as a crusted or ulcerated, melanotic or amelanotic tumour.

Plantar melanoma with acral lentiginous histology usually grows slowly, as witnessed by the fact that, compared to nodular melanoma of the sole of the foot, there is a longer clinical history before diagnosis, while the average thickness and level of invasion are less (Scrivner et al., 1987). Most plantar melanomas arise in the weight-bearing areas of the sole.

Subungual melanoma occurs with almost equal frequency on the hands and feet, the thumbs and big toes being most commonly affected; there is probably a female preponderance (Daly et al., 1987). There was presumably patient selection in the series from the Armed Forces Institute of Pathology, in which there was a 2:1 male preponderance (Patterson and Helwig, 1980). In an early phase, a dark discolouration of the nail and nail bed may be noticed, which may take the form of melanonychia striata, a longitudinal streak of pigmentation (Kato et al., 1989) or may involve the whole nail. Clinically, remnants of previous

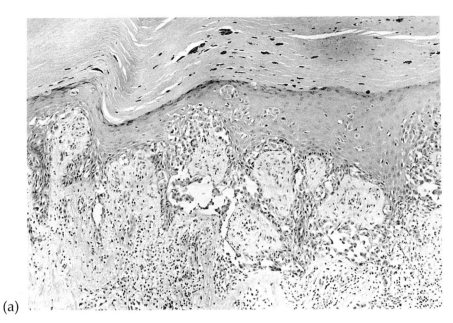

(a)

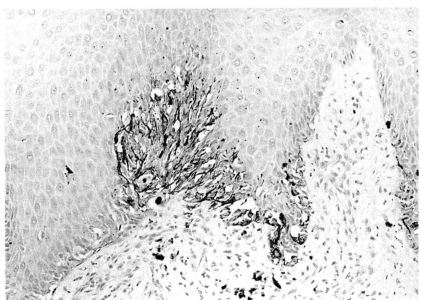

(b)

Figure 9.20 Early acral lentiginous melanoma. (a) Atypical melanocytes extend along the irregular dermoepidermal junction, resulting in a 'moth-eaten' appearance; tumour cells ascend into upper layers of the epidermis (HE, × 90). (b) A group of heavily pigmented dendritic melanocytes is present at the dermoepidermal junction (HE/Masson Fontana, × 185).

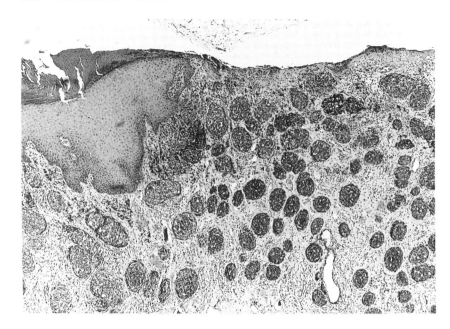

Figure 9.21 Acral lentiginous melanoma. There is ulceration and a distinctive growth pattern with formation of compact round nests (HE, × 35).

subungual haemorrhage may produce a very similar appearance, so that a biopsy is required to distinguish between the two. Later, pain, loss or destruction of the nail, ulceration of the nailbed and involvement of the surrounding skin may ensue. There is often substantial patient and doctor delay, which was more than 2 years in 40% of cases in the series of Patterson and Helwig (1980).

9.7.2 Histological features

Initially acral lentiginous melanoma consists of a proliferation of atypical melanocytes arranged singly along the epidermal basement membrane and often extending along sweat gland ducts. The cells are medium-sized, often dendritic, and show mild to moderate nuclear enlargement, pleomorphism and hyperchromasia. Usually some of these atypical melanocytes ascend into the upper layers of the epidermis and become entrapped in the thick cornified layer (Figure 9.20). However, ascending cells may be rare or even absent. In the absence of dermal invasion, it may then be very difficult indeed to ascertain that the lesion is malignant. Larger epithelioid melanocytes may sometimes

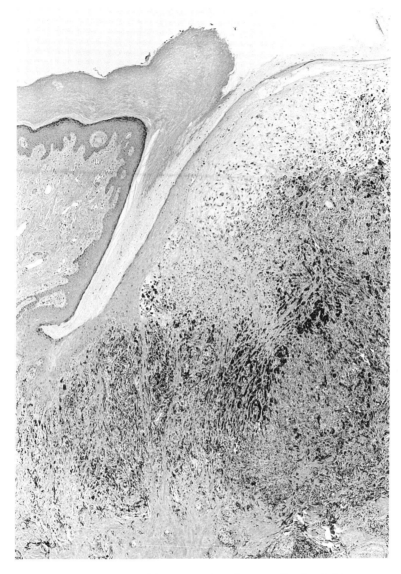

Figure 9.22 Subungual (acral lentiginous) melanoma. To the right, an extensive proliferation of elongated, variably pigmented melanocytes is present. To the left, the nail fold is seen (HE, × 45).

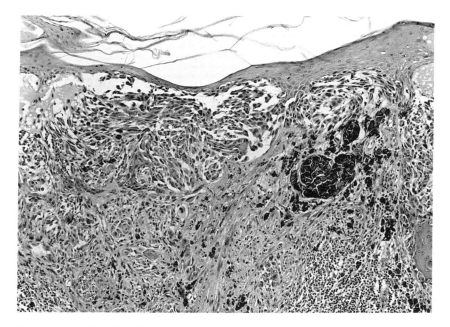

Figure 9.23   Spindle cell melanoma. Irregular architecture with horizontally and vertically orientated nests. One nest is heavily pigmented (HE, × 90).

be present also and more often exhibit a pagetoid pattern of spread. In contrast to lentigo maligna melanoma, in which the epidermis is atrophic, the epidermis shows some degree of acanthosis and hyperkeratosis.

When the tumour invades the dermis, this takes the form of thin strands and ill-defined aggregates and bundles or compact nodules (Figure 9.21). A desmoplastic melanoma type (p. 253) may also occur. Varying degrees of fibrosis and a predominantly lymphocytic inflammatory response are usually seen. In larger tumours, ulceration, areas of regression and deep penetration of subcutaneous tissues are common, especially in subungual locations (Figure 9.22), where the tumour often invades deeply and reaches the underlying periosteum.

9.8   Spindle cell melanoma

Some melanomas consist largely or wholly of spindled tumour cells (Figures 9.23–9.25). Although many of these tumours can be subclassified as one of the four main types of melanoma discussed above, the diagnosis of these spindle cell tumours has its own difficulties, so that it is helpful to discuss them under a separate heading. Those

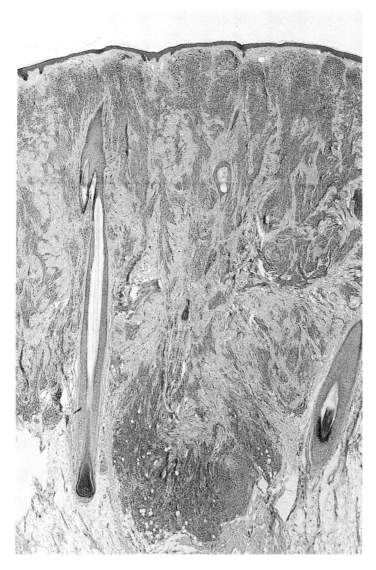

Figure 9.24   Spindle cell melanoma of scalp. At low magnification, this tumour shows some resemblance to congenital naevus. However, the tumour does not grow preferentially along adnexae and forms compact sheets, also at the base (HE, × 25).

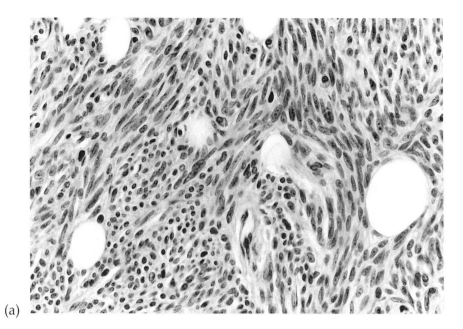

(a)

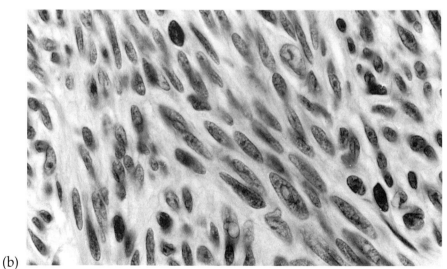

(b)

Figure 9.25 Spindle cell melanoma, same case as in Figure 9.24. (a) In deep areas, a highly cellular proliferation of slightly pleomorphic spindle cells engulfs scattered pre-existent adipocytes of the subcutis (HE, × 370). (b) There is mild to moderate anisonucleosis and a moderately fine chromatin pattern. The tumour, located on the scalp of a young adult, later metastasized (HE, × 920).

spindle cell melanomas which are associated with prominent des-moplasia will be discussed in the next section.

Spindle cell melanomas are more common in some extracutaneous sites such as the uvea and various mucous membranes. They are usually pigmented, at least focally, but some are amelanotic or contain very little pigment. Most are obviously malignant tumours, but in a minority, the distinction from Spitz naevus and other spindle cell naevi can be difficult; such 'Spitzoid' melanomas are discussed later in this chapter (p. 264).

Important hallmarks of malignancy include a *compact appearance of cellular bundles*, which often traverse the entire thickness of the dermis, cellular *pleomorphism*, mitoses deep within the tumour (but these by themselves are insufficient proof of malignancy), absence of maturation (but this is also absent in blue naevi) and, perhaps most importantly, an intraepidermal component exhibiting the character-istics of malignancy such as marked asymmetry, ascent of melanocytes and, most importantly, *pagetoid lateral spread* of tumour cells.

Apart from melanocytic lesions, the tumour should be distinguished from a variety of cutaneous spindle cell tumours, including spindle cell carcinoma and some cases of angiosarcoma with a solid growth pattern. Thorough sampling, in search of a focal junctional tumour component, or evidence of neoplastic vascular structures or carcinomatous tumour nodules as well as immunostains are of aid in this differential diagnosis (Figure 9.26). In certain sites like the vulva, where spindle cell mel-anoma is relatively common, one must be especially careful before diagnosing squamous carcinoma on the basis of continuity with the epidermis: amelanotic spindle cell melanoma may mimic squamous carcinoma closely by exhibiting such continuity.

9.9   Desmoplastic and neurotropic melanoma

Desmoplastic melanoma is characterized by spindle-shaped invasive tumour cells accompanied by an increase in collagen. Neurotropic melanoma is a variant showing conspicuous growth along nerves, often visible macroscopically as thickening of the nerves (Reed and Leonard, 1979; Jain and Allen, 1989).

The first detailed description of the tumour was provided by Conley and colleagues (1971); a number of recent series have brought the total of reported cases to well over a hundred (Kossard *et al.*, 1987; Reiman *et al.*, 1987; Egbert *et al.*, 1988; Walsh *et al.*, 1988; Jain and Allen, 1989). Scattered examples have been reported in the literature as cutaneous or superficial malignant schwannoma.

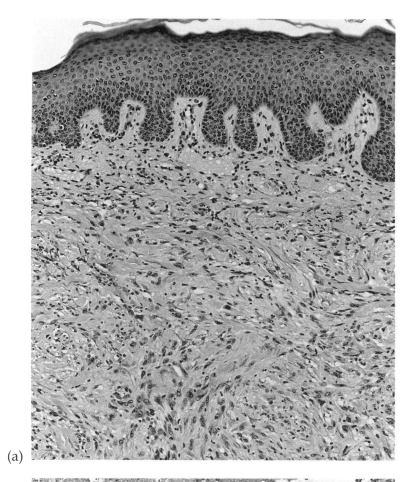

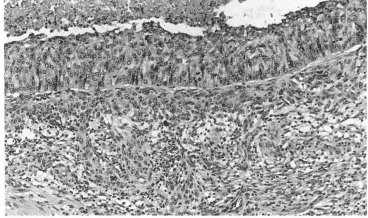

9.9.1   Clinical features

Desmoplastic melanoma often arises in sun-exposed skin, often in the head and neck region, particularly the face, where it may be associated with lentigo maligna. Other sites are distributed over the trunk and extremities; occasional examples are encountered in mucous membranes and perianal skin. The tumour usually occurs in later adult life, although cases have been reported in early adolescence. In most series there is a male preponderance. The clinical appearance, a dermal nodule or tumour up to several centimetres in diameter, is not very distinctive, unless a pre-existent pigmented lesion such as lentigo maligna is present. We have seen cases diagnosed clinically as banal or benign conditions like epidermoid cyst and neurofibroma.

There is a marked tendency to local recurrence, related to inadequate initial surgery, and recurrences are especially ominous in the neurotropic variant, which spreads along nerves and may reach the neurocranium. In one series of 45 desmoplastic melanomas, tumour recurred locally in 55% of cases (Jain and Allen, 1989). Regional and distant metastases often occur also in the course of the disease.

Although some workers have suggested that this melanoma variant carries a better prognosis (Walsh *et al.*, 1988), most authors agree that the desmoplastic melanoma is an aggressive neoplasm, leading to a high percentage of tumour recurrences and metastases. The mortality rate varies between series and was as high as 66% in one recent series (Reiman *et al.*, 1987). In the series of Jain and Allen (1989), 36% of patients had died or were terminally ill after a mean follow-up period of only 4.6 years; this figure rose to 64% for the 11 nerve-centred cases. Neurotropic melanoma of the head and neck with macroscopical involvement of nerves appears to carry an exceptionally poor prognosis (Jain and Allen, 1989). It has been suggested that desmoplastic melanoma is more aggressive than lentigo maligna melanoma (Egbert *et al.*, 1988), but it should be realized that the latter is also an aggressive tumour, notwithstanding its reputation for indolent behaviour in the earlier literature. As with other histological types of melanoma, the head and neck region is a prognostically unfavourable site (p. 306; Gussack *et al.*, 1983).

◄ **Figure 9.26**   Spindle cell squamous carcinoma. (a) In this subepidermal portion, the tumour shows a close resemblance to spindle cell melanoma. Note the absence of atypical melanocytes in the overlying epidermis (HE, × 115). (b) Other areas show distinct epithelial differentiation; the tumour was positive for keratins and negative for S-100 (HE, × 90).

Radical surgery offers the best chance of cure (Reiman *et al.*, 1987), but responses to chemotherapy and radiotherapy have been observed (Jain and Allen, 1989).

9.9.2   Histological features

The tumour consists of a poorly demarcated, moderately cellular proliferation of atypical elongated cells, intermingled with varying amounts of collagen, located within the greatly thickened dermis and often extending into the subcutis (Figure 9.27). The tumour cells are arranged in bundles, often oriented haphazardy, or form vague storiform or cartwheel patterns. Long vertical bundles often reach from the upper dermis to the subcutis, while laterally, individual tumour cells infiltrate singly between the pre-existent dermal collagen bundles. Circumferential growth around skin appendages is sometimes seen. Some predominantly lymphocytic inflammatory infiltrate is often present. Necrosis is sometimes seen; occasionally there is myxoid change as well.

In some cases there is distinct neurotropism, i.e. the tumour cells grow preferentially within and around nerves at a distance from the tumour mass (Figure 9.28), leading to macroscopically detectable thickening of these nerves; such cases are designated *neurotropic melanoma*.

The tumour cells are greatly elongated, with pale, indistinct eosinophilic to amphophilic cytoplasm and elongated, hyperchromatic nuclei. The intradermal tumour cells only rarely contain melanin pigment; most tumours are completely amelanotic. Multinucleate cells are seen in about half of the cases (Jain and Allen, 1989). Nuclear grooves and invaginations of cytoplasm into the nucleus, which may occasionally contain a small amount of melanin, are helpful features indicating that the lesion is melanocytic in origin (Su *et al.*, 1985). Mitoses are often scanty, but may occasionally be frequent. There is a close intermingling of tumour cells and collagen fibres (From *et al.*, 1983).

In some cases the melanocytic nature of the tumour becomes apparent when the epidermis is scrutinized: it may exhibit the classical features of lentigo maligna or, when this is not apparent, there is often a mild degree of lentiginous or irregularly nested proliferation of slightly

---

Figure 9.27   Desmoplastic melanoma. (a) An extensive proliferation of elongated atypical melanocytes is present throughout the dermis (HE, × 45). (b) There is an intermingling of spindled tumour cells and newly formed collagen bundles (HE, × 185).

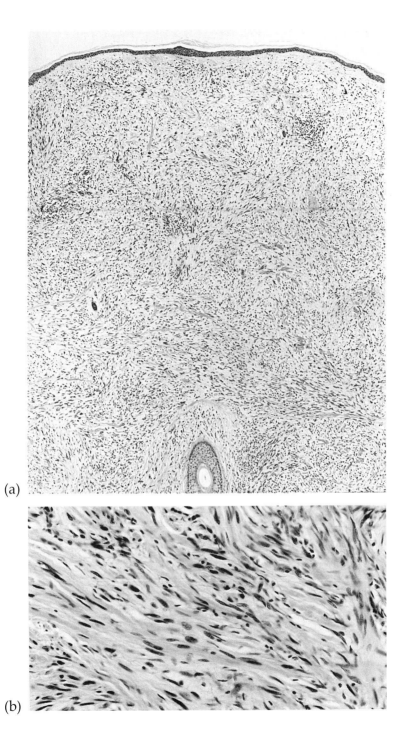

(a)

(b)

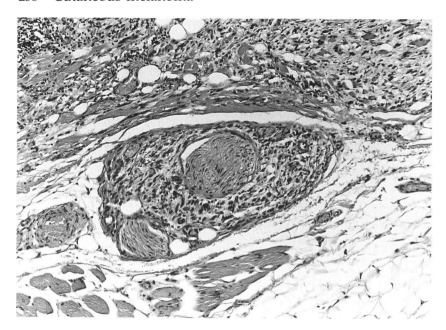

Figure 9.28   Neurotropic melanoma. A nerve in the vicinity of the main mass of the tumour is enveloped by a sheath of tumour cells (HE, × 90).

atypical melanocytes, which may extend along skin appendages. This important diagnostic feature is relatively inconspicuous compared to the extensive intradermal tumour cell proliferation, and should therefore be specifically looked for. The presence of intraepidermal atypical melanocytes was one of the original diagnostic criteria of Conley and co-workers (1971). However, in the experience of others (Tuthill *et al.*, 1988; Jain and Allen, 1989) and ourselves, they may be absent; whether such tumours have arisen *de novo* within the dermis (Reed and Leonard, 1979; Jain and Allen, 1989) or whether the intra-epidermal component has regressed or has been missed in incompletely sampled lesions, remains a moot point.

The tumour can be confused with a large variety of cutaneous spindle cell lesions: these include reactive fibrosis, dermatofibroma, dermato-fibrosarcoma protuberans, malignant schwannoma, malignant fibrous histiocytoma, leiomyosarcoma, fibrosarcoma, spindle cell squamous carcinoma (Figure 9.26), angiosarcoma, desmoplastic Spitz naevus (Table 9.2), cellular blue naevus, and melanoma of soft parts (Barr *et al.*, 1980; Egbert *et al.*, 1988).

In most cases, the tumour cells exhibit moderate or strong *positivity for S-100* (Warner *et al.*, 1984). This feature is very helpful, since it distinguishes the tumour from spindle cell squamous carcinoma and

Table 9.2 Desmoplastic Spitz naevus *vs* desmoplastic melanoma

	Desmoplastic Spitz naevus	*Desmoplastic melanoma*
Site	most often extremities	most often head and neck
Age peak incidence	early adulthood	late adulthood
Atypical intraepidermal melanocytes	absent	often present
Atypia dermal component	mild	mild – marked
Mitoses	rare	rare – frequent
Necrosis	absent	sometimes
'Maturation'	often present	absent

fibroblastic proliferations. Immunostaining for keratin is useful in order to exclude spindle cell squamous carcinoma. Ultrastructurally, the tumour cells are said to combine the features of fibroblasts (prominent rough endoplasmic reticulum, intercellular collagen; From *et al.*, 1983) with a resemblance to Schwann cells (basal laminae, interdigitating cell processes, microtubules, intercellular junctions; Warner *et al.*, 1981; DiMaio *et al.*, 1982; Dardick and Rippstein, 1987). Melanosomes are often absent. The ultrastructural Schwann cell features should not lead to a diagnosis of malignant schwannoma: as discussed previously (p. 71), a resemblance to Schwann cells is seen at the base of many naevi, and occasionally also in primary and metastatic melanoma, and this may be related to the close embryologic relationship of melanocytes and Schwann cells. Importantly, *desmoplastic melanoma preferentially metastasizes to regional lymph nodes, thereby exhibiting metastatic behaviour more in keeping with melanoma than with malignant schwannoma.* Interestingly, some of these metastases show the histological features of conventional melanoma, while local recurrences usually retain the distinctive appearance of desmoplastic melanoma (Walsh *et al.*, 1988).

Rarely, cutaneous metastases of a conventional melanoma exhibit a spindle cell type and an associated increase in collagen, similar to that of desmoplastic melanoma. In such cases the ultrastructural features of the tumour cells show a resemblance to Schwann cells (DiMaio *et al.*, 1982; Dabbs and Bolen, 1984; Nyong'o *et al.*, 1986; Dardick and Rippstein, 1987).

9.10   Borderline and minimal deviation melanoma

Some melanomas show only mild cytological atypia and a rather regular architecture, and thus resemble benign naevi. Some authors have used the terms 'borderline melanoma' and 'minimal deviation melanoma' to indicate these tumours, the former being limited to the epidermis and papillary dermis, while the latter extend into the reticular dermis (Reed *et al.*, 1975; Muhlbauer *et al.*, 1983; Barr *et al.*, 1984), but not into the subcutis (Mihm and Googe, 1990).

The concept implicitly suggests that 'borderline' morphology may be associated with a biological behaviour intermediate between that of benign naevi and melanomas. Indeed, a less aggressive behaviour of such melanomas was claimed (Phillips *et al.*, 1986), but the statistical validity of this claim was subsequently questioned (Vollmer, 1987) and cases which behaved aggressively have been documented (Becker *et al.*, 1979; Warner *et al.*, 1980a).

In view of the difficulties in differentiating these tumours from benign lesions, one would need strong arguments that each case of a series has been diagnosed correctly, since an admixture with benign lesions would obviously also result in a spurious impression of a less aggressive behaviour of the group as a whole.

We have encountered several melanomas with little cytological atypia which did not give rise to clinically evident metastases until after 10 years or more. However, such a protracted course can also be seen in melanomas with more marked cytological atypia, and, conversely, in some melanomas with little atypia the disease runs a rapid clinical course. Indeed, such anecdotal observations cannot form the basis for any generalization about behaviour.

Histologically, the common denominator of these melanomas is the absence of immediately obvious cytological atypia; however, a subtle degree of nuclear enlargement, nucleolar prominence and lack of maturation, as well as subtle architectural features of malignancy are present (Figures 9.29 and 9.30). The presence of mitoses near the base

---

Figure 9.29   So-called borderline melanoma. (a) At this magnification, the lesion appears symmetrical and well demarcated (HE, × 20). (b) At a higher magnification, at one side of the tumour, there is a predominantly lentiginous spread of melanocytes over a distance of a dozen rete ridges (HE, × 90). (c) Throughout the tumour, compact, closely apposed nests of slightly atypical oval or polygonal melanocytes are seen. Mitoses are also found at the base (one is seen left of centre). The tumour metastasized after several years (HE, × 370).

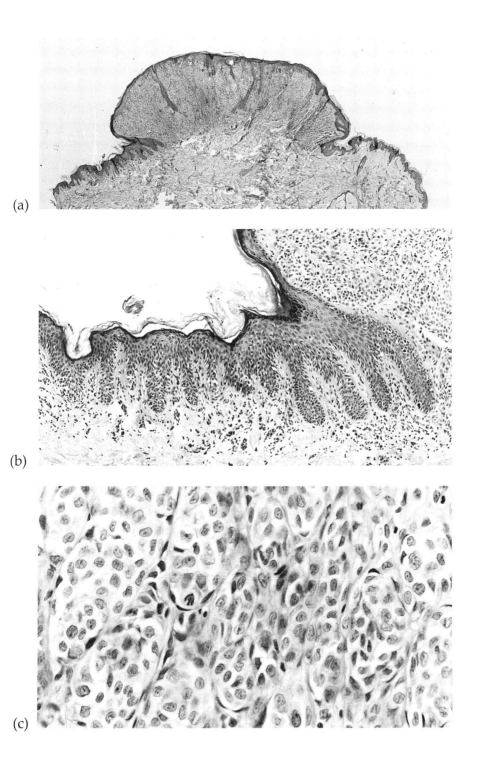

(a)

(b)

(c)

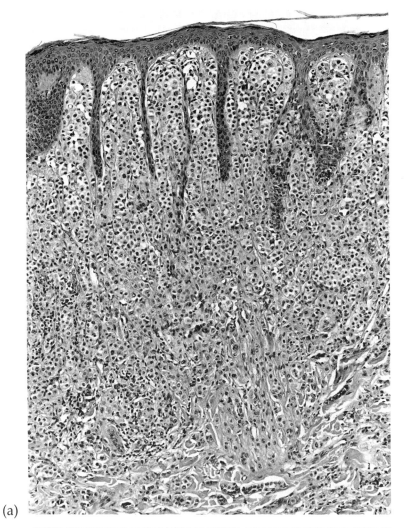

of the tumour is an important feature in the diagnosis of malignancy.

In practice, the diagnosis of borderline and minimal deviation melanomas as a separate subgroup is fraught with difficulties. To begin with, the terminology is unfortunate: a melanoma with mild cytological atypia would start out as a borderline melanoma, and then become a minimal deviation melanoma when the reticular dermis is invaded, and subsequently become a conventional melanoma type after invasion of the subcutis. It is not logical to change the designation of melanoma subtype merely on the basis of the level of invasion. Also, there is no clear demarcation between 'common' melanoma and minimal deviation melanoma: the difference is a matter of degree, and it is very difficult to establish reproducible diagnostic criteria, i.e. to formulate precisely how much cytological atypia is compatible with minimal deviation melanoma, or when it is enough for the diagnosis to be one of the common melanoma types.

The problem has been accentuated by the fact that some experts in the field have subdivided these melanomas into no fewer than seven subtypes and 18 sub-subtypes (Muhlbauer *et al.*, 1983; Phillips *et al.*, 1986), a division which will appeal to the splitters but not to the lumpers! Some have spoken of 'minimal deviation patterns' in areas of otherwise obvious melanomas (Reed *et al.*, 1975). The benefit of identifying sub-subgroups in terms of prognosis has not been demonstrated. In view of the problems of demarcating the group as a whole from conventional melanoma, no purpose is served by the general pathologist attempting these subdivisions. It is certainly possible to identify melanomas with only minor degrees of cytological atypia, but this somewhat ill-defined entity continues to constitute a diagnostic challenge. At present, in view of the many unresolved problems, we do not advocate the diagnosis of borderline and minimal deviation melanoma as subgroups of melanoma in a routine setting of diagnostic histopathology. However, some melanoma types, described in the next subsections, would fall under the general heading of minimal deviation melanoma, but, in our opinion, they are sufficiently distinctive to be discussed separately.

◀ **Figure 9.30**   So-called minimal deviation melanoma. (a) There is a relatively bland, largely intradermal proliferation of monomorphic, rather small, polygonal melanocytes. Abrupt changes in cellular features or growth pattern are absent. Within the reticular dermis, the growth is infiltrating rather than pushing, the latter being more common in melanomas (HE, × 115). (b) The cytological features of these atypical epithelioid cells forming compact strands are indicative of malignancy. The tumour later metastasized (HE, × 370).

9.10.1   Verrucous naevoid melanoma

Under the name of 'verrucous pseudonaevoid melanoma', a rare type of melanoma has been described, which shows a *close architectural resemblance to the common benign papillomatous compound naevus*; this may lead to a misdiagnosis of benignity if insufficient attention is paid to the subtle signs of malignancy which distinguish it from its benign counterpart (Levene, 1980; Suster *et al.*, 1987). We have abbreviated the term 'pseudonaevoid' to 'naevoid', since the latter means 'naevus-like', whereas the former constitutes something of a tautology.

Verrucous naevoid melanoma is generally larger than benign papillomatous naevi: unusually large, acquired papillomatous melanocytic tumours should therefore be viewed with suspicion, and should be scrutinized for signs of malignancy. Like the papillomatous naevus, verrucous naevoid melanoma shows a papillomatous surface, with keratinous plugs trapped between the papillomatous projections (Figure 9.31). The epidermis is usually thin, but forms long, irregular rete ridges between which the markedly thickened papillary dermis contains nests and sheets of polygonal or oval melanocytes, which exhibit varying degrees of cytological atypia. Often there are readily apparent differences in cellular and nuclear size of melanocytes in different areas of the lesion, although within individual areas the tumour cells may appear rather monomorphic. Mitoses are present in the dermal part of the lesion, usually also at its base. Areas of continuous junctional proliferation of atypical melanocytes are seen, in contrast to benign papillomatous naevi, although this may also be a feature in dysplastic naevi (p. 193). Melanocyte ascent is often difficult to evaluate because of the marked epidermal thinning; it should be specifically looked for at the edges of the lesion, where the epidermis is often thickened. Pagetoid lateral intraepidermal spread is sometimes present, and we have seen several examples in which small subepidermal microsatellites were present at some distance from the primary tumour (Table 9.3).

Verrucous naevoid melanoma should not be confused with 'polypoid melanoma', a conventional, usually ulcerating, melanoma with exophytic growth pattern (p. 240).

9.10.2   Spindle cell melanoma resembling Spitz naevus ('spitzoid melanoma')

Some melanomas consisting largely or wholly of spindled tumour cells may exhibit a striking resemblance to the spindle cell type of Spitz naevus (Figures 9.32 and 9.33); they are sometimes referred to colloquially as 'spitzoid melanomas'. This is a heterogeneous group of tumours, in which the resemblance to Spitz naevus is attributable to different features in different cases.

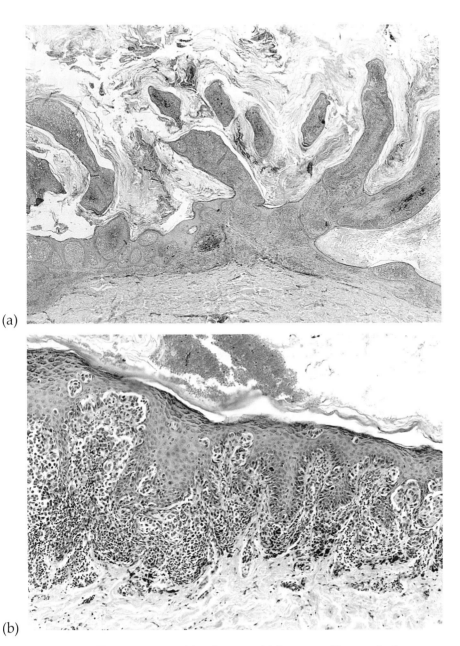

(a)

(b)

Figure 9.31 Verrucous naevoid melanoma. (a) Large papillary projections are covered by a very thick horn layer. An extensive proliferation of melanocytes is present mainly within the papillary dermis (HE, × 20). (b) Irregularly distributed melanocytes at the dermoepidermal junction; some ascend into the upper parts of the epidermis. In this case, satellites were present at the time of diagnosis (HE, × 90).

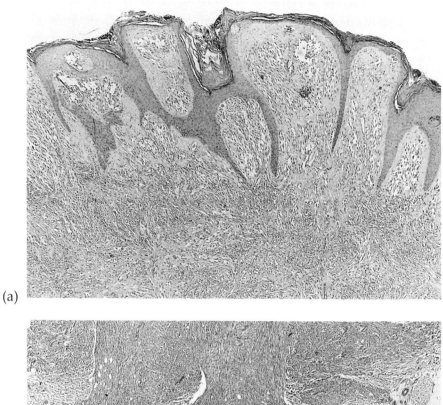

(a)

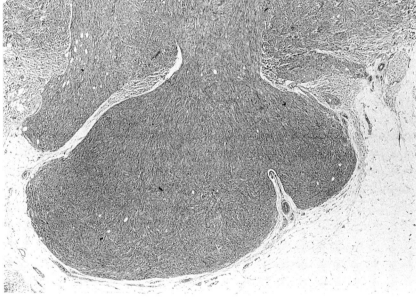

(b)

Figure 9.32 'Spitzoid' melanoma ('malignant Spitz naevus'). (a) The superficial portion shows a distinct resemblance to Spitz naevus (HE, × 45). (b) Unlike Spitz naevus, the deep portion extends into the subcutis with a pushing, nodular growth pattern (HE, × 20).

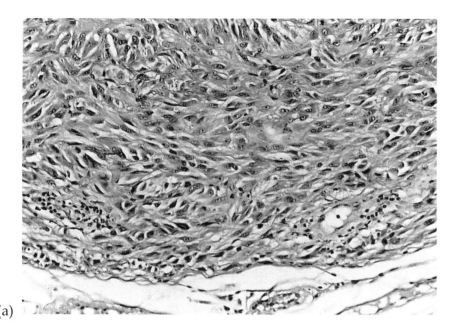

(a)

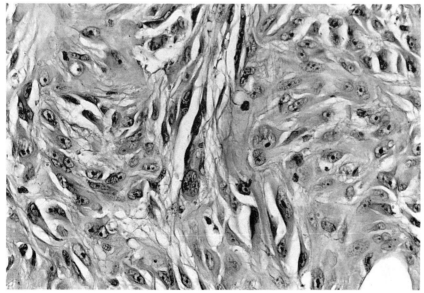

(b)

Figure 9.33 'Spitzoid' melanoma, same case as Figure 9.32. Tell-tale signs of malignancy in this tumour are found at the base: (a) A compact, densely cellular, pushing growth pattern is seen (HE, × 185). (b) At the base, the tumour cells remain large and pleomorphic, with vesicular nuclei containing a prominent nucleolus (HE, × 370).

Table 9.3 Verrucous naevoid melanoma *vs* papillomatous naevus

	Verrucous naevoid melanoma	*Papillomatous naevus*
Size	usually large	usually <0.6 cm
Shape	often asymmetrical	symmetrical
Epidermal melanocytic atypia	often present	absent
Continuous junctional proliferation	present	absent
Ascent of melanocytes	often present especially at margins	absent
Mitoses in dermal melanocytes	usually present	absent
Satellitosis	not uncommon	absent

NB: Despite the large number of differences of detail, on low power, verrucous naevoid melanoma is easily confused with a benign naevus.

The histological differences between Spitz naevi and 'spitzoid melanomas' may be subtle, requiring a very careful and detailed evaluation of many features (Okun, 1979; Peters and Goellner, 1986). It is only of limited value to point out the many differences between Spitz naevi and, say, superficial spreading melanoma; the much greater difficulty for the pathologist is the differentiation between Spitz naevus and these 'spitzoid' melanomas.

The differential diagnosis between Spitz naevus and melanoma has been discussed in Chapter 7 (p. 174; Table 7.2) and will be summarized only briefly here. Some important potential or definite indicators of malignancy are: large size, ulceration, extensive and confluent junctional activity, ascent of atypical melanocytes at the lateral margins of the lesion, distinct nuclear atypia, lack of 'maturation' at the base of the tumour, high mitotic rate, mitoses deep within the dermal component, presence of long, highly cellular fascicles within the dermis which often reach the subcutis, compact groups of cells and pushing borders at the base, irregular pigmentation, and the presence of many plasma cells in the inflammatory infiltrate (Okun, 1979; Smith *et al.*, 1989).

Oedema and telangiectasia in the upper dermis are often absent, but in Spitz naevi of adolescence and adulthood they are also often absent,

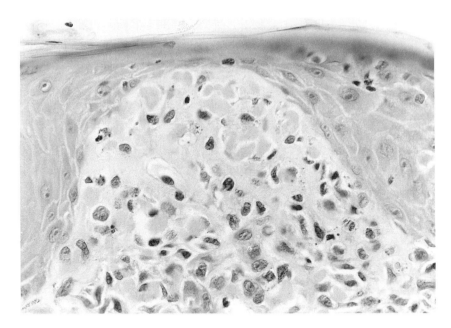

Figure 9.34 Small amorphous eosinophilic globules at the dermoepidermal interface and subepidermal region (Kamino bodies) are found in a minority of melanomas. They are usually smaller than those in Spitz naevi and show less tendency to become confluent. This melanoma showed unequivocal features of malignancy in other areas (HE, × 185).

so that as a negative feature this is of limited value. Furthermore, teleangiectasia is found in an appreciable proportion of melanomas so that its presence does not rule out malignancy. Its importance as a diagnostic feature must not be exaggerated.

It should be remembered that Kamino bodies (p. 164), commonly found in Spitz naevi, are occasionally present in melanoma, although in the latter case they tend to be smaller (Figure 9.34).

Spindle cell melanoma can be distinguished from other types of melanoma by the following features: the tumour is composed entirely of spindle cells, it involves the epidermis but does not possess a radial intraepidermal growth phase, and there is no pre-existent blue naevus or congenital naevus (Ainsworth *et al.*, 1979). In contrast to desmoplastic melanoma, there is no associated extensive collagen formation (Egbert *et al.*, 1988).

Once one is dealing with a subtype of melanoma which closely resembles Spitz naevus, itself notorious for its resemblance to melanoma, it will be apparent that diagnostic distinctions are refined to a degree which impinges on the limits of what it is practically possible to achieve. Indeed, it may occasionally be impossible to decide confidently whether a lesion is a Spitz naevus or a 'spitzoid' melanoma; it is then wise to explain this difficulty to the clinician and to decide on the optimal treatment on an individual basis, rather than to force oneself to make an unwarranted diagnosis.

Recently, Smith and colleagues (1989) described a group of tumours which they designated *malignant Spitz naevi*. These tumours, which occurred mainly under the age of 30, and which were located mostly on the head and neck and extremities, differed from Spitz naevus in their large size (usually over 1 cm), extension into the subcutis with an expansile growth pattern, and their capacity to metastasize to lymph nodes, which occurred in six out of 32 cases. In these six instances, only one node was involved. However, all 30 patients of whom follow-up data were available, including all six with nodal metastases, were alive without disease after a mean interval of six years. Consequently, the possibility of 'benign metastasis' similar to that encountered with some cellular blue naevi (p. 124) was raised. Indeed, in retrospect, some of the data of the series of 'minimal deviation melanomas' published by Phillips *et al.* (1986) may support this notion: of this series of 21 patients, nine had a 'Spitz variant' tumour, and all of these patients, eight of whom were under 25 years of age, were without evidence of disease at last follow-up, whereas three of the other 12 patients had died of disease or had a recurrence. These data appear to confirm the idea that such spitzoid tumours, even in the presence of deep penetration and a pushing growth pattern, and even nodal metastases, carry an excellent prognosis.

However, a note of caution should immediately be added at this point: the number of cases with nodal metastases in the report of Smith and colleagues (1989) is small and the folow-up is short; moreover, others have provided convincing reports of lethal widespread tumour metastasis in young patients with tumours greatly resembling Spitz naevus (e.g. Okun, 1979). Therefore, it is certainly premature to conclude that a close histological resemblance to Spitz naevus, in the presence of deep, pushing growth and regional lymph node involvement, indicates a benign course of disease in all instances. The matter clearly requires further study. We recently encountered a similar case (Figures 9.32 and 9.33) where a large regional lymph node metastasis, destroying the nodal parenchyma, developed after about one year. We would be hesitant to predict that this patient will not develop distant metastases.

9.11   Balloon cell melanoma
Balloon cell change, which has been described before in the context of balloon cell naevus (p. 90), may occur also in melanoma (Gardner and

Vazquez, 1970; Aloi *et al.*, 1988); melanocytes with balloon cell change are large and possess copious amounts of pale, finely vacuolated cytoplasm, which often contains a small amount of dust-like melanin pigment (Figure 9.35). Ultrastructurally, the cytoplasmic ballooning corresponds to enlargement, degeneration and fusion of melanosomes (p. 92).

Architectural features of malignancy include pagetoid lateral spread within the epidermis, marked variation in architectural and cellular features of the dermal component and irregular pigmentation. In balloon cell melanoma, nuclear atypia is variable and may be mild. Mitoses may be scarce, whereas mitoses are consistently absent in balloon cell naevi (Su *et al.*, 1985). In some balloon cell naevi, the nuclear size is similar to that in some balloon cell melanomas. The tumour often extends deeply into the reticular dermis or into the subcutis, forming lobated cell masses (Table 9.4).

More commonly than other melanoma types, balloon cell melanoma gives rise to multiple cutaneous and subcutaneous metastases (Peters and Su, 1985). Balloon cell change is often more prominent in metas-

Table 9.4 Balloon cell melanoma *vs* balloon cell naevus

	Balloon cell melanoma	*Balloon cell naevus*
Pagetoid upward and lateral spread	often	absent
Ulceration	present or absent	absent
Dermal penetration	often deep reticular dermis or subcutis	papillary or superficial reticular dermis
Size	small or large	usually <1 cm
Nests	irregular size/shape	less irregular
Nuclear atypia	various degrees, nuclei may be small	absent
Mitoses	usually some present, but may be rare	absent
'Maturation'	absent	present
Pigmentation	may be markedly irregular	usually regular, faint
Multinucleate cells	not uncommon	uncommon (among balloon cells)

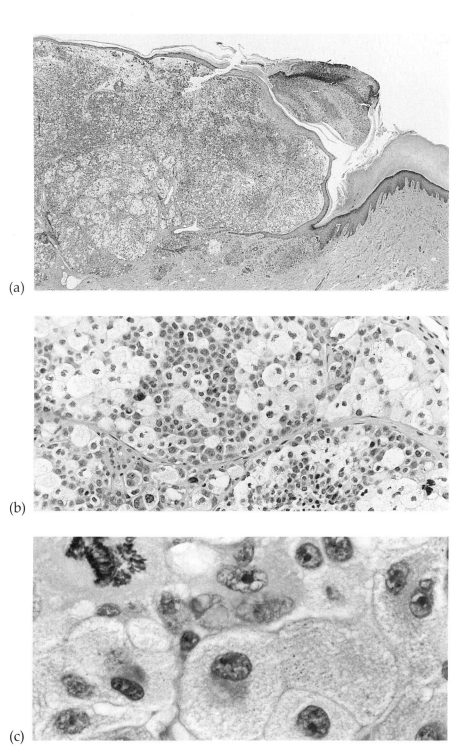

(a)

(b)

(c)

tases or in local recurrences, and may be present in metastases of melanomas not showing this phenomenon (Friedman *et al.*, 1982). Rarely, balloon cell melanoma presents with a metastatic lesion (Akslen and Myking, 1989). When such a lesion is totally amelanotic, the differential diagnosis may pose problems. Immunostaining for S-100 can then be of help.

9.12   Intradermal melanoma arising in intradermal naevus

Rarely a primary melanoma is wholly confined to the dermis while the overlying epidermis is normal and uninvolved; in or adjacent to some of these melanomas, a pre-existent acquired intradermal naevus may be recognized (Okun and Bauman, 1965; Okun *et al.*, 1974; Benisch *et al.*, 1980). Histologically these tumours may be mistaken for cutaneous metastases of melanoma of unknown origin, especially when a pre-existent intradermal naevus is not present in the slides or is not recognized as such.

Not surprisingly, the clinical appearance is usually deceptively benign, the lesion presenting as a regularly shaped lightly pigmented nodule, often without irregularities in pigmentation and without ulceration. Numbers of reported cases are small, but there may be a predilection for the head. As a result of the intradermal origin and late detection, the tumour often extends into the subcutis (Benisch *et al.*, 1980).

Histologically, the melanoma and intradermal naevus are found side by side or closely intermingled. Tumour cells are epithelioid or fusiform; balloon cell change was seen in one case (Okun *et al.*, 1974). The appearance of the malignant component may be very similar to a cutaneous metastasis. Step sections throughout the lesion are needed in order to exclude the presence of a small malignant intraepidermal component, or to detect a small remnant of an intradermal naevus. Obviously, meticulous clinical investigation of the skin is needed to exclude the presence of a partially or completely regressed primary melanoma elsewhere.

◀ **Figure 9.35**   Balloon cell melanoma. (a) Exophytic tumour, partly covered by a crust; irregular nests and aggregates of pale tumour cells (HE, × 20). (b) Intermingling of conventional epithelioid tumour cells and large cells with copious, pale cytoplasm. Note tendency to necrosis (bottom right) (HE, × 185). (c) These tumour cells show a large amount of finely granular or microvacuolar cytoplasm; cellular borders are clearly defined. Nuclei show variation in size and shape, contain a prominent nucleolus and are partly hyperchromatic. Note atypical mitotic figure (HE, × 920).

9.13   Malignant blue naevus

Malignant blue naevus (Goldenhersh *et al.*, 1988; Nakano *et al.*, 1988; Temple-Camp *et al.*, 1988) is very rare type of melanoma which arises in a cellular blue naevus or, less restrictively, exhibits a striking architectural and cytological resemblance to cellular blue naevus. The tumour has to be distinguished from cellular blue naevus, deep penetrating naevus, spindle cell and desmoplastic melanoma, and melanoma of soft parts (Kuhn *et al.*, 1988). Since the number of well-documented cases is small, diagnostic criteria are not as well established as is desirable. Goldenhersh and colleagues (1988) reviewed 10 well documented cases and added one case.

The tumour occurs in a wide age range (10–80 years; mean, 40 years). The scalp is the most common single site, while the foot also appears to be a favoured site; other sites are scattered over the body. Almost all reported cases concern white patients. There appears to be no sex preference.

Most commonly, the tumour appears as a bluish or black cutaneous nodule, often 3 cm or more in diameter, and there may be a history of recent growth of a long-standing nodule.

Histologically, the lesion resembles cellular blue naevus, but there are *areas of markedly increased nuclear atypia, frequent mitoses including atypical ones and, in about half of the cases, necrosis.* An epithelioid cell type may occur in places. Tumour cells sometimes palisade around necrotic foci (Hernandez, 1973). The overlying epidermis is uninvolved. S-100 positivity is seen in the majority of tumours (Kuhn *et al.*, 1988).

Sometimes, but not always, the disease runs a protracted course, regional lymph node metastases becoming clinically evident after many years, and there may be prolonged survival after that. Metastases have to be distinguished from the commoner lymph node deposits ('benign metastases') occurring with cellular blue naevus (p. 124). In genuine malignant blue naevus, widespread distant metastasis leading to death has been reported in about one-third of cases (Ginzburg *et al.*, 1986).

9.14   Congenital melanoma; materno-fetal metastasis

Very rarely malignancy develops in a giant congenital naevus while the baby is still *in utero* (Campbell *et al.*, 1987; Schneiderman *et al.*, 1987). Eight cases of congenital melanoma without an associated congenital naevus are on record (reviewed by Prose *et al.*, 1987). Some of these metastasized; long survival of four of these patients with either lymph node metastasis or local recurrence suggests that the course is not always as aggressive as these findings might lead one to expect. To our knowledge, feto-maternal metastasis of fetal melanoma has not been reported. Giant congenital naevi are occasionally associated with naevus cell aggregates within the placental tissue (p. 154); it is very important that this is not confused with metastatic congenital melanoma.

A small number of cases of advanced metastatic melanoma during pregnancy, giving rise to metastasis to the placenta and fetus, and leading to death of both mother and child shortly after birth, have been reported (Trozak *et al.*, 1975; Campbell *et al.*, 1987). This very dramatic course of disease is extremely rare and all reported cases concerned patients with advanced metastatic melanoma.

9.15 Childhood melanoma

Melanomas occurring before puberty have been estimated at about 0.3–0.4% of all melanomas (data reviewed by Trozak *et al.*, 1975); cases before the age of 20 years amount to almost 2% (Reintgen *et al.*, 1989).

The earlier literature on childhood melanoma is often unreliable because many reported cases were actually Spitz naevi. Saksela and Rintala (1968), revising 17 cases initially diagnosed as childhood melanoma, were able to confirm the diagnosis only twice; 13 other lesions were reclassified as various types of benign naevus, and the remaining two cases as malignant tumours of uncertain nature.

Clinical features of melanoma occurring before the age of 20 years were assessed recently (Bader *et al.*, 1985; Reintgen *et al.*, 1989). There is no sex preference; in boys, predominant sites are the head, neck and trunk; in girls, the arms and legs. A significant number of childhood melanomas arise within giant congenital naevi and, as indicated in the previous section, these melanomas may rarely arise even before birth. Some childhood melanomas occur in patients with xeroderma pigmentosum (Boddie and McBride, 1985) or the familial dysplastic naevus syndrome (Roth *et al.*, 1990).

When controlled for tumour thickness and ulceration, overall survival of patients under the age of 20 years with stage I melanoma does not differ significantly from that in adults (Roth *et al.*, 1990); an overall 5-year survival rate of 77% was reported (Reintgen *et al.*, 1989).

The main histological differential diagnosis of melanoma in childhood is Spitz naevus, which at this age is much more common than melanoma. The histological features of melanoma in childhood are usually the same as in adulthood. However, 'Spitz-like' melanomas appear to be more common before adulthood (Smith *et al.*, 1989) and this adds to the difficulty of distinguishing the two in young individuals.

9.16 Melanoma arising in congenital naevus

Malignant tumours arising within congenital naevi form a heterogeneous group of tumours. Those occurring in small and intermediate-

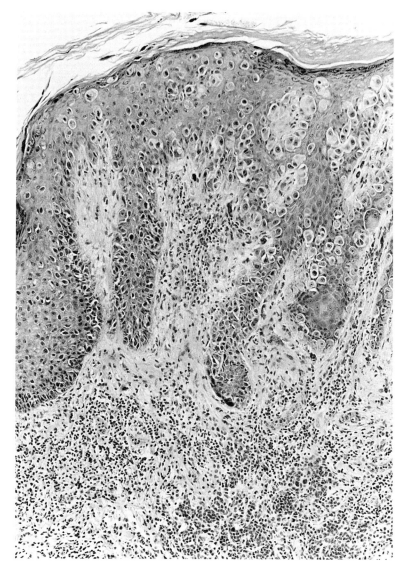

Figure 9.36   *In situ* melanoma overlying intradermal congenital naevus (HE, ×
115).

sized congenital naevi originate in the superficial portion of the naevus
(Figure 9.36) and show the features of common types of melanoma. In
contrast, malignant transformation in giant congenital naevi often
occurs deep within the dermal component and may show a large

variety of appearances: they may resemble malignant blue naevus, malignant schwannoma, undifferentiated small round cell tumours, or may consist of undifferentiated spindle cells, sometimes with the formation of lamellar formations resembling meissnerian corpuscles; heterologous mesenchymal (rhabdo-, lipo-) differentiation has also been reported (Hendrickson and Ross, 1981; Weidner et al., 1985).

9.17 Multiple melanoma

About 5% of melanoma patients develop more than one primary melanoma (Moseley et al., 1979). There is no obvious sex preference. The prognosis appears to depend on the thickness and stage of the thickest melanoma (Moseley et al., 1979). Obviously, the possibility of a cutaneous metastasis rather than a second primary tumour should be envisaged (section 9.16.1). The possibility of multiple epidermotropic metastases should be considered very seriously before diagnosing multiple primary melanomas (Warner et al., 1980b), especially when multiple tumours occur within a short time span or involve the same region of the body.

Rarely there may be very large numbers of tumours, even totalling over a hundred (Kahn and Donaldson, 1970; Sigg et al., 1988). Most of these cases occur in the context of the dysplastic naevus syndrome (p. 188).

An extraordinary case of over a hundred small melanomas arising from hair follicles on the face and trunk of a 79-year-old man with a history of long-term cutaneous exposure to insecticides was reported in the German literature (Sigg et al., 1988). This report mentions three similar unreported cases also involving elderly patients. Histologically, a proliferation of medium-sized or large atypical melanocytes arranged in lentiginous or pagetoid pattern within the hair follicles and extending into the surrounding adventitial and reticular dermis was present. The possibility of multiple epidermotropic metastases must be excluded (see below).

9.17.1 The differential diagnosis of primary and secondary cutaneous melanoma

The histological distinction between a cutaneous metastasis and a primary melanoma can usually be made with reasonable confidence (Table 9.5). Cutaneous metastases (including satellites and in transit metastases) usually lie totally within the dermis or subcutis without involvement of the overlying epidermis. However, in a minority of cases, there is involvement of the overlying epidermis; such cases are

Table 9.5 Primary cutaneous melanoma *vs* cutaneous metastasis

	Primary melanoma	*Cutaneous metastasis*
Epidermal involvement	usually present, equals or exceeds dermal component	usually absent; if present, <dermal component
Ascending tumour cells	usually present	usually absent
Epidermal collarette	usually absent	sometimes present
Cellular atypia	may be prominent	may be prominent
Cellular pleomorphism	often considerable	often monotonous cytology
Inflammatory infiltrate	usually present	often absent
Reactive fibrosis	may be prominent	usually mild
Tumour cells in vascular lumina	usually not seen	often present

designated *epidermotropic melanoma metastases* (Kornberg *et al.*, 1978). When the epidermis is involved, the lateral extension of the dermal component exceeds that of the epidermal component. Ascent and pagetoid spread of tumour cells is occasionally seen and the epidermis may be thinned, while the dermal papillae are widened. In superficially located dermal metastases, elongated epidermal rete ridges and the skin appendages at the lateral borders are often turned inward, resulting in the formation of a *collarette*. Not infrequently groups of tumour cells are seen in vascular lumina, a feature which is only seldom present in primary melanomas (Kornberg *et al.*, 1978). Repigmentation of cutaneous amelanotic metastases at the site of contact with the epidermis was reported by Botha and Lennox (1954).

At least as important for the distinction is the *relatively bland appearance of cutaneous metastases*, as compared to primary lesions; this difference is especially helpful when small lesions are concerned. Primary tumours generally show much more variation in morphology of the tumour cells, as well as an inflammatory and fibrotic host response (Elder *et al.*, 1979). A typical small cutaneous metastasis usually consists of an ill-defined intradermal aggregate of tumour cells, which are often highly abnormal but all of which show a similar appearance and which are associated with no or very mild dermal reactive changes (Figure 9.37). In some lesions there may be inflamma-

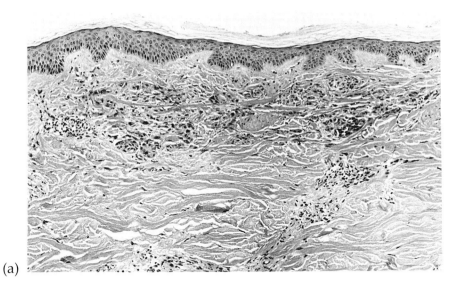

(a)

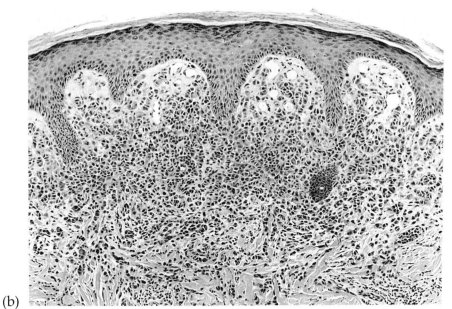

(b)

Figure 9.37 *In transit* metastases of melanoma. (a) An ill-defined aggregate of tumour cells is present in the superficial reticular dermis. Note the virtual absence of an inflammatory or fibrotic response (HE, × 35). (b) Subepidermal *in transit* metastasis. In this case the epidermis is slightly elevated but uninvolved, and rete ridges are slightly curved inward at the sides. There is some oedema, but there is only a slight inflammatory and fibrotic response (HE, × 35).

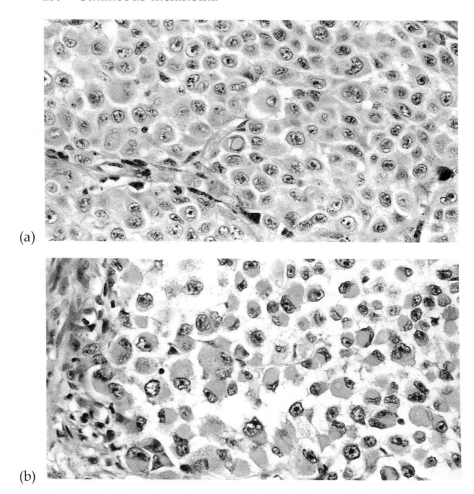

(a)

(b)

Figure 9.38   Metastatic melanoma, epithelioid cell type. (a) Large, loosely cohesive aggregates are formed; cellular borders are ill-defined, and the nuclei possess large nucleoli. Note nuclear pseudoinclusion near centre. Such features are highly suggestive of melanoma rather than carcinoma (HE, × 370). (b) The tumour cells dissociate from one another and possess a relatively large amount of dense, homogeneous, ground glass-like eosinophilic cytoplasm (HE, × 370).

tion or regression, but the overall aspect is still less varied than in primary lesions.

In some cases, a cutaneous metastasis has to be differentiated from an intradermal naevus, a distinction mainly based on cytological features and the absence of 'maturation'.

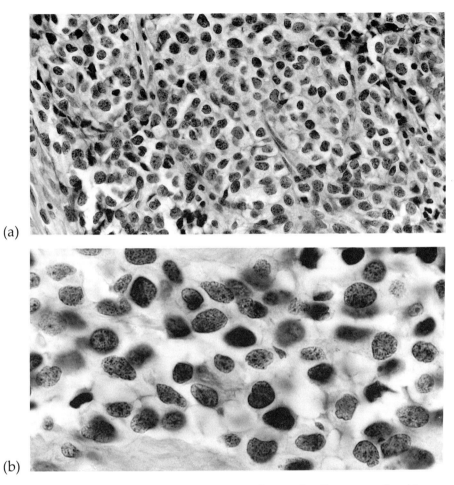

(a)

(b)

Figure 9.39 Metastatic melanoma, small cell type. Small tumour cells with ovoid hyperchromatic nuclei, inconspicuous nucleoli and a small amount of pale, poorly defined cytoplasm. (a) HE, × 370. (b) HE, × 920.

9.18   Primary and metastatic melanoma simulating other neoplasms

The cell type most commonly seen in metastatic melanoma is the epithelioid type, which usually exhibits a large atypical nucleus and well-developed cytoplasm (Figure 9.38), although in some instances the nucleus is small and the cytoplasm inconspicuous (Figure 9.39). There is usually a diffuse growth pattern, but the pattern is also dependent on the architecture of the tissue involved (Figures 9.40–9.42).

Melanoma may simulate a wide variety of tumours, including

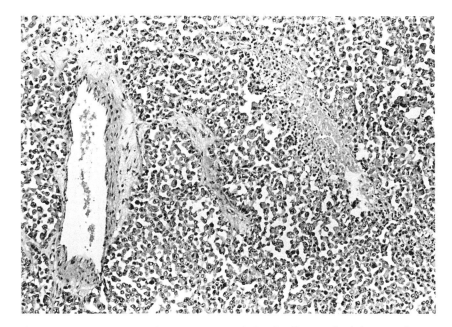

Figure 9.40 Metastasis of melanoma, epithelioid cell type. Such large and dissociating sheets of round tumour cells, with areas of necrosis, are suggestive of melanoma (HE, × 90).

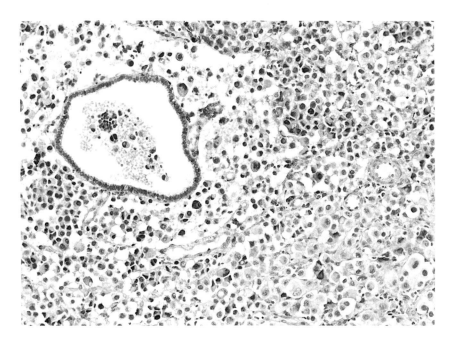

Figure 9.41 Melanoma metastasis in endometrium. Endometrial gland is engulfed by epithelioid tumour cells within the stroma (HE, × 185).

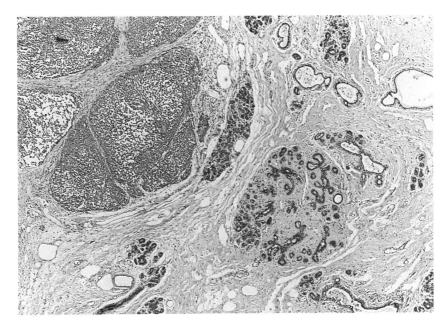

Figure 9.42 Metastasis of melanoma in breast. Well-defined large nodules of dissociated tumour cells are seen; there is no contiguity with lobular or ductal epithelium. Metastases in the breast are often misdiagnosed initially as primary carcinomas (HE, × 20).

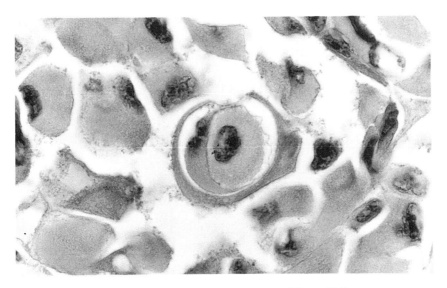

Figure 9.43 Tumour cell-tumour cell 'cannibalism' (HE, × 920).

lymphoma, undifferentiated carcinoma, adenocarcinoma, a variety of sarcomas and many others. When the case presents with an amelanotic metastasis, the diagnosis poses even greater difficulties. In general, once the possibility of melanoma is seriously considered and investigated, the diagnosis can usually be established conclusively, by means of melanin stains together with a panel of antibodies such as HMB-45 and antibodies to S-100, vimentin, keratins, epithelial membrane antigen and leukocyte common antigen. The danger lies in the fact that the possibility of melanoma may not be considered at all, because at first glance the cytological or architectural features of the tumour suggest a totally different diagnosis.

In the paragraph on cytological features of melanoma (p. 227), the spectrum of the more common appearances of melanoma cells has been discussed. Here, we shall focus on those metastatic melanomas which, because of uncommon cytological or architectural features, may lead to confusion with other malignant tumours.

Tumour cell cannibalism (Figure 9.43) results in concentrically arranged cells which may at first glance resemble a small horn pearl, indicative of squamous carcinoma.

A conspicuous *signet-ring cell appearance* is found in some primary and metastatic melanomas (Figure 9.44; Sheibani and Battifora, 1988; Nahkleh *et al.*, 1990). In some instances, cytoplasmic diastase-resistant PAS-positivity is detected, increasing the resemblance to metastatic adenocarcinoma. Mucicarmine stains are negative and on immunohistochemistry and electron microscopy, the centres of the tumour cells are found to contain accumulated vimentin filaments (Sheibani and Battifora, 1988). Usually, the tumour cells are at least faintly positive for S-100 and HMB-45, while no reactivity is found with epithelial markers and leukocyte common antigen.

As described previously (p. 259), metastatic melanoma rarely consists exclusively of *spindled cells* (Figures 9.45 and 9.46), with ultrastructural features resembling Schwann cells, and with associated collagen production, even when the primary tumour does not show any resemblance to desmoplastic melanoma. A search for scattered inconspicuous epithelioid cells and intranuclear cytoplasmic pseudo-inclusions may be rewarding; since they can usually be found, and aid in the differentiation from several spindle cell neoplasms.

Rarely, melanoma may be composed largely of *bizarre giant cells* (Figure 9.47), resulting in a resemblance to malignant fibrous histiocytoma or liposarcoma (Lodding *et al.*, 1990). A dense *infiltrate of neutrophils*, which may accumulate and degenerate within tumour giant cells, is occasionally seen in such cases.

A small number of melanomas with *metaplastic cartilage and bone* formation have been reported (Grunwald *et al.*, 1985; Moreno *et al.*,

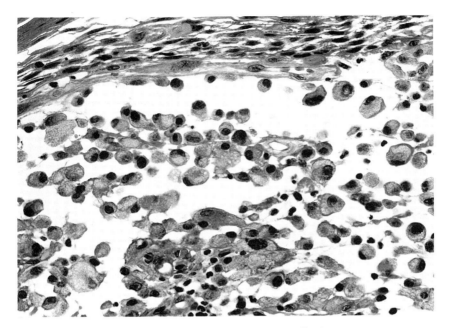

Figure 9.44 Melanoma cells simulating signet-ring cell adenocarcinoma (HE, × 370).

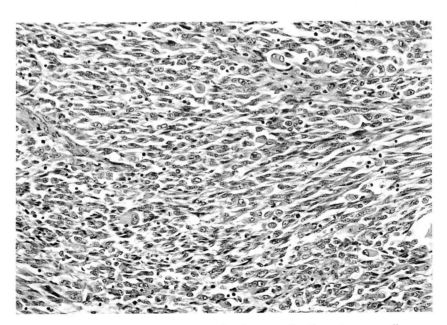

Figure 9.45 Lymph node metastasis of melanoma. Fusiform tumour cells predominate, but there are also scattered polygonal and round tumour cells with more copious cytoplasm, highly suggestive of melanoma (HE, × 185).

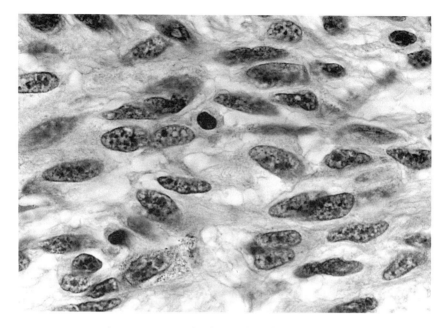

Figure 9.46 Fusiform tumour cells of spindle cell melanoma, one of which contains a scatter of small melanin granules (HE, × 920).

1986; Nakagawa *et al.*, 1990). Most of these tumours were of the desmoplastic variety.

Occasionally, *balloon cell change* is seen in a melanoma metastasis, even when this was not present in the primary tumour (Figure 9.48). Marked cytoplasmic pallor may result in appearances suggestive of metastatic renal carcinoma, while very marked macrovacuolar change of the cytoplasm may occasionally lead to a close resemblance to liposarcoma (Lodding *et al.*, 1990).

A conspicuous growth pattern of *compact ribbons with transversely oriented nuclei* (Levene, 1980) may simulate metastatic neuroendocrine carcinoma.

Prominent branching thin-walled blood vessels, superficially mimicking a 'staghorn' appearance, occurs in some melanomas, both primary and metastatic, and may lead to confusion with haemangiopericytoma (Nahkleh *et al.*, 1990).

Extensive *dissociation of tumour cells* with adherence of tumour cells to the surrounding stroma may architecturally simulate alveolar rhabdomyosarcoma (Figure 9.49). *Pseudopapillary patterns* may be produced by tumour cells adhering to fibrovascular stalks. Large

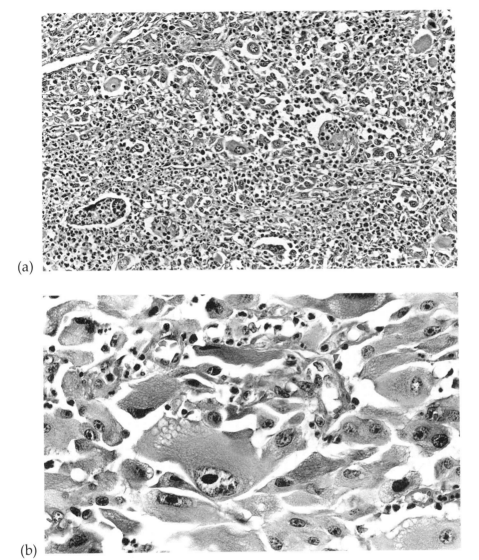

(a)

(b)

Figure 9.47 Metastatic melanoma with large, bizarre tumour cells and an admixture of neutrophils, some of which accumulate within tumour giant cells. (a) HE, × 90. (b) HE, × 370.

sheets of tumour cells with extensive dissociation occasionally mimic malignant lymphoma with diffuse architecture. In such instances, the

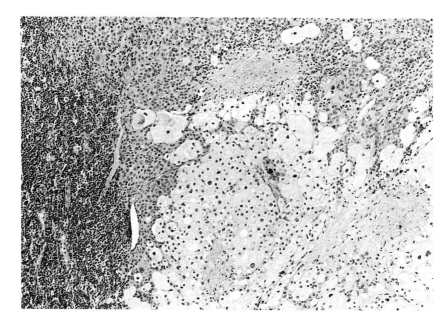

Figure 9.48 Lymph node metastasis of melanoma with focal balloon cell change. This may occur in the absence of balloon cell change in the primary tumour (HE, × 90).

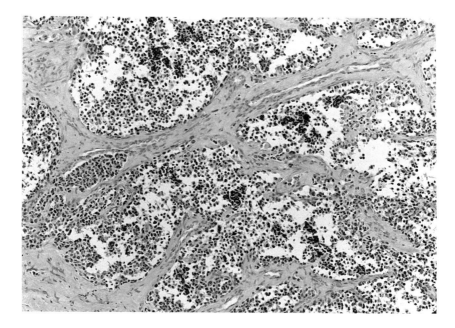

Figure 9.49 Metastatic melanoma, 'pseudoalveolar' pattern resulting in a resemblance to alveolar rhabdomyosarcoma. Tumour cells line stromal septa and dissociate within irregular spaces. Cytological features, clinical data and additional stains distinguish the tumour from rhabdomyosarcoma (HE, × 90).

cytological features and clinical context, as well as additional immunocytochemistry will establish the correct diagnosis.

Primary and metastatic melanoma may rarely induce a conspicuous
myxoid stromal reaction, so that various myxoid tumours (myxoid
variants of malignant fibrous histiocytoma, liposarcoma, rhabdomyosarcoma and chondrosarcoma, malignant sweat gland tumours,
pleomorphic adenoma, etc.) may be mimicked (Bhuta *et al.*, 1986;
Nottingham and Slater, 1988; Urso *et al.*, 1990). Large amounts of
connective tissue-type mucin, PAS-negative and strongly positive for
Alcian blue and colloidal iron, and sensitive to hyaluronidase treatment, accumulate between tumour cells and reactive stromal cells.
Myxoid malignant schwannoma, which may also be S-100 positive,
should be considered when there is no history of melanoma, and when
the tumour is large, solitary and deeply located without cutaneous involvement, and blends intimately with nerve bundles (Bhuta *et al.*, 1986).
Dissociation of tumour cells may lead to irregular empty spaces and
sometimes a *pseudoglandular pattern* (Figure 9.50). Melanin may be
difficult to demonstrate; however, the tumour cells are S-100 positive
and melanosomes may be identified on electron microscopy (Bhuta *et
al.*, 1986; Rocamora *et al.*, 1988).

Melanoma has been reported to present with an ovarian metastasis
consisting of large epithelioid cells or of smaller oval cells with oval to
spindle-shaped nuclei, the histology being suggestive of an ovarian
stromal tumour (Fitzgibbons *et al.*, 1987). There is usually, but not
always, a history of previous cutaneous melanoma. S-100, usually
positive in melanoma metastases but negative in granulosa cell tumours,
is useful in this differential diagnosis.

9.18.1 *Immunohistological diagnosis of melanoma*

In view of the difficulties that may occur in diagnosing amelanotic
metastatic melanoma, especially in the absence of an obvious primary,
it appears appropriate to discuss in some detail the usefulness of
immunohistochemistry in this diagnosis.

As discussed in Chapter 2, it is imperative to use a panel of antibodies rather than one only; furthermore, *the total pattern of immuno-
reactivities should be weighed against the clinical and histological data*,
in order to minimize the chance of a faulty diagnosis. As a routine, we
use a panel of antibodies to S-100 protein, vimentin, various keratins
and leukocyte common antigen, and HMB-45. Depending on the given
context, this panel is supplemented with other antibodies.

Anti S-100 antibodies, which are applicable to paraffin sections, are
perhaps the most important ones in the diagnosis of metastatic mel-

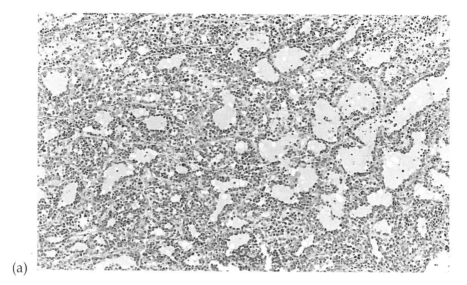

(a)

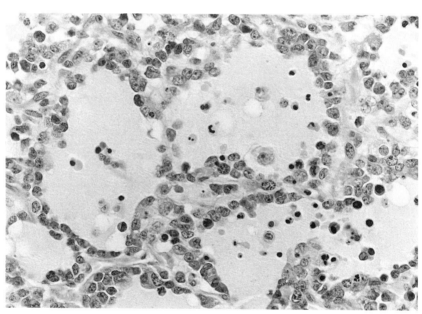

(b)

Figure 9.50 Melanoma metastasis, 'pseudoglandular' pattern. (a) There is a conspicuous pattern of irregular gland-like spaces, due to accumulation of mesenchymal-type mucins (HE, × 90). (b) Tumour cells line thin stromal septa, from which some dissociate and degenerate within the pools of mucin (HE, × 370).

anoma. Most melanomas, including the amelanotic ones, are immuno-reactive with antibodies to S-100 (p. 23 Gaynor *et al.*, 1981; Springall *et al.*, 1983). Other S-100 positive tumours include peripheral nerve tumours, granular cell tumour, chondroma, chordoma, lipoma and liposarcoma, paraganglioma, several salivary gland tumours, myo-epithelial tumours of various organs, histiocytosis X (Schmitt and Bacchi, 1989) and a variety of adenocarcinomas, especially those of the salivary gland, breast, kidney, endometrium and ovary (Drier *et al.*, 1987; Herrera *et al.*, 1988). However, this cross-reactivity with non-melanocytic tumours is rarely a major problem, since the latter can usually be distinguished from melanoma on clinical and morphological grounds. S-100 immunohistochemistry has also been advocated for the detection of small numbers of melanoma cells in regional lymph nodes (p. 321).

Monoclonal antibody HMB-45 (Gown *et al.*, 1986; Duray *et al.*, 1988) is much more specific for melanocytic tumours (Colombari *et al.*, 1988; Ordónez *et al.*, 1988); if the differential diagnosis includes a non-melanocytic S-100 positive tumour, e.g. in the case of a salivary gland tumour (Podesta *et al.*, 1989), HMB-45 is a very useful antibody. However, although HMB-45 recognizes some melanomas that are S-100 negative (Bonetti *et al.*, 1989), it is on the whole less sensitive for melanoma. The antibody recognizes a premelanosomal glycoprotein (Zarbo *et al.*, 1990) explaining its high specificity for cells producing melanin (p. 23); however, in amelanotic melanoma only scattered cells are positive or the tumour is completely negative. Antibody NKI/beteb recognizes a different epitope of the same antigen (Vennegoor *et al.*, 1988), but in addition to the limitations of HMB-45, its sensitivity is greatly reduced in paraffin-embedded material.

Monoclonal antibody NKI/C3 (Van Duinen *et al.*, 1984; Vennegoor *et al.*, 1985) has also been used in the diagnosis of melanocytic tumours: however, in view of its considerable cross-reactivity with many non-melanocytic tumour types, we do not advocate its use for diagnostic purposes.

Anti-neuron specific enolase (Dhillon *et al.*, 1982), PGP 9.5, as well as a large number of other, less well-known monoclonal antibodies, often raised against incompletely characterized antigens, have also been used for the diagnosis of melanoma; we do not find these of significant additional diagnostic value, compared to the panel mentioned above.

Intermediate filaments are of interest mainly in the differential diag-nosis of melanoma *vs* carcinoma. Melanoma is usually strongly positive for vimentin, whereas most carcinomas are negative or show only weak positivity, but contain keratin filaments (Ramaekers *et al.*, 1983). Importantly, a minority of melanomas are also positive with a variety of antikeratin antibodies, especially on frozen sections (Gatter *et al.*, 1985; Miettinen and Franssila, 1989). The pattern of immunoreactivity with a series of antikeratin antibodies with restricted specificities and two-dimensional Western blot analysis indicates that such keratin expression is restricted to low molecular weight keratins (Zarbo *et al.*, 1990). The finding of keratin expression in some melanomas under-scores the importance of the use of panels of antibodies in tumour typing.

Epithelial membrane antigen (EMA) is occasionally expressed in melanocytic tumours; it may be especially apparent in type C cells of compound and intradermal naevi (Cramer, 1990), and very rarely it may be found in melanoma (Toublanc *et al.*, 1990).

Strong positivity with antisera to immunoglobulin heavy and light chains in tumour cells of a melanoma was reported by Montero (1987), which underscores the danger of basing the diagnosis on a very few antibodies or one only.

9.18.2   Ultrastructure of metastatic melanoma

Although the large majority of amelanotic melanoma metastases are diagnosable by means of a combination of clinical, histological and immunohistochemical data, there remain a few cases where only the ultrastructural demonstration of *melanosomes* provides the definitive diagnosis (Gibson and Goellner, 1988). It should be realized that in melanoma, abnormal melanosomes (Cesarini, 1971; Mintzis and Silvers, 1978; Mazur and Katzenstein, 1980) may be the only ones present, so that familiarity with the classic types of melanosome does not suffice (Figure 9.51). Such abnormal forms of melanosome in melanoma may be difficult to distinguish from other intracytoplasmic granules and vesicles unrelated to melanin synthesis, notably myelin figures and various types of secondary lysosome (Erlandson, 1987). Also, melanosomes may have been transferred to tumour cells from pre-exisiting melanocytes (Szpak *et al.*, 1988), a pitfall which must be borne in mind. Spindle cell melanoma and desmoplastic melanoma may show ultrastructural features of Schwann cells (p. 259).

Irregular microvillus-like cytoplasmic projections may be seen in melanoma cells (Mazur and Katzenstein, 1980). Melanoma cells rarely contain irregular cytoplasmic invaginations and lumina lined by slender, microvillus-like cytoplasmic extensions (Yum *et al.*, 1984). Features of Schwann cells, such as interdigitating cytoplasmic folds, may be present.

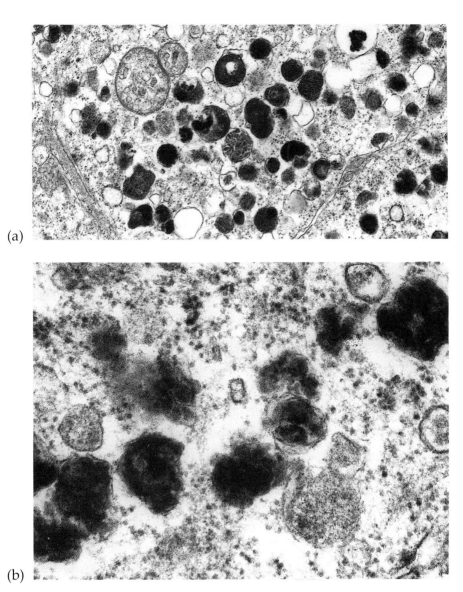

(a)

(b)

Figure 9.51 Metastatic melanoma. Melanosomes, with a granular, irregularly clumped content. Electron micrograph (a) × 17 400; (b) × 63 400.

9.19   Cutaneous and generalized melanosis in metastatic melanoma

Metastatic melanoma may rarely lead to generalized or focal pigmentation of the skin. Lysis of heavily pigmented tumour cells and hyperactivity of epidermal melanocytes (Rowden, 1980) probably both play a
role. Histologically, epidermal hyperpigmentation may be seen, and/or
dermal and subcutaneous histiocytes contain melanin which is
presumably synthesized by the tumour cells, carried and deposited *via*
the circulation (Silberberg *et al.*, 1968; Piérard, 1988). A variety of
internal organs may likewise become melanin-laden and there may be
accompanying melanuria, melanoptysis (black sputum) and dark-
brown discolouration of the serum (Eide, 1981).

References

Ackerman, A. B. (1980) Malignant melanoma, a unifying concept. *Hum. Pathol.*, **11**, 591–5.

Ackerman, A. B. (1982) Disagreements with the current classification of malignant melanomas. *Am. J. Surg. Pathol.*, **6**, 733–43.

Ackerman, A. B. (1984) Histopathologists can diagnose malignant melanoma *in situ* correctly and consistently. *Am. J. Dermatopathol.*, **6** (Suppl.), 103–7.

Ackerman, A. B. and David, K. M. (1986) A unifying concept of malignant melanoma: biologic aspects. *Hum. Pathol.*, **17**, 438–40.

Ainsworth, A. M., Folberg, R., Reed, R. J. and Clark, W. H. (1979) Melanocytic nevi, melanocytomas, melanocytic dysplasias, and uncommon forms of melanoma. In *Human Malignant Melanoma* (eds W. H. Clark, L. I. Goldman and M. J. Mastrangelo). New York: Grune & Stratton, pp. 167–208.

Akslen, L. A. and Myking, A. O. (1989) Balloon cell melanoma mimicking clear cell carcinoma. *Pathol. Res. Pract.*, **184**, 548–50.

Albino, A. P., Nanus, D. M., Mentle, I. R. *et al.* (1989) Analysis of *ras* oncogenes in malignant melanoma and precursor lesions: correlation of point mutations with different phenotype. *Oncogene*, **4**, 1363–74.

Aloi, F. G., Coverlizza, S. and Pippione, M. (1988) Balloon cell melanoma: a report of two cases. *J. Cutan. Pathol.*, **15**, 230–3.

Arrington, J. H., III, Reed, R. J., Ichinose, H. and Krementz, E. T. (1977) Plantar lentiginous melanoma: a distinctive variant of human cutaneous malignant melanoma. *Am. J. Surg. Pathol.*, **1**, 131–43.

Bader, J. L., Li, F. P., Olmstead, P. M., Strickman, N. A. and Green, D. M.(1985) Childhood malignant melanoma. Incidence and etiology. *Am. J. Pediatr. Hematol. Oncol.*, **7**, 341–5.

Bale, S. J., Dracopoli, N. C., Tucker, M. A. *et al.* (1989) Mapping the gene for hereditary cutaneous malignant melanoma-dysplastic nevus to chromosome 1p. *New Engl. J. Med.*, **320**, 1367–72.

Barr, R. J., Morales, R. V. and Graham, J. H. (1980) Desmoplastic nevus: a distinct histologic variant of mixed spindle cell and epithelioid cell nevus. *Cancer*, **46**, 557–64.

Barr, L. H., Goldman, L. I., Solomon, J. A., Sanusi, D. I. and Reed, R. J. (1984) Minimal deviation melanoma. *Surg., Gynecol. Obstet.*, **159**, 546–8.

Becker, D. W., Miller, C. J. and Keller, H. B. (1979) Metastatic minimal deviation melanoma. *Ann. Plast. Surg.*, **4**, 230–7.

Benisch, B., Peison, B., Kannerstein, M. and Spivack, J. (1980) Malignant melanoma originating from intradermal nevi. A clinicopathologic entity. *Arch. Dermatol.*, **116**, 696–8.

Bhuta, S., Mirra, J. M. and Cochran, A. J. (1986) Myxoid malignant melanoma: a previously undescribed histologic pattern noted in metastatic lesions and report of four cases. *Am. J. Surg. Pathol.*, **10**, 203–11.

Boddie, A. W. and McBride, C. M. (1985) Melanoma in childhood and adolescence. In *Cutaneous Melanoma* (eds C. M. Balch and G. W. Milton). Philadelphia: Lippincott Co., pp. 64–70.

Bonetti, F., Colombari, R., Zamboni, G., Chilosi, M. and Legnani, F. (1989) Signet ring melanoma, S-100 negative. *Am. J. Surg. Pathol.*, **13**, 522–3.

Botha, M. C. and Lennox, B. (1954) Re-pigmentation of amelanotic metastases of malignant melanoma by contact with epidermis. *J. Pathol. Bacteriol.*, **67**, 99–104.

Briggs, J. C. (1980) Reticulin impregnation in the diagnosis of malignant melanoma. *Histopathology*, **4**, 507–16.

Campbell, W. A., Storlazzi, E., Vintzileos, A. M., Wu, A., Schneiderman, H. and Nochimson, D. J. (1987) Fetal malignant melanoma: ultrasound presentation and review of the literature. *Obstet. Gynecol.*, **70**, 434–9.

Cesarini, J. P. (1971) Recent advances in the ultrastructure of malignant melanoma. *Rev. Eur. Etudes Clin. Biol.*, **16**, 316–22.

Chapman, P., Banerjee, A., Anderson, J. R. and Lamberty, B. G. H. (1987) Digital volar amelanotic malignant melanoma in a child. *J. Hand Surg.*, **12**, 117–19.

Clark, W. H., From, L., Bernardino, E. and Mihm, M. C., (1969) The histogenesis and biologic behavior of primary human malignant melanomas of the skin. *Cancer Res.*, **29**, 705–26.

Clark, W. H., Ten Heggler, B. and Bretton, R. (1972) Electron microscopic observations of human cutaneous melanomas correlated with their biologic behaviour. In *Melanoma and Skin Cancer* (ed. W. H. McCarthy). Sydney: VCN Blight, pp. 121–41.

Clark, W. H., Ainsworth, A. M., Bernardino, E. A., Yang, C.-H., Mihm, M. C. and Reed, R. J. (1975) The developmental biology of primary human malignant melanomas. *Semin. Oncol.*, **2**, 83–103.

Clark, W. H., Elder, D. E. and Van Horn, M. (1986) The biologic forms of malignant melanoma. *Hum. Pathol.*, **17**, 443–50.

Clemente, C., Cascinelli, N. and Rilke, F. (1980) Monomorphic cellular proliferation of malignant melanomas of the skin as a prognostic morphologic parameter. *Hum. Pathol.*, **11**, 299–300.

Coleman, W. P., Davis, R. S., Reed, R. J. and Krementz, E. T. (1980) Treatment of lentigo maligna and lentigo maligna melanoma. *J. Dermatol. Surg. Oncol.*, **6**, 476–9.

Colombari, R., Bonetti, F., Zamboni, G. *et al.* (1988) Distribution of melanoma specific antibody (HMB-45) in benign and malignant melanocytic tumors. An immunohistochemical study on paraffin sections. *Virchows Arch. A. (Pathol. Anat.)*, **413**, 17–24.

Conley, J., Lattes, R. and Orr, W. (1971) Desmoplastic malignant melanoma (a variant of spindle cell melanoma). *Cancer*, **28**, 914–36.

Cooke, K. R. and Fraser, J. (1985) Migration and death from malignant melanoma. *Int. J. Cancer.*, **36**, 175–8.

Cramer, S. F. (1990) Epithelial membrane staining of melanocytic nevi. *Hum. Pathol.*, **21**, 121–2.

Dabbs, D. J. and Bolen, J. W. (1984) Superficial spreading malignant melanoma with neurosarcomatous metastasis. *Am. J. Clin. Pathol.*, **82**, 109–14.

Daly, J. M., Berlin, R. and Urmacher, C. (1987) Subungual melanoma: a 25-year review of cases. *J. Surg. Oncol.*, **35**, 107–12.

Dardick, I. and Rippstein, P. (1987) Subcutaneous metastatic spindle cell tumor. *Ultrastruct. Pathol.*, **11**, 745–50.

Davis, J., Pack, G. T. and Higgins, G. K. (1967) Melanotic freckle of Hutchinson. *Am. J. Surg.*, **113**, 457–63.

Dhillon, A. P., Rode, J. and Leathem, A. (1982) Neurone specific enolase: an aid to the diagnosis of melanoma and neuroblastoma. *Histopathology*, **6**, 81–92.

DiMaio, S., MacKay, B., Smith, L. *et al.* (1982) Neurosarcomatous transformation in malignant melanoma, an ultrastructural study. *Cancer*, **50**, 2345–54.

Drier, J. K., Swanson, P. E., Cherwitz, D. L. and Wick, M. R. (1987) S100 protein immunoreactivity in poorly differentiated carcinomas. Immunohistochemical comparison with malignant melanoma. *Arch. Pathol. Lab. Med.*, **111**, 447–52.

Drzewiecki, K. T., Frydman, H., Andersen, K., Poulsen, H., Ladefoged, C. and Vibe, P. (1990) Malignant melanoma. Changing trends in factors influencing metastasis-free survival from 1964 to 1982. *Cancer*, **65**, 362–6.

Dubreuilh, W. (1894) Lentigo malin des vieillards. *Ann. Derm. Syph. (Paris)*, **5** (ser. 3), 1092–9.

Duray, P. H., Palazzo, J., Gown, A. M. and Ohuchi, N. (1988) Melanoma cell heterogeneity. A study of two monoclonal antibodies compared with S-100 protein in paraffin sections. *Cancer*, **61**, 2460–8.

Egbert, B., Kempson, R. and Sagebiel, R. (1988) Desmoplastic malignant melanoma. A clinicohistopathologic study of 25 cases. *Cancer*, **62**, 2033–41.

Eide, J. (1981) Pathogenesis of generalized melanosis with melanuria and melanoptysis secondary to malignant melanoma. *Histopathology*, **5**, 285–94.

Elder, D. E., Ainsworth, A. M. and Clark, W. H. (1979) The surgical pathology of cutaneous malignant melanoma. In *Human Malignant Melanoma* (eds W. H. Clark, *et al.*). New York: Grune & Stratton, pp. 55–108.

Elwood, J. M., Gallagher, R. P., Davison, J. and Hill, G. B. (1985) Sunburn, suntan and the risk of cutaneous malignant melanoma — the Western Canada Melanoma Study. *Br. J. Cancer*, **51**, 543–9.

English, J. S. C. and Swerdlow, A. J. (1987) The risk of malignant melanoma, internal malignancy and mortality in xeroderma pigmentosum patients. *Br. J. Dermatol.*, **117**, 457–61.

Erlandson, R. A. (1987) Ultrastructural diagnosis of amelanotic malignant melanoma: aberrant melanosomes, myelin figures or lysosomes? *Ultrastruct. Pathol.*, **11**, 191–208.

Fallowfield, M. E. and Cook, M. G. (1989) Vascular invasion in malignant melanomas. An independent prognostic variable? *Am. J. Surg. Pathol.*, **13**, 217–20.

Feibleman, C. E., Stoll, H. and Maize, J. C. (1980) Melanomas of the palm, sole, and nailbed: a clinicopathologic study. *Cancer*, **46**, 2492–2504.

Fitzgibbons, P. L., Martin, S. E. and Simmons, T. J. (1987) Malignant melanoma metastatic to the ovary. *Am. J. Surg. Pathol.*, **11**, 959–67.

Fitzpatrick, T. B. (1988) The validity and practicality of sun-reactive skin types I through VI. *Arch. Dermatol.*, **124**, 869–71.

Friedman, M., Roa, U and Fox, S. (1982) The cytology of metastatic balloon cell melanoma. *Acta Cytol.*, **26**, 39–43.

From, L., Hanna, W., Kahn, H. J., Gruss, J., Marks, A. and Baumal, R. (1983) Origin of desmoplasia in desmoplastic malignant melanoma. *Hum. Pathol.*, **14**, 1072–80.

Gallagher, R. P., Elwood, J. M., Threlfall, W. J., Spinelli, J. J., Fincham, S. and Hill, G. B. (1987) Socioeconomic status, sunlight exposure, and risk of malignant melanoma: the Western Canada Melanoma Study. *J. Natl. Cancer Inst.*, **79**, 647–52.

Gardner, W. and Vazquez, M. (1970) Balloon cell melanoma. *Arch. Pathol.*, **89**, 470–2.

Gatter, K. C., Ralfkiaer, E., Skinner, J. *et al.* (1985) An immunocytochemical study of malignant melanoma and its differential diagnosis from other malignant tumours. *J. Clin. Pathol.*, **38**, 1353–7.

Gaynor, R., Herschman, H. R., Irie, R., Jones, P., Morton, D. and Cochran, A. (1981) S100 protein: a marker for human malignant melanomas? *Lancet*, **i**, 869–71.

Gibson, L. E. and Goellner, J. R. (1988) Amelanotic melanoma: cases studied by Fontana stain, S-100 immunostain, and ultrastructural examination. *Mayo Clin. Proc.*, **63**, 777–82.

Ginzburg, A., Hodak, E. and Sandbank, M. (1986) Malignant blue nevus. Letter to the editor. *J. Dermatol. Surg. Oncol.*, **12**, 1252, 1328.

Goldenhersh, M. A., Sarin, R. C., Barnhill, R. L. and Stenn, K. S. (1988) Malignant blue nevus. Case report and literature review. *J. Am. Acad. Dermatol.*, **19**, 712–22.

Goldman, L. (1951) Some investigative studies of pigmented nevi with cutaneous microscopy. *J. Invest. Dermatol.*, **16**, 407–10.

Gown, A. M., Vogel., A. M., Hoak, D., Gough, F. and McNutt, M. A. (1986) Monoclonal antibodies specific for melanocytic tumors distinguish subpopulations of melanocytes. *Am. J. Pathol.*, **123**, 195–203.

Grunwald, M. H., Rothem, A. and Feuerman, E. J. (1985) Metastatic malignant melanoma with cartilaginous metaplasia. *Dermatologica*, **170**, 249–52.

Gussack, G. S., Reitgen, D., Cox, E., Fisher, S., Cole, T. and Seigler, H. (1983) Cutaneous melanoma of the head and neck: a review of 399 cases. *Arch. Otolaryngol.*, **109**, 803–8.

Hartley, L., Birch, J. M., Marsden, H. B. and Harris, M. (1987) Malignant melanoma in families of children with osteosarcoma, chondrosarcoma, and adrenal cortical carcinoma. *J. Med. Genet.*, **24**, 664–8.

Hendrickson, M. R. and Ross, J. C. (1981) Neoplasms arising in congenital giant naevi. Morphologic study of seven cases and a review of the literature. *Am. J. Surg. Pathol.*, **5**, 109–35.

Hernandez, F. J. (1973) Malignant blue nevus. A light and electron microscopic study. *Arch. Dermatol.*, **107**, 741–4.

Herrera, G. A., Turbat-Herrera, E. A. and Lot, R. L. (1988) S-100 protein expression by primary and metastatic adenocarcinomas. *Am. J. Clin. Pathol.*, **89**, 168–76.

Holly, E. A., Kelly, J. W., Shpall, S. N. and Chiu, S.-H. (1987) Number of melanocytic nevi as a major risk factor for malignant melanoma. *J. Am. Acad. Dermatol.*, **17**, 459–68.

Hutchinson, J. (1890) On senile moles and senile freckles and on their relation-

298 Cutaneous melanoma

ship to cancerous processes. *Arch. Surg.*, **2**, 218.

Hutchinson, J. (1894) Lentigo-melanosis. A further report. *Arch. Surg. (Lond.)*, **5**, 253–6.

Inbar, M., Matzkin, H., Rozin, R. R., Chaitik, S. and Klauzner, J. M. (1988) Malignant melanoma developing in an irradiation field. *Br. J. Radiol.*, **61**, 519–20.

Jain, S. and Allen, P. W. (1989) Desmoplastic malignant melanoma and its variants. A study of 45 cases. *Am. J. Surg. Pathol.*, **13**, 358–73.

Kahn, L. B. and Donaldson, R. C. (1970) Multiple primary melanoma — case report and study of tumor growth in vitro. *Cancer*, **25**, 1162–9.

Kamino, H., Tam, S. T. and Alvarez, L. (1990) Malignant melanoma with pseudocarcinomatous hyperplasia — an entity that can simulate squamous cell carcinoma. A light-microscopic and immunohistochemical study of four cases. *Am. J. Dermatopathol.*, **12**, 446–51.

Kato, T., Usuba, Y., Takematsu, H. *et al.* (1989) A rapidly growing pigmented nail streak resulting in diffuse melanosis of the nail. A possible sign of subungual melanoma *in situ*. *Cancer*, **64**, 2191–7.

Kefford, R. F. (1990) Genetics of melanoma. In *Cutaneous Melanoma, Biology and Management* (eds N. Cascinelli, M. Santinami and U. Veronesi). Milano: Masson, pp. 39–43.

Koh, H., Michalik, E., Sober, A. J. *et al.* (1984) Lentigo maligna melanoma has no better prognosis than other types of melanoma. *J. Clin. Oncol.*, **2**, 994–1001.

Kopf, A. W., Mintzis, M. and Bart, R. S. (1975) Diagnostic accuracy in malignant melanoma. *Arch. Dermatol.*, **111**, 1291–2.

Kornberg, R., Harris, M. and Ackerman, A. B. (1978) Epidermotropically metastatic malignant melanoma. *Arch. Dermatol.*, **114**, 67–69.

Kossard, S., Doherty, E. and Murray, E. (1987) Neurotropic melanoma. A variant of desmoplastic melanoma. *Arch. Dermatol.*, **123**, 907–12.

Krementz, E. T., Sutherland, C. M., Carter, R. D. and Ryan, R. F. (1976) Malignant melanoma in the American black. *Ann. Surg.*, **183**, 533–42.

Kuehnl-Petzold, C. H., Berger, H. and Weibelt, H. (1982) Verrucous-keratotic variations of malignant melanoma. A clinicopathologic study. *Am. J. Dermatopathol.*, **4**, 403–10.

Kuhn, A., Groth, W., Gartmann, H. and Steigleder, G. K. (1988) Malignant blue nevus with metastases to the lung. *Am. J. Dermatopathol.*, **10**, 436–41.

Kuo, T.-T., Chan, H.-L. and Hsueh, S. (1987) Clear cell papulosis of the skin. A new entity with histogenetic implications for cutaneous Paget's disease. *Am. J. Surg. Pathol.*, **11**, 827–34.

Ledwig, P. A. and Robinson, J. K. (1990) Should the excisional biopsy of clinically probable melanomas include a margin that might also serve as adequate for treatment? *Arch. Dermatol.*, **126**, 877–8.

Lee, J. A. H. (1985) The rising incidence of cutaneous malignant melanoma. *Am. J. Dermatopathol.*, **7**, 35–39.

Levene, A. (1980) On the histological diagnosis and prognosis of malignant melanoma. *J. Clin. Pathol.*, **33**, 101–24.

Lodding, P., Kindblom, L.-G. and Angervall, L. (1990) Metastases of malignant melanoma simulating soft tissue sarcoma. A clinicopathological, light- and electron microscopic and immunohistochemical study of 21 cases. *Virchows Arch. A (Pathol. Anat.)*, **417**, 377–88.

MacKie, R. M., Elwood, J. M. and Hawk, J. L. M. (1987) Links between exposure to ultraviolet radiation and skin cancer. A report of the Royal College of Physicians. *J. R. Coll. Physicians London*, **21**, 1–6.

Mazur, M. T. and Katzenstein, A. L. (1980) Metastatic melanoma: the spectrum of ultrastructural morphology. *Ultrastruct. Pathol.*, **1**, 337–56.

McGovern, V. J. (1982) The nature of melanoma. A critical review. *J. Cutan. Pathol.*, **9**, 61–81.

McGovern, V. J. (1983) *Melanoma, Histological Diagnosis and Prognosis* (ed. A. Blaustein). Biopsy Interpretation Series. New York: Raven Press.

McGovern, V. J. and Murad, T. M. (1985) Pathology of melanoma: an overview. In *Cutaneous Melanoma. Clinical Management and Treatment Results Worldwide* (eds C. M. Balch, G. W. Milton, H. M. Shaw and S. Soong). Philadelphia: J. B. Lippincott Co., pp. 29–54.

McGovern, V. J., Shaw. H. M. Milton, G. W. and Farago, G. A. (1980) Is malignant melanoma arising in a Hutchinson's melanotic freckle a separate disease entity? *Histopathology*, **4**, 235–42.

McGovern, V. J., Cochran, A. J., Van der Esch, E. P., Little, J. H. and MacLennan, R. (1986) The classification of malignant melanoma, its histologic reporting and registration. A revision of the 1972 Sydney classification. *Pathology*, **18**, 12–21.

Mehregan, A. H. and Pinkus, H. (1966) Artifacts in dermal histopathology. *Arch. Dermatol.*, **94**, 218–25.

Mérot, Y. and Frenk, E. (1989) Spitz nevus (large spindle cell and/or epithelioid cell nevus). Age-related involvement of the suprabasal epidermis. *Virchows Arch. A (Pathol. Anat.)*, **415**, 97–101.

Michalik, E. E., Fitzpatrick, T. B. and Sober, A. J. (1983) Rapid progression of lentigo maligna to deeply invasive lentigo maligna melanoma. Report of two cases. *Arch. Dermatol.*, **119**, 831–5.

Miettinen, M. and Franssila, K. (1989) Immunohistological spectrum of malignant melanoma. The common presence of keratins. *Lab. Invest.*, **61**, 623–8.

Mihm, M. C. and Googe, P. B. (1990) *Problematic Pigmented Lesions. A Case Method Approach*. Philadelphia: Lea & Febiger, p. 242.

Mintzis, M. M. and Silvers, D. N. (1978) Ultrastructural study of superficial spreading melanoma and benign simulants. *Cancer*, **42**, 502–11.

Montero, C.(1987) Endocytosis of immunoglobulin heavy and light chains by melanoma cells. *Hum. Pathol.*, **18**, 970.

Moreno, A., Lamarca, J., Martinez, R. and Guix, M. (1986) Osteoid and bone formation in desmoplastic malignant melanoma. *J. Cutan. Pathol.*, **13**, 128–34.

Moseley, H. S., Giuliano, A. E., Storm, F. K., Clark, W. H., Robinson, D. S. and Morton, D. L. (1979) Multiple primary melanoma. *Cancer*, **43**, 939–44.

Muhlbauer, J. E., Margolis, R. J., Mihm, M. C. *et al.* (1983) Minimal deviation melanoma: a histologic variant of cutaneous melanoma in its vertical growth phase. *J. Invest. Dermatol.*, **80**, 63S–65S

Nahkleh, R. E., Wick, M. R., Rocamora, A., Swanson, P. E. and Dehner, L. P. (1990) Morphologic diversity in malignant melanomas. *Am. J. Clin. Pathol.*, **93**, 731–40.

Nakagawa, H., Imakado, S., Nogita, T. and Ishibashi, Y. (1990) Osteosarcomatous changes in malignant melanoma: immunohistochemical and ultrastructural studies of a case. *Am. J. Dermatopathol.*, **12**, 162–8.

Nakano, S., Groth, W, Gartmann, H. and Steigleder, G. K. (1988) Malignant blue nevus with metastases to lung. *Am. J. Dermatopathol.*, **10**, 436–41.

Nottingham, J. F. and Slater, D. N. (1988) Malignant melanoma: a new mimic of colloid carcinoma. *Histopathology*, **13**, 576–8.

Nyong'o, A. O., Huntrakoon, M., Parsa, C. and Raja, A. (1986) Superficial spreading malignant melanoma with neurosarcomatous metastasis. *Pathology*, **18**, 473–7.

Okun, M. R. (1979) Melanoma resembling spindle and epithelioid cell nevus. *Arch. Dermatol.*, **115**, 1416–20.

Okun, M. R. and Bauman, L. (1965) Malignant melanoma arising from an intradermal nevus. *Arch. Dermatol.*, **92**, 69–72.

Okun, M. R., DiMattia, A., Thompson, J. and Pearson, H. (1974) Malignant melanoma developing from intradermal nevi. *Arch. Dermatol.*, **110**, 599–601.

Ordóñez, N. G., Xiaolong, J. and Hichey, R. C. (1988) Comparison of HMB-45 monoclonal antibody and S-100 protein in the immunohistochemical diagnosis of melanoma. *Am. J. Clin, Pathol.*, **90**, 385–90.

Patterson, R. H. and Helwig, E. B. (1980) Subungual malignant melanoma: a clinical-pathologic study. *Cancer*, **46**, 2074–87.

Penneys, N. S. (1987) Microinvasive lentigo maligna melanoma. *J. Am. Acad. Dermatol.*, **17**, 675–80.

Peters, M. S. and Goellner, J. R. (1986) Spitz naevi and malignant melanomas of childhood and adolescence. *Histopathology*, **10**, 1289–1302.

Peters, M. S. and Su, W. P. D. (1985) Balloon cell malignant melanoma. *J. Am. Acad. Dermatol.*, **13**, 351–4.

Phillips, M. E., Margolis, R. J., Mérot, Y. *et al.* (1986) The spectrum of minimal deviation melanoma: a clinicopathologic study of 21 cases. *Hum. Pathol.*, **17**, 796–806.

Piérard, G. E. (1988) Melanophagic dermatitis and panniculitis. A condition revealing an occult metastatic malignant melanoma. *Am. J. Dermatopathol.*, **10**, 133–6.

Podesta, A., Wagner-Reiss, K. and Duray, P. H. (1989) Distinction between metastatic melanoma and primary parotid gland carcinoma using monoclonal HMB45 antimelanoma antibody: report of a case. *Hum. Pathol.*, **20**, 77–80.

Prose, N. S., Laude, T. A., Heilman, E. R. and Coren, C. (1987) Congenital malignant melanoma. *Pediatrics*, **79**, 967–70.

Ralfkiaer, E., Hou-Jensen, K., Gatter, K. C., Drzewiecki, K. T. and Mason, D. Y. (1987) Immunohistological analysis of the lymphoid infiltrate in cutaneous malignant melanomas. *Virchows Arch. A.*, **410**, 355–61.

Ramaekers, F. C. S., Puts, J. J. G., Moesker, O., Kant, A., Vooijs, G. P. and Jap, P. H. K. (1983) Intermediate filaments in malignant melanomas. Identification and use as marker in surgical pathology. *J. Clin. Invest.*, **71**, 635–43.

Rampen, F. H. and Fleuren, E. (1987) Melanoma of the skin is not caused by ultraviolet radiation but by a chemical xenobiotic. *Med. Hypoth.*, **22**, 341–6.

Reed, R. J. (1976) Acral lentiginous melanoma. In *New Concepts in Surgical Pathology of the Skin*, New York: J. Wiley & Sons, pp. 89–97.

Reed, R. J. (1984) A classification of melanocytic dysplasias and malignant melanomas. *Am. J. Dermatopathol.*, **6**, 195–206.

Reed, R. J. (1985) The histological variance of malignant melanoma: the inter-relationship of histological subtype, neoplastic progression and biological behavior. *Pathology*, **17**, 301–12.

Reed, R. J. and Leonard, D. D. (1979) Neurotropic melanoma (a variant of desmoplastic melanoma). *Am. J. Surg. Pathol.*, **3**, 301–11.

Reed, R. J., Ichinose, H., Clark, W. H. and Mihm, J. C. (1975) Common and uncommon melanocytic nevi and borderline melanomas. *Semin. Oncol.*, **2**, 119–47.

Reiman, H. M., Goellner, J. R., Woods, J. E. and Mixter, R. C. (1987) Desmoplastic melanoma of the head and neck. *Cancer*, **60**, 2269–74.

Reintgen, D. S., Vollmer, R. and Seigler, H. F. (1989) Juvenile malignant melanoma. *Surg. Gynecol. Obstetr.*, **168**, 249–53.

Rocamora, A., Carrillo, R., Vives, R. and Solera, J. C. (1988) Fine needle aspiration biopsy of myxoid metastasis of malignant melanoma. *Acta Cytol.*, **32**, 94–100.

Roth, M. E., Grant-Kels, J. M., Kuhn, K., Greenberg, R. D. and Hurwitz, S. (1990) Melanoma in children. *J. Am. Acad. Dermatol.*, **22**, 265–74.

Rowden, G., Sulica, V. I., Butler, T. P. and Manz, H. J. (1980) Malignant melanoma with melanosis. Ultrastructural and histological studies. *J. Cutan. Pathol.*, **7**, 125–39.

Saksela, E. and Rintala, A. (1968) Misdiagnosis of prepubertal malignant melanoma. Reclassification of a cancer registry material. *Cancer*, **22**, 1308–14.

Salomon, J., Donald, J., Shaw, H., McCarthy, W. and Kefford, R. (1989) Linkage analysis of Australian hereditary melanoma kindreds using RFLP loci on chromosome 1p. *2nd Internat. Conference on Melanoma*, Abs, 152.

Sarkany, I. (1972) Malignant melanoma in lymphoedematous arm following radical mastectomy for breast carcinoma (an extension of the syndrome of Stewart and Treves). *Proc. Royal Soc. Med.*, **65**, 253–4.

Schmitt, F. C. and Bacchi, C. E. (1989) S-100 protein: is it a useful tumour marker in diagnostic immunocytochemistry? *Histopathology*, **15**, 281–8.

Schneiderman, H., Yu-Yuan, A., Campbell, W. A. *et al.* (1987) Congenital melanoma with multiple prenatal metastases. *Cancer*, **60**, 1371–7.

Scrivner, D., Oxenhandler, R. W., Lopez, M. and Perez-Mesa, C. (1987) Plantar lentiginous melanoma. A clinicopathologic study. *Cancer*, **60**, 2502–9.

Seiji, M. and Takahashi, M. (1974) Malignant melanoma with adjacent intraepithelial proliferation. *Tohoku J. Exp. Med.*, **114**, 93–107.

Sheibani, K. and Battifora, H. (1988) Signet-ring cell melanoma. A rare morphologic variant of malignant melanoma. *Am. J. Surg. Pathol.*, **12**, 28–34.

Shukla, V. K., Hughes, D. C., Hughes, L. E., McCormick, F. and Padua, R. A. (1989) *Ras* mutations in human melanotic lesions: K-*ras* activation is a frequent and early event in melanoma development. *Oncogene Res.*, **5**, 121–7.

Sigg, C., Pelloni, F. and Hardmeier, T. (1988) Multiple primäre Melanome der Haarfollikel — eine Sonderform des malignen Melanomas der Haut. *Hautarzt*, **39**, 447–51.

Silberberg, I., Kopf, A. W. and Gumport, S. L. (1968) Diffuse melanosis in malignant melanoma. *Arch. Dermatol.*, **97**, 671–7.

Silverman, J. F., Blahove, M., Collins, J. L. and Norris, H. T. (1988) Cutaneous malignant melanoma in a black patient with neurofibromatosis (von Recklinghausen's disease). *Am. J. Dermatopathol.*, **10**, 536–40.

Smith, K. J., Skelton, H. G., Lupton, G. P. and Graham, J. H. (1989) Spindle cell and epithelioid cell nevi with atypia and metastasis (malignant Spitz nevus). *Am. J. Surg. Pathol.*, **13**, 931–9.

Soyer, H.-P,. Smolle, J., Kerl, H. and Stettner, H. (1987) Early diagnosis of malignant melanoma by surface microscopy. *Lancet*, **ii**, 803.

Soyer, H.-P., Smolle, J., Hödl, S., Pachernegg, H. and Kerl, H. (1989) Surface microscopy. A new approach to the diagnosis of cutaneous pigmented tumors. *Am. J. Dermatopathol.*, **11**, 1–10.

Specht, C. S. and Smith, T. W. (1988) Uveal malignant melanoma and von Recklinghausen's neurofibromatosis. *Cancer*, **62** 812–7.

Springall, D. R., Gu, J., Cocchia, D. *et al.* (1983) The value of S-100 immuno-staining as a diagnostic tool in human malignant melanomas. A comparative study using S-100 and neuron-specific enolase antibodies. *Virchows Arch. A. (Pathol. Anat.)*, **400**, 331–43.

Su, W. P. D., Goellner, J. R. and Peters, M. S. (1985) Unusual histopathologic variants of cutaneous malignant melanoma. In *Pathology of Unusual Malignant Cutaneous Tumors* (ed. M. R. Wick). New York: Marcel Dekker, pp. 281–98.

Suster, S., Ronnen, M and Bubis, J. J. (1987) Verrucous pseudonevoid melanoma. *J. Surg. Oncol.*, **36**, 134–7.

Swerdlow, A. J., English, J., MacKie, R. M. *et al.* (1986) Benign melanocytic naevi as a risk factor for malignant melanoma. *Br. Med. J.*, **292**, 1555–9.

Szpak, C. A., Shelburne, J., Linder, J. and Klintworth, G. K. (1988) The presence of stage II melanosomes (premelanosomes) in neoplasms other than melanomas. *Modern Pathol.*, **1**, 35–43.

Takematsu, H., Obata, M., Tomita, Y., Kato, T., Takahashi, M. and Abe, R. (1985) Subungual melanoma. A clinicopathologic study of 16 Japanese cases. *Cancer*, **55**, 2725–31.

Temple-Camp, C. R. E., Saxe, N. and King, H. (1988) Benign and malignant cellular blue nevus. A clinicopathologic study of 30 cases. *Am. J. Dermatopathol.*, **10**, 289–96.

Tindall, B., Finlayson, R., Ven, D. *et al.* (1989) Malignant melanoma associated with human immunodeficiency virus infection in three homosexual men. *J. Am. Acad. Dermatol.*, **20**, 587–91.

Toker, C. (1970) Clear cells of the nipple epidermis. *Cancer*, **25**, 601–10.

Toublanc, M., Grossin, M., Benrejeb, N. *et al.* (1990) Un cas de mélanome malin exprimant les marqueurs des cellules épithéliales en immunohisto-chimie sur coupes en paraffine. *Ann. Pathol. (Paris)*, **10**, 34–36.

Trent, J. M., Meyskens, F. L., Salmon, S. E. *et al.* (1990) Relation of cytogenetic abnormalities and clinical outcome in metastatic melanoma. *New Engl. J. Med.*, **322**, 1508–11.

Trozak, D. J., Rowland, W. D. and Hu, F. (1975) Metastatic malignant melanoma in prepubertal children. *Pediatrics*, **55**, 191–204.

Tuthill, R. J., Weinzweig, N. and Yetman, R. J. (1988) Desmoplastic melanoma: a clinicopathologic study of ten cases with electron microscopy and immuno-histology. *J. Cutan. Pathol.*, **15**, 348.

Urso, C., Giannotti, B. and Bondi, R. (1990) Myxoid melanoma of the skin. *Arch. Pathol. Lab. Med.*, **114**, 527–8.

Van Duinen, S. G., Ruiter, D. J., Hageman, Ph. *et al.* (1984) Immunohisto-chemical and histochemical tools in the diagnosis of amelanotic melanoma. *Cancer*, **53**, 1566–73.

Van Haeringen, A., Bergman, W., Nelan, M. R. *et al.* (1989) Exclusion of the dysplastic nevus syndrome locus from the short arm of chromosome 1 by linkage analysis studies in Dutch families. *Genomics*, **5**, 61–4.

Van 't Veer, L. J., Burgering, B. M. T., Versteeg, R. *et al.* (1989) N-*ras* mutations in human cutaneous melanoma from sun-exposed body sites. *Mol. Cell. Biol.*, **9**, 3114–6.

Vennegoor, C., Calafat, J., Hageman, Ph. *et al.* (1985) Biochemical character-ization and cellular localization of a formalin-resistant melanoma-associated antigen reacting with monoclonal antibody NKI/C-3. *Int. J. Cancer*, **35**, 287–95.

Vennegoor, C., Hageman, Ph., Van Nouhuijs, H. *et al.* (1988) A monoclonal antibody specific for cells of the melanocyte lineage. *Am. J. Pathol.*, **130**, 179–92.

Vollmer, R. T. (1987) Minimal deviation melanoma. *Hum. Pathol.*, **18**, 869–70.

Walsh, N. M. G., Roberts, J. T., Orr, W. and Simon, G. T. (1988) Desmoplastic malignant melanoma. A clinicopathologic study of 14 cases. *Arch. Pathol. Lab. Med.*, **112**, 922–7.

Warner, T. F. C. S., Seo, I. S. and Bennett, J. E. (1980a) Minimal deviation melanoma with epidermotropic metastases arising in a congenital nevus. *Am. J. Surg. Pathol.*, **4**, 175–83.

Warner, T. F. C. S., Gilbert, E. F. and Ramirez, G. (1980b) Epidermotropism in melanoma. *J. Cutan. Pathol.*, **7**, 50–54.

Warner, T. F. C. S., Hafez, G. R., Finch, R. E. and Brandenberg, J. H. (1981) Schwann cell features in neurotropic melanoma. *J. Cutan. Pathol.*, **8**, 177–87.

Warner, T. F. C. S., Lloud, R. V., Hafez, G. R. and Angevine, J. M. (1984) Immunohistochemistry of neurotropic melanoma. *Cancer*, **53**, 254–7.

Wayte, D. M. and Helwig, E. B. (1968) Melanotic freckle of Hutchinson. *Cancer*, **21**, 893–911.

Weidner, N., Flanders, D. J., Jochimsen, P. R. and Stamler, F. W. (1985) Neurosarcomatous malignant melanoma arising in a neuroid giant congenital melanocytic nevus. *Arch. Dermatol.*, **121**, 1302–6.

Weinstock, M. A. and Sober, A. J. (1987) The risk of progression of lentigo maligna to lentigo maligna melanoma. *Br. J. Dermatol.*, **116**, 303–10.

Yum, M., Goheen, M. and Mandelbaum, I. (1984) Intracytoplasmic lumina in metastatic melanoma cells. *Arch. Pathol. Lab. Med.*, **108**, 183–4.

Zarbo, R. J., Gown, A. M., Nagle, R. B., Visscher, D. W. and Crissman, J. D. (1990) Anomalous cytokeratin expression in malignant melanoma: one- and two-dimensional Western blot analysis and immunohistochemical survey of 100 melanomas. *Modern Pathol.*, **3**, 494–501.

10 Prognostic factors in cutaneous melanoma

In the previous chapter the spectrum of histological appearances of cutaneous melanoma was described; here, we shall discuss the features related to prognosis, with an emphasis on those which are assessed histologically. We shall focus mainly on clinically localized disease and briefly discuss the prognosis of metastatic disease at the end of the chapter.

A number of recent large series and reviews provides detailed information on prognosis of melanoma (Sondergaard and Schou, 1985a, 1985b; Braun-Falco *et al.*, 1986; Vollmer, 1989); survival data from many centres around the world were presented in a volume edited by Balch and colleagues (1985a). A critical review of the literature on multivariate analyses of prognostic factors in cutaneous melanoma was recently presented by Vollmer (1989).

The most important prognostic parameters identified are: clinical and pathological tumour stage, maximal thickness, level of cutaneous invasion, presence of ulceration, mitotic index, the presence of satellites and site of the primary tumour. It should be noted that these are not independent variables. A large number of additional prognostic factors has been suggested; again, some of these are related to the ones mentioned above, especially tumour thickness (McGovern *et al.*, 1979; Kopf *et al.*, 1987). Their impact on survival, therefore, generally diminishes or even disappears when cases are stratified for thickness.

To estimate cure rates of melanoma, it is important that follow-up periods are sufficiently long. It is not uncommon that metastases become clinically manifest after more than 5 or even 10 years, and as a result of this, initial differences in survival may disappear.

The prognosis is similar in the four main *histological subtypes* (superficial spreading, nodular, lentigo maligna and acral lentiginous melanoma), after correction for the main prognostic parameters mentioned above (Schmoeckel *et al.*, 1983; Bonett *et al.*, 1986; Sondergaard and Schou, 1985a). Initially, lentigo maligna melanoma was thought to carry a better prognosis (McGovern *et al.*, 1980), but in most subsequent series this was not confirmed (Gussack *et al.*, 1983; Koh *et al.*, 1984a). Prognosis of acral lentiginous melanoma is generally unfavourable, but this is related to the fact that many of these melanomas are thick, probably as a result of considerable patient and doctor delay which is not uncommon in this tumour type (p. 248).

A *polypoid growth pattern* which is seen in about one-fifth of primary melanomas, most commonly in the nodular variant, is associated with a poor prognosis (Manci *et al.*, 1981), but these tumours are often ulcerated, over 3 mm in thickness, and more commonly occur in males; after stratification for these unfavourable prognostic factors, the polypoid growth pattern *per se* does not influence survival (McGovern *et al.*, 1983a; Schmoeckel *et al.*, 1983; Reed *et al.*, 1986). There is still uncertainty about the prognostic relevance of some rare melanoma types such as Spitz-like spindle cell melanoma (p. 270). Neurotropic melanoma (p. 253) has a very high local recurrence potential related to its distinctive invasive growth pattern.

10.1   Clinical and pathological tumour stage

To allow optimal assessment of prognosis and comparison of treatment results, various staging systems have been developed. None of these has been universally adopted.

Most commonly, melanoma is divided into three stages: stage I represents localized disease; stage II, regional cutaneous (satellite or *in transit*) metastasis or regional lymph node metastasis; stage III, distant metastasis. However, in view of the large differences in prognosis of clinically localized disease, several more elaborate staging systems have further subdivided localized disease. The staging systems of the UICC, American Joint Committee and M. D. Anderson (Smith, 1976; International Union Against Cancer, 1978; Beahrs and Myers, 1983), are given in Table 10.1. Because of these different systems, some confusion exists in melanoma staging, and it is therefore important to indicate which staging system is used whenever one speaks of a specific stage.

10.2   Site, sex and age

These three parameters provide significant information about prognosis partly, but not wholly, because of their association with tumour thickness and ulceration. As a consequence, part of the impact of site, sex and age on prognosis is lost when cases are stratified for these two powerful prognostic factors.

Table 10.1 Staging systems of cutaneous melanoma

UICC staging system	
Stage	*Criteria*
IA	Primary melanoma Clark level II or III, ≤1.5 mm in thickness
IB	Primary melanoma Clark level IV or V, or ≥1.5 mm in thickness
II	Regional lymph node spread
III	'Juxtaregional' lymph node spread (e.g. involvement of iliac lymph nodes in case of a melanoma of the leg)
IV	Distant metastasis

M.D. Anderson staging system	
Stage	*Criteria*
I	Primary tumour only (IA: intact primary melanoma; IB: locally excised melanoma; IC: multiple primary melanomas)
II	Local recurrence or metastasis, within 3 cm of the site of the primary tumour
III	Regional metastases (IIIA: extranodal tissues; IIIB: lymph node metastases; IIIAB: both extranodal and nodal metastasis)
IV	Distant metastasis (IVA: cutaneous metastases only; IVB: visceral metastases)

American Joint Committee on Cancer staging system	
Stage	*Criteria*
IA	Localized melanoma, ≤0.75 mm, or level II
IB	Localized melanoma, 0.76–1.5 mm, or level III
IIA	Localized melanoma, 1.5–4 mm or level IV
IIB	Localized melanoma >4 mm, or level V
III	Limited nodal metastases, involving one regional lymph node basin, or <5 *in transit* metastases in the absence of nodal metastases
IV	Advanced regional metastases or distant metastases

10.2.1   Site

On the basis of 5-year survival figures of a series of 971 patients with clinically localized melanoma, Rogers and colleagues (1983) identified the following high risk sites: scalp, mandibular area, midline of trunk (anterior and posterior), medial side of upper thighs, hands and feet (except arches), popliteal fossae and genitalia. Lower arms and upper legs were associated with a favourable prognosis. The impact on prognosis remained significant in a model of eight other predictive variables including thickness, age, sex, level, mitotic index and ulceration. It may be that patient delay (scalp, midline of back), high vascularity of the tissue (hands and feet, genitalia), bilateral lymphatic drainage (midline of trunk) and resection with narrow margins (face, genitalia) play a role in these differences in prognosis. Many other workers also found that melanomas located on the limbs have a better prognosis than those on the trunk or head and neck region (e.g. Reintgen *et al.*, 1987). The upper limbs appear to be a slightly more favourable site than the lower limbs.

The *BANS region* (upper Back, posterior Arm, posterior Neck and posterior Scalp region) has been associated with an unfavourable course of disease in melanomas between 0.76 and 1.69 mm thick (Day *et al.*, 1982; Weinstock *et al.*, 1988); however, this was not found in large series of melanomas of various thicknesses (Balch *et al.*, 1985b; Cascinelli *et al.*, 1986). Melanomas of the scalp and ear were associated with an especially poor prognosis in one series (Wanebo *et al.*, 1988).

Subungual melanomas as a group have a relatively unfavourable prognosis, which is at least partly accounted for by their relative late detection: in one series, 10-year survival rates of stage I and stage II were 55 and 0%, respectively (Daly *et al.*, 1987).

10.2.2   Sex

In clinical stage I melanoma, females have a better prognosis (Cascinelli *et al.*, 1980), largely because the tumours are more often located on the extremities, and are thinner and less often ulcerated (Balch *et al.*, 1985b; O'Doherty *et al.*, 1986). However, *prognosis in females remains somewhat better after correction for site and thickness* (Kuehnl-Petzoldt *et al.*, 1984). In a study in the United Kingdom, this difference was prominent in the 50–79-year age group (O'Doherty *et al.*, 1986).

In a large Swedish series the relative hazard of tumour recurrence in men was significantly increased during the first eight years after diagnosis only, whereas in the group of female patients there was excess mortality throughout a much longer follow-up period (Thörn *et al.*, 1987). Late recurrence of cutaneous melanoma is seen most commonly in females with tumours of intermediate thickness (p. 320). These data emphasize the importance of long follow-up periods in estimates of cure rates of melanoma: a follow-up period of 5 years will provide important indications, but a period of 10 years is much to be preferred.

10.2.3   Age

In males but not in females, younger age is associated with a more favourable prognosis (Thörn *et al.*, 1987). Old age is associated with an unfavourable prognosis (Cohen *et al.*, 1987), partly due to the increased thickness of melanomas diagnosed in these patients. Also, melanomas of the face and ear are more common in the elderly, whereas those of

Table 10.2 Levels of cutaneous invasion (Clark)

Level I:	Melanoma *in situ*: all melanoma cells above the basement membrane
Level II:	Melanoma cells within the papillary dermis and/or periadnexal adventitial dermis; an occasional cell or even a strand or small nest of cells may extend into the upper reticular dermis
Level III:	Melanoma fills the papillary dermis completely, forming almost a straight line at the base, and impinging upon the reticular dermis without significant invasion of it
Level IV:	Distinct invasion well into the reticular dermis
Level V:	Invasion into subcutaneous tissues

the trunk decrease in incidence, those of the extremities remaining more or less constant (Cohen *et al.*, 1987).

10.3   Levels of invasion

In 1965, Mehnert and Heard proposed a histological staging system of cutaneous melanoma: stage 0 (melanoma *in situ*), stage I (invasion of papillary dermis), stage II (invasion of reticular dermis) and stage III (invasion of subcutis). A modified system, which distinguishes also between invasion of the papillary dermis and total filling of the papillary dermis by tumour, was proposed four years later by Clark and colleagues (1969) and this system became generally accepted.

According to Clark and colleagues (1969), five levels of invasion are distinguished (Table 10.2). Briefly, level I constitutes melanoma *in situ*; level II, invasion of the papillary dermis; level III, filling of the papillary dermis by tumour; level IV, invasion of the reticular dermis; level V, invasion of the subcutaneous tissues. A further refinement of this system into no fewer than 12 sub-levels was used by Sondergaard and Schou (1985a).

Different levels of cutaneous invasion are associated with substantial differences in survival. Survival figures vary between series, sometimes considerably; however, to give some indication of prognosis, figures which are based on averages of the large series obtained from many centres around the world and reported in the volume by Balch *et al.* (1985a), are given in Table 10.3.

There are theoretical and practical drawbacks to the assessment of levels of invasion proposed by Clark and colleagues (1969). The distinction between these levels is not always straightforward. The difference between levels II and III is not absolute and may result in observer variability (Wanebo *et al.*, 1975); the border between the papillary and reticular dermis is indistinct or absent in some sites (Breslow, 1977) and

Table 10.3 Survival figures in cutaneous melanoma according to level (Clark's)

Clark's level	5-year survival (%)	10-year survival (%)
Level II	96	93
Level III	83	71
Level IV	71	59
Level V	52	36

may be obscured by tumour-induced fibrosis; melanomas may invade the reticular dermis without first filling the papillary dermis, i.e. may skip level III. It is unclear in some cases whether the penetration of the reticular is enough to qualify for level IV disease; the distinction then becomes somewhat arbitrary and interobserver variation results.

10.4   Tumour thickness

The maximal thickness of a melanoma, as measured according to the recommendations by Breslow (1970; 1975; 1980), is the most important single prognostic parameter. Maximal thickness is best measured with an *ocular micrometer*, at right angles to the surface of the adjacent normal skin, from the top of the granular layer of the overlying epidermis or from the ulcer base over the deepest point of invasion, in the case of an ulcerated melanoma. The lower reference point is formed by the deepest invasive tumour cells, whether they be connected to the main tumour mass or separated from it, as is the case in microsatellitosis (p. 314). If the deepest tumour cells are within the epithelial compartment, as may occur when there is prominent epidermal hyperplasia, these are not taken into account. About 10% of melanomas extend along skin appendages, intraepithelially or within the immediately surrounding adventitial dermis (Figure 10.1): such thin but sometimes deep extensions, which sometimes would even double the thickness, should not be included in the measurements (Breslow, 1980). Indeed, follow-up data support this rule (Sondergaard and Schou, 1985a). When an ocular micrometer is not available thickness measurements can be performed with an accuracy of 0.1 mm with the *Vernier scale* present on almost all microscopes (Kirkham and Cotton, 1984).

Some indication of 5- and 10-year overall survival figures of clinical stage I melanoma of various thicknesses, again based on the major series reported in the volume by Balch *et al.* (1985a) are given in Table 10.4.

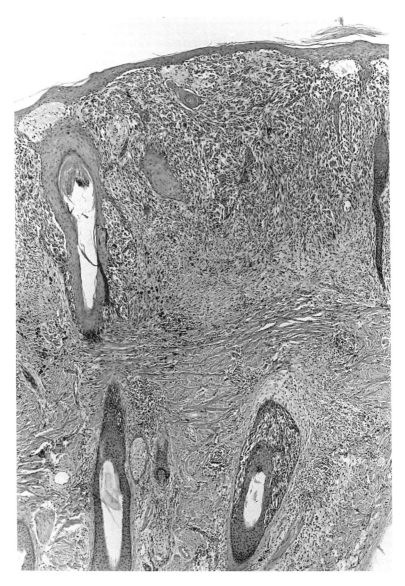

Figure 10.1 Spindle cell melanoma extending within the follicular epithelium and perifollicular adventitial dermis (lower half). Intra- and periadnexal extension is not included in the measurement of tumour thickness (HE, × 45).

Table 10.4 Survival figures in cutaneous melanoma according to thickness

Maximal thickness (mm)	5-year survival (%)	10-year survival (%)
<0.76	97	94
0.76–1.49	88	82
1.5–2.49	77	63
2.5–3.99	71	61
≥4	47	40

Tangential sectioning results in an overestimation of tumour thickness; however, in practice, this is rarely a significant problem, unless gross mistakes are made in tissue orientation during embedding. A deviation of 22.5 degrees leads to an increase in apparent thickness of only 9% (Breslow, 1977).

Thickness measurement has several important theoretical and practical advantages over the assessment of levels of invasion as proposed by Clark and colleagues (1969). First, intra- and interobserver reproducibility is better, and it can be applied to those sites in which there is no clear distinction between papillary and reticular dermis, or when there is reactive fibrosis. Also, in each of Clark's levels, there are considerable differences in thickness which correspond with differences in prognosis, e.g. level IV melanomas ranged in thickness from 0.6 to 12.6 mm in a series of Balch and colleagues (1985b). Therefore, tumour thickness is a more powerful prognostic parameter than level of invasion (Balch *et al.*, 1978; Breslow *et al.*, 1978). Nevertheless, most authors found that the level of invasion retains prognostic significance even after taking thickness into account (Day *et al.*, 1982; Kelly *et al.*, 1985a; Sondergaard and Schou, 1985a), although this was not found by all (Balch *et al.*, 1985b).

While the prognostic significance of tumour thickness has been repeatedly demonstrated, there is disagreement about the optimal cut-off points to yield the most meaningful subgroups. Three subgroups were originally proposed by Breslow (1975); 0–0.75 mm; 0.76–1.5 mm, and >1.5 mm. However, the prognosis of melanomas between 0.76 and 0.85 mm was not worse than that of melanomas under 0.76 mm, and therefore, an upper limit of 'thin' melanomas of 0.85 mm was proposed (Day *et al.*, 1981c; Briggs *et al.*, 1984). Some authors even found that thickness does not influence prognosis in the group of melanomas under 1.5 mm (Kuehnl-Petzoldt and Fisher, 1987). However, most large series do report some differences, as indicated by the survival data summarized above.

The cut-off point between 'intermediate' and 'thick' melanomas has also varied: Balch and colleagues (1978) found more significant differences in survival when 4 mm rather than 1.5 mm was used as a cut-off point. Day and colleagues (1981c) proposed four rather than three groups (cut-off points: 0.85, 1.70, and 3.60 mm). However, the suggestion of these authors of 'natural break-points' and 'increase in quantum jumps' of metastasis risk is not borne out by survival data in large patient groups. On the basis of a literature review and his own data, Vollmer (1989) concluded that a continuous function of thickness rather than a breakdown into three or four categories provides optimal prognostic information. Several mathematical formulae using thickness as continuous function have been put forward (Soong, 1985; Karakousis *et al.*, 1988; 1989). The 'prognostic index' (thickness times number of mitoses per square millimetre) recommended by Schmoeckel and colleagues (1983; p. 313) is also such a continuous function of thickness.

It is important to note that *tumour thickness cannot be assessed adequately on the basis of frozen sections*. This is one of the important reasons why frozen section diagnosis of melanoma should be discouraged. Tumour thickness is often greater in frozen sections, but contrary to earlier claims (Shafir *et al.*, 1983), there is no constant relationship between thickness in frozen sections and in paraffin sections, so that tumour thickness cannot be reliably calculated from measurements on frozen sections (Nield *et al.*, 1988).

10.4.1 Thin melanoma

Because of the increased awareness and earlier detection of melanoma, the number of very thin melanomas which rarely metastasize has risen disproportionately. As a consequence, the clinician and pathologist are now often asked whether they can predict accurately if a patient is indeed cured after definitive excision of such a tumour.

Prognostic factors were assessed in a series of 846 patients by Shaw and colleagues (1987), but minimum follow-up time was only 2 years. In this study and in several others (Kelly *et al.*, 1985a; Naruns *et al.*, 1986; Slingluff *et al.*, 1988; Kuehnl-Petzoldt and Fisher, 1987; Blessing *et al.*, 1990) the following factors were associated with unfavourable prognosis: male sex, location on head and neck (especially scalp) and axial sites of the trunk, the presence of ulceration, high mitotic rate, Clark's levels III and IV and regression. The thickness of the uninvolved dermis was prognostically significant in the series of Blessing and co-workers (1990). The prognostic significance of regression in thin melanomas was not found by all workers: this issue will be discussed in detail below (section 10.8, p. 316).

Although melanomas increase in thickness during the course of the disease, *thin melanoma cannot be equated with early melanoma*: due to substantial differences in growth rate, there is no obvious correlation between duration of symptoms and tumour thickness (Retsas *et al.*, 1986).

10.5   Mitotic rate, and related prognostic index

The number of mitoses per square millimetre is a significant prognostic indicator. Mitoses should be counted in areas in which they are most numerous and necrotic areas should be discarded (Schmoeckel and Braun-Falco, 1978); figures should be given per square millimetre rather than per high power field (HPF), in view of the differences in size of the latter.

Schmoeckel and co-workers (Schmoeckel and Braun-Falco, 1978; Schmoeckel *et al.*, 1983) and Kopf and colleagues (1987) proposed the use of the 'prognostic index', which equals thickness in millimetres times number of mitoses per square millimetre. A prognostic index of <19 *vs* ≥19 distinguished prognostically different subgroups of patients in melanomas of intermediate thickness (Kopf *et al.*, 1987). The mitotic rate of melanomas is higher in thicker melanomas, so that the two are not independent variables; indeed, Vollmer (1989) found that in his material, thickness taken to the third power was an even better predictor of lymph node metastases than thickness alone or in combination with ulceration or mitotic rate!

A high ^{3}H-thymidine labelling index was associated with early tumour recurrence in stage II melanomas (Costa *et al.*, 1987). Immunostaining with monoclonal antibody *Ki-67*, which detects an antigen present in proliferating cells, correlated poorly with mitotic rate in one study of primary melanoma, possibly because of poor signal-to-background ratio, and therefore is not advocated as an alternative to mitotic counts (Ostmeier and Suter, 1988). Moreover, it can only be used on frozen sections.

10.6   Ulceration

It has long been recognized that ulceration, which is present in about one-quarter of stage I melanomas, is an important prognostically unfavourable sign (Allen and Spitz, 1953; Tompkins, 1953). Roughly, 5- and 10-year overall survival figures of melanomas with ulceration are 65 and 55%, contrasting with 85 and 80% for nonulcerated tumours (Balch *et al.*, 1985b). Ulceration is closely associated with tumour thickness and stage but, even after correcting for these, it portends a significantly worse prognosis in tumours of intermediate or high thickness

(Balch *et al.*, 1980). Conversely, within the group of ulcerated melanomas, thickness remains of diagnostic importance. The influence of ulceration on prognosis appears to be particularly marked in females (McGovern *et al.*, 1982).

The prognostically unfavourable effect of ulceration does not result from underestimation of tumour thickness due to the depth of the ulcer crater: in the study of Balch and colleagues (1980), mean estimated ulcer depth was only 0.08 mm.

It is less often realized that *the diameter of the ulcer is a prognostically important factor, and therefore,* that *this should be measured whenever there is ulceration.* Ulceration of more than 3 mm in width was prognostically unfavourable in stage I melanomas over 1.5 mm in thickness; however, when ulceration was less than 3 mm in width, prognosis did not differ from nonulcerated tumours, whereas those with ulceration of 3–6 mm had survival rates comparable to those with ulceration extending over more than 6 mm (Day *et al.*, 1981a); therefore, 3 mm seems to be the best cut-off point to use.

10.7 Satellites

Satellites can be defined as cutaneous metastases of melanoma occurring within the reticular dermis or subcutis at a distance of less than 5 cm from the primary tumour. The margin of 5 cm is an arbitrary one; others have used 2 and 3 cm as cut-off points. Those located at a greater distance, but in the region of skin draining to the same lymph node basin, are termed *in transit* metastases. Thus, satellites and *in transit* metastases are very similar lesions pathologically, but their distinction has a practical basis: satellites are the lesions the surgeon is aiming to prevent by means of re-excision. Both satellites and *in transit* metastases are about 1.5 times more common in females than in males (Rampen *et al.*, 1987).

Microscopic satellites, or *'microsatellites'*, are tumour nests at least 0.5 mm in diameter, located within the reticular dermis or subcutis, or within vessels, and separated from the melanoma by normal tissue in the section used for assessment of maximal thickness; *they should be included in the thickness measurement* (Breslow, 1980; Day *et al.*, 1981a; Harrist *et al.*, 1984). Microsatellites may represent any of three situations: true dermal or subcutaneous metastases, tumour emboli in vessels, or continuous extensions of the tumour mass which are not continuous in the plane of section (Harrist *et al.*, 1984).

The presence of microsatellites is bad news. In clinical stage I melanoma, the presence of microsatellites was associated with a 5-year disease-free survival of 36%, as opposed to 89% in cases without microsatellites (Day *et al.*, 1981a). Since they are included in thickness measurements, the presence of microsatellites is obviously associated with increased melanoma thickness: microsatellites were seen in only 2.8% of melanomas under 3 mm but in 37% of thicker tumours (Kelly *et al.*, 1984). However, the difference in survival remains significant after stratification for thickness and presence of ulceration (Day *et al.*, 1981a). In a series of melanomas over 1.5 mm in thickness, the presence of microsatellites was associated with a prevalence of 53% of occult lymph node metastases (as detected at subsequent elective lymph node dissection), as opposed to 12% of cases without microsatellites (Harrist *et al.*, 1984).

Tumour thickness influences decision on excision width. There has been much debate about the optimal width of resection margins of primary melanoma (Breslow and Macht, 1977; Ackerman and Scheiner, 1983; Aitken *et al.*, 1984; Kelly *et al.*, 1984). Margins of clinically uninvolved skin of 5 cm or more have been used by many in the past. In contrast, Ackerman and Scheiner (1983) advised that 'surgery for a primary cutaneous melanoma should be no different from surgery for any other malignant neoplasm that is primary in the skin. . . . The surgeon should excise what he or she judges clinically to be the entire neoplasm and only little more than that'. However, this standpoint does not do justice to the fact that the chance of clinically undetectable microsatellitosis determining the local cure rate, is typically a problem of melanoma and not, at any rate not to the same extent, of other malignant neoplasms of the skin. The chance of the presence of clinically undetectable satellites is obviously an important factor in the decision on optimal margins of the definitive excision of the primary tumour. Since the incidence of satellites is closely related to tumour thickness, it is reasonable to take tumour thickness into account in the choice of the width of the margin for the definitive excision. As a guideline, at our hospital, a margin of 1 cm is used for melanomas under 1 mm, a margin of 2 cm for those between 1 and 2 mm, and a margin of 3 cm for those thicker than 2 mm. Others use different margins, varying from 2 to 5 cm, for the latter group of tumours. Some sites of the body necessitate narrower surgical margins: the theoretical ideal may clash with practical realities.

In the past, the possible occurrence of a 'field change effect', i.e. an increase in number of normal and atypical intraepidermal melanocytes, the latter of unknown malignant potential, involving the peritumoural epidermis, has also played a role in the discussion of optimal surgical resection margins; however, a recent study (Fallowfield and Cook, 1990) has indicated that such a 'field change' probably does not exist (p. 2).

10.8   Regression

Some degree of host reponse in the form of an inflammatory infiltrate and fibrosis is very common in primary cutaneous melanoma. This host response is often irregularly distributed, thus contributing to the architectural irregularity and asymmetry characteristic of melanoma. In some cases groups of tumour cells degenerate and disappear and a focus of active inflammation followed by scarring is all that remains; usually this happens only focally (*'partial regression'*), but less commonly the whole tumour may disappear in this way.

Whereas the extremes of this spectrum (focal mild host reponse, and total regression of the tumour) are easily distinguished, *it is much more difficult to arrive at reproducible criteria of partial regression*; this problem is illustrated by the fact that reported figures for prevalence of regression in melanoma have varied between 10 and 70% (Cooper *et al.*, 1985; Shaw *et al.*, 1989). *This is relevant to the controversy on the prognostic significance of partial regression in melanoma in general and in thin melanoma in particular.*

According to Cooper and co-workers (1985), regression is present when one or more segments within the tumour show a marked reduction or absence of intradermal tumour cells; instead, this area shows a lymphocytic infiltrate and/or fibrosis, melanophages, and telangiectasia.

In general it appears that the presence of partial regression has no great impact on survival (McLean *et al.*, 1979, McGovern *et al.*, 1983b; Kelly *et al.*, 1985b; Cooper *et al.*, 1985). One could envisage that in melanomas with regression, thickness measurements may be performed at a time when maximum thickness has decreased because of regression; indeed, there is discussion as to whether regression constitutes an unfavourable sign in *thin melanomas*: in an early series, five out of 23 thin melanomas showing regression metastasized within 6 years, contrasting with only two of 98 cases without regression (Gromet *et al.*, 1978). Paladugu and Yonemoto (1983) found regression in 11 out of 36 thin melanomas; five of these metastasized, in contrast to only three of the other 25. Shaw and colleagues (1989) found signs of regression in all 28 thin melanomas presenting with stage II disease, as opposed to 61% of 735 cases with stage I disease who remained free of disease during follow-up. Kuehnl-Petzold and colleagues (1987) found that thin melanomas with regression were often larger, were more often located on the trunk and head, and were more common in males, which may account for at least part of the difference in survival found by several authors.

Balch and colleagues (1985b) found a slight initial unfavourable influence of regression in thin melanoma, but after 10 years this difference disappeared. McGovern and colleagues (1983b) reported 8% metastasis in thin melanoma with regression *vs* 5% in those without regression, but cumulative 10-year survival figures of both groups were the same. Briggs and colleagues (1984) failed to find a correlation between regression and death due to metastatic melanoma in their series of 90 thin melanomas.

It may be that histological assessment of regression should be quantitated rather than scored as either present or absent: Ronan and colleagues (1987) found that, out of a total of 30 thin melanomas with regression, metastases developed in six out of seven tumours with more than 77% regression, the other 23 cases showing less than 77% regression.

In conclusion, unfavourable prognostic influence of regression in thin melanoma was found in some but not in all studies. Reported numbers of metastatic thin melanoma are usually quite small, and some referral bias or other problems in case selection may have influenced the results. In some series an index case leading to the study was included, biasing the statistics. At present it is not completely clear whether regression carries a slight unfavourable prognostic significance in thin melanomas.

In contrast to thin melanoma, in *melanomas of intermediate thickness* (between 0.76 and 1.5 mm), regression was associated with a slightly more favourable course (Balch *et al.*, 1985b). Others also reported a favourable influence in *thick melanomas* (Sondergaard and Schou, 1985a, 1985b).

Apart from melanoma regression, which often results in an irregular focus of depigmentation within the melanoma, circumscribed areas of *cutaneous hypopigmentation at a distance* from the melanoma, or a depigmented 'halo' surrounding the tumour, are found in some cases: in this group, 5-year survival figures are slightly more favourable than in an otherwise similar group (Bystryn *et al.*, 1987). This may link up with the tendency for slightly more favourable prognosis of stage II melanomas with unknown (probably completely regressed) primary tumour, as compared to other stage II melanomas (p. 322).

10.9   Vascular invasion

With routine stains, vascular invasion is detected in some primary melanomas. In a multivariate analysis, vascular invasion was dependent on tumour thickness and was not an independent prognostic factor (Sondergaard and Schou, 1985a). Tissue shrinkage artifacts can simulate vascular lumina; staining the endothelium of lymphatics and blood vessels with *Ulex europaeus* I lectin (UEA-I) aids in the identification of thin-walled vessels, so that vascular invasion is seen more commonly, though still very rarely in melanomas under 1.61 mm (Fallowfield and Cook, 1989). Whether this results in significant prognostic information is not yet known.

10.10   Pre-existent naevus

A significantly better survival has been reported in patients whose melanomas were associated histologically with a pre-existent benign naevus (Friedman *et al.*, 1983; Rogers *et al.*, 1983). This influence of prognosis remained significant after taking into account tumour thickness and other prognostic parameters. However, Schmoeckel and colleagues (1983) and Sondergaard and Schou (1985b) did not find such a significance; the issue therefore remains controversial.

10.11   Dermal inflammatory infiltrate

The presence of a dense lymphocytic infiltrate is associated with a favourable prognosis (Sondergaard and Schou, 1985a); however, thick melanomas have significantly less lymphocytic infiltrate than thin lesions. *The prognostic significance of lymphocytic infiltrate diminishes, but does not disappear completely, after correction for tumour thickness.* The amount of lymphocytic infiltrate can be semiquantitatively assessed according to Sondergaard and Schou (1985a): 0, no lymphocytic reaction; 1, a few small patches of lymphocytes; 2, many large patches; 3, a discontinuous band beneath the tumour, leaving one to two islands of melanoma, each measuring less than 0.5 mm, without lymphocytes beneath; 4, continuous band of infiltrate beneath the tumour.

In contrast to lymphocytic infiltrates, the presence of a marked *plasmocellular infiltrate* has been incriminated as a sign of the presence of lymph node metastasis (Weissmann *et al.*, 1984). Mascaro and colleagues (1987) found abundant plasma cells in 29 out of 132 melanomas; their presence was related to thickness, ulceration and location, and an unfavourable prognosis. Further study is needed to substantiate the value of this feature.

10.12   Cytological features

Severe cellular atypia and, surprisingly, also the small cell lymphocyte-like cell type of melanoma are associated with a poor prognosis

(Schmoeckel *et al.*, 1983). Nuclear pleomorphism and large nucleoli are indicative of unfavourable prognosis, but are related to mitotic activity (Sondergaard and Schou, 1985a). Large nuclei were more common in thick melanomas; a large nuclear size, measured as nuclear area or volume (Heenan *et al.*, 1989; Sørensen, 1989; Tosi *et al.*, 1989), as well as marked variation in nuclear area and 'form factor' (Lindholm *et al.*, 1988) were related to an unfavourable prognosis.

Van der Esch and colleagues (1981), and Baak and Tan (1986) reported a better prognosis in melanomas with spindle-shaped nuclei as opposed to those with predominantly round nuclei. A spindle-shaped cell type as the predominant cell type in the invasive component was also found to indicate a relatively low risk of metastasis (Sondergaard and Schou, 1985a).

Amelanotic melanomas tend to be thick, perhaps due to a rapid growth rate and/or late diagnosis. The unfavourable prognosis is accounted for by this greater thickness as compared to pigmented melanomas.

In most studies *aneuploidy* is correlated with an increased chance of recurrence and a shorter disease-free survival in stage I melanoma (Von Roenn *et al.*, 1986; Coon *et al.*, 1987; Heenan *et al.*, 1989); after stratification for tumour thickness, aneuploidy was actually the most significant prognostic factor in one series of 177 stage I melanomas (Kheir *et al.*, 1988). In contrast, Lindholm and colleagues (1990), studying 50 stage I melanomas with a minimum follow-up period of 10 years, did not find a significant correlation with prognosis. Further study will be required to ascertain the possible usefulness of aneuploidy as a prognostic marker.

Structural abnormalities of chromosomes 7 and 11, as assessed by chromosome banding analysis of 62 cases of metastatic melanoma, was associated with a significantly shorter survival in one recent study (Trent *et al.*, 1990).

There is controversy regarding the prognostic significance of strong *immunoreactivity for S-100*. Rode and Dhillon (1984) reported an unfavourable prognostic significance of strong S-100 positivity. However, Kernohan and Rankin (1987) found strong immunoreactivity for S-100 in only two out of 13 melanomas leading to death within 1 year, but in 12 out of 14 cases surviving longer than 10 years. Hagen and colleagues (1986) did not find a significant difference in clinical behaviour of melanomas expressing high and low levels of S-100. Assessment of S-100 reactivity was semiquantitative and subjective in all three studies; staining methods as well as assessment methods were different. The matter remains unresolved.

HLA-DR expression in melanoma cells is seen most commonly in tumours invading the reticular dermis, is often strongest at the invasion front, and is associated with an increased inflammatory infiltrate. Indeed, expression of HLA-DR and also the intercellular adhesion molecule ICAM-1 can be induced by lymphokines and may therefore be a result of the presence of the inflammatory infiltrate (Johnson *et al.*, 1989). Early tumour recurrence was more common in melanomas expressing HLA-DR, but there is dependence on stronger prognostic parameters such as thickness (Bröcker *et al.*, 1984; 1985). In metastatic melanoma, different patterns of HLA class I and II expression have also been associated with differences in prognosis (Van Duinen *et al.*, 1988).

The presence of *oestrogen receptors* as assessed with an oestrogen-binding assay, has been related to a more protracted clinical course (Walker *et al.*, 1987). Prognostic significance of immunoreactivity with a variety of monoclonal antibodies has been reported (Natali *et al.*, 1987); further studies will be needed to ascertain their possible usefulness in routine surgical pathology.

10.13   Late recurrence of melanoma

Rarely, cutaneous melanoma recurs after a disease-free interval of more than 10 years; *often, such cases concern female patients with melanomas of intermediate thickness* (Koh *et al.*, 1984b; Khanna *et al.*, 1986). Late tumour recurrence is somewhat more common in ocular melanoma; relapses occur most commonly in the liver (Gatchell and Minor, 1972). Long-term spontaneous regression of melanoma followed by late recurrence has rarely been reported (Bulkley *et al.*, 1975).

10.14   Prognosis of metastatic melanoma

10.14.1   *Melanoma with regional lymph node metastasis*

Regional lymph node metastases may be clinically evident at the time of diagnosis of the primary tumour, they may develop later, or they may be found in the absence of a clinically evident primary tumour. The prognosis is similar in all three situations; overall 5-year survival at the time of diagnosis of the regional lymph node metastasis is of the order of 30–40%.

The tumour burden in the regional lymph node station (number and percentage of nodes involved) is an important prognostic factor. In one study, four or more involved lymph nodes were associated with an 8-year survival of 25%, as opposed to 50–55% for cases with one to three involved nodes (Cohen et al., 1977). In the series of Balch and colleagues (1981), 5-year survival rates with one, two to four, and more than four positive nodes were 58, 27 and 10%, respectively. Cochran and colleagues (1989) demonstrated that additional prognostic information is obtained when, in addition to the number of nodes involved, the sectional area of nodes involved by tumour is expressed as a percentage of the total nodal sectional area (up to 15%, favourable; over 15%, unfavourable).

Small numbers of tumour cells in lymph nodes are more easily detected with S-100 immunostaining: in a study of 2227 lymph nodes, 16 nodes, from 14 patients, were found to contain tumour which had passed unnoticed at routine histology (Cochran et al., 1988). Six of these 14 patients died, as opposed to 18 out of 86 patients without such metastases, apparently indicating that even such very small metastases carry prognostic significance. However, the number of tumour deaths in the group with occult tumour cells in this series was rather high, when compared to other survival figures of stage II melanoma with a small tumour burden. The clinical significance of detection of very small numbers of tumour cells therefore remains to be confirmed. The tumour cells have to be distinguished from interdigitating reticulum cells, some sinus macrophages, naevus cells occasionally found in lymph node capsule (p. 362), and Schwann cells of perinodal nerves, all of which are S-100 positive.

Surprisingly, *several prognostic features of the primary tumour retain considerable prognostic significance even in the presence of regional lymph node metastases*. The maximal thickness of the primary tumour (Day et al., 1981b; Callery et al., 1982), the level of invasion (Cohen et al., 1977), the presence of ulceration (Balch et al., 1980; 1981) and the site of the primary tumour are all significant in this respect. Ulceration in particular appears to be important: ulcerated and non-ulcerated stage II melanomas are associated with 5-year survival rates of around 25 and 50%, respectively.

A combination of prognostic factors of the primary tumour and tumour burden in the regional lymph nodes will probably allow an optimal prediction of clinical outcome. In a group of 325 patients with clinical stage I melanomas who underwent elective regional lymph node dissection, Day and co-workers (1981b) found metastases in 46 cases; these could be subdivided into a high risk group (at least 20% of identified lymph nodes positive, or primary tumour thickness at least 3.5 mm; 5-year disease-free survival 17.5%), and a low risk group (less than 20% positive nodes and tumour under 3.5 mm in thickness; 5-year survival 80%).

10.14.2   Melanoma with distant metastases

Prognosis of melanoma with distant metastases is poor. Overall 2-year survival is around 10–20%; very few patients survive 5 years or longer. In a series of 102 cases with distant metastases, the median survival after removal of all clinically detectable tumour was 18 months (Feun et al., 1982). The most commonly involved sites of clinically evident distant metastases are, in decreasing order: lung, subcutis, bone, brain and liver (Nambisan et al., 1987). According to some, multiple organ involvement is associated with even poorer survival, and involvement of the liver, which is disproportionately common in melanoma of the eye and mucous membranes, appears to be associated with a worse survival than lung and brain involvement (Nambisan et al., 1987). However, in another series (Feun et al., 1982), there were no major differences in survival according to the sites involved or the number of resected metastases.

Very rarely, spontaneous regression of metastatic melanoma has led to long-term disease-free survival. It seems likely that in such cases an antitumour immune response was involved (Bulkley et al., 1975; Sroujieh, 1988).

10.15   Metastatic melanoma with unknown primary

In about 4–12% of patients with metastatic melanoma, the primary tumour is not clinically apparent (Das Gupta et al., 1963; Smith and Stehlin, 1965; Baab and McBride, 1975; Pellegrini, 1980; Balch et al., 1981); presumably, complete regression of a cutaneous melanoma has occurred in most of these cases. Such cases of metastatic melanoma with unknown primary tumour concern males about twice as commonly as females (Chang and Knapper, 1982), which is in accordance with the higher frequency of regression of melanoma found in men. Meticulous clinical examination of the skin drained by the lymph node, with the aid of a Wood's lamp, may reveal a small scar indicating the site of the primary tumour (McGovern, 1975); this should be excised and examined for possible residual tumour. In rare instances the primary tumour is found in an extracutaneous site.

The prognosis of cases with unknown primary tumour is similar to that of metastatic melanoma with known and resected primary tumour, or perhaps even slightly better: in one series, 5- and 10-year survival figures, in cases with involvement of one lymph node station only, were 46 and 41% (Chang and Knapper, 1982). Accordingly, similar treatment strategies are advocated for these patients (Giuliano *et al.,* 1980; Balch *et al.,* 1981; Chang and Knapper, 1982; Jonk *et al.,* 1990).

References

Ackerman, A. B. and Scheiner, A. M. (1983) How wide and deep is wide and deep enough? A critique of surgical practice in excisions of primary cutaneous malignant melanoma. *Hum. Pathol.,* **14**, 743–4.

Aitken, D. R., James, A. G. and Carey, L. C. (1984) Local cutaneous recurrence after conservative excision of malignant melanoma. *Arch. Surg.,* **119**, 643–6.

Allen, A. C. and Spitz, S. (1953) Malignant melanoma. A clinicopathological analysis of the criteria for diagnosis and prognosis. *Cancer,* **6**, 1–45.

Baab, G. H. and McBride, C. M. (1975) Malignant melanoma. The patient with an unknown site of primary origin. *Arch. Surg.,* **110**, 896–900.

Baak, J. P. A. and Tan, G. J. K. H. (1986) The adjuvant prognostic value of nuclear morphometry in stage I malignant melanoma of the skin. A multivariate analysis. *Anal. Quant. Cytol. Histol.,* **8**, 241–4.

Balch, C. M., Murad, T. M., Soong, S.-J., Ingalls, A. L., Halpern, N. B. and Maddox, W. A. (1978) A multifactorial analysis of melanoma: prognostic histopathological features comparing Clark's and Breslow's staging methods. *Ann. Surg.,* **188**, 732–42.

Balch, C. M., Wilkerson, J. A., Murad, T. M., Soong, S.-J., Ingalls, A.L. and Maddox, W. A. (1980) The prognostic significance of ulceration of cutaneous melanoma. *Cancer,* **45**, 3012–7.

Balch, C. M., Soong, S.-J., Murad, T. M., Ingalls, A. L. and Maddox, W. A. (1981) A multifactorial analysis of melanoma. III. Prognostic factors in melanoma patients with lymph node metastases (stage II). *Ann. Surg.,* **193**, 377–88.

Balch, C. M., Milton, G. W., Shaw, H. M. and Soong, S.-J. (eds) (1985a) *Cutaneous Melanoma. Clinical Management and Treatment Results Worldwide.* Philadelphia: J. B. Lippincott.

Balch, C. M., Soong, S.-J., Shaw, H. M. and Milton, G. W. (1985b) An analysis of prognostic factors in 4000 patients with cutaneous melanoma. In *Cutaneous Melanoma. Clinical Management and Treatment Results Worldwide.* Philadelphia: J. B. Lippincott, pp. 321–52.

Beahrs, O. H. and Myers, M. H. (1983) *Manual for Staging of Cancer.* American Joint Committee on Cancer, Philadelphia: J. B. Lippincott, p. 117.

Blessing K., McLaren, K. M., McLean, A. and Davidson, P. (1990) Thin malignant melanomas (≤1.5 mm) with metastasis: a histological study and survival analysis. *Histopathology,* **17**, 389–95.

Bonett, A., Roder, D. and Esterman, A. (1986) Melanoma case survival rates in South Australia by histological type, thickness and level of tumour at diagnosis. *Med. J. Aust.,* **144**, 680–2.

Braun-Falco, O., Landthaler, M., Hölzel, D., Konz, B. and Schmoeckel, C.

(1986) Therapie und Prognose maligner Melanome der Haut. *Dtsch. Med. Wschr.*, **111**, 1750–6.

Breslow, A. (1970) Thickness, cross-sectional areas and depth of invasion in the prognosis of cutaneous melanoma. *Ann. Surg.*, **172**, 902–8.

Breslow, A. (1975) Tumor thickness, level of invasion and node dissection in stage I cutaneous melanoma. *Ann. Surg.*, **182**, 572–5.

Breslow, A. (1977) Problems in the measurement of tumor thickness and level of invasion in cutaneous melanoma. *Hum. Pathol.*, **8**, 1–2.

Breslow, A. (1980) Prognosis in cutaneous melanoma: tumor thickness as a guide to treatment. *Pathol. Ann.*, **15-I**, 1–22.

Breslow, A. and Macht, S. D. (1977) Optimal size of resection margins for thin cutaneous melanoma. *Surg. Gyn. Obstet.*, **145**, 691–2.

Breslow, A., Cascinelli, N., Van der Esch, E. P. and Morabito, A. (1978) Stage I melanoma of the limbs: assessment of prognosis by levels of invasion and maximum thickness. *Tumori*, **64**, 273–84.

Briggs, J. C., Ibrahim, N. B. N., Hastings, A. G. and Griffiths, R. W. (1984) Experience of thin cutaneous melanomas (<0.76 mm and <0.85 mm thick) in a large plastic surgery unit: a 5 to 17-year follow-up. *Br. J. Plast. Surg.*, **37**, 501–6.

Bröcker, E.-B., Suter, L. and Sorg, C. (1984) HLA-DR antigen expression in primary melanomas of the skin. *J. Invest. Dermatol.*, **82**, 244–7.

Bröcker, E.-B., Suter, L., Brüggen, J., Ruiter, D. J., Macher, E. and Sorg, C. (1985) Phenotypic dynamics of tumor progression in human malignant melanoma. *Int. J. Cancer*, **36**, 29–35.

Bulkley, G. B., Cohen, M. H., Banks, P. M., Char, D. H. and Ketcham, A. S. (1975) Long-term spontaneous regression of malignant melanoma with visceral metastases. Report of a case with immunologic profile. *Cancer*, **36**, 485–94.

Bystryn, J.-C., Rigel, D., Friedman, R. J. and Kopf, A. (1987) Prognostic significance of hypopigmentation in malignant melanoma. *Arch. Dermatol.*, **123**, 1053–5.

Callery, C., Cochran, A. J., Roe, D. J. *et al.* (1982) Factors for survival in patients with malignant melanoma spread to the regional lymph nodes. *Ann. Surg.*, **196**, 69–75.

Cascinelli, N., Morabito, A., Bufalino, R. *et al.* (1980) Prognosis of stage I melanoma of the skin. *Int. J. Cancer.*, **26**, 733–9.

Cascinelli, N., Vaglini, M., Bufalino, R. and Morabito, A. (1986) BANS. A cutaneous region with no prognostic significance in patients with melanoma. *Cancer*, **57**, 441–4.

Chang, P. and Knapper, W. H. (1982) Metastatic melanoma of unknown primary. *Cancer*, **49**, 1106–11.

Clark, W. H., From, L., Bernardino, E. A. and Mihm, M. C. (1969) The histogenesis and biologic behavior of primary human malignant melanoma of the skin. *Cancer Res.*, **29**, 705–15.

Cochran, A. J., Wen, D.-R. and Morton, D. L. (1988) Occult tumor cells in the lymph nodes of patients with pathological stage I malignant melanoma. An immunohistological study. *Am. J. Surg. Pathol.*, **12**, 612–8.

Cochran, A. J., Lana, A. M. A. and Wen, D.-R. (1989) Histomorphometry in the assessment of prognosis in stage II malignant melanoma. *Am. J. Surg. Pathol.*, **13**, 600–4.

Cohen, M. H., Ketcham, A. S., Felix, E. L. *et al.* (1977) Prognostic factors in patients undergoing lymphadenectomy for malignant melanoma. *Ann. Surg.*, **186**, 635–42.

Cohen, H. J., Cox, E., Manton, K. and Woodbury, M. (1987) Malignant melanoma in the elderly. *J. Clin. Oncol.*, **5**, 100–6.

Coon, J. S., Bines, S., Kheir, S. *et al.* (1987) DNA flow cytometry in stage I cutaneous melanoma. *Cytometry*, **1**, 55S.

Cooper, P. H., Wanebo, H. J. and Hagar, R. W. (1985) Regression in thin malignant melanoma. Microscopic diagnosis and prognostic importance. *Arch. Dermatol.*, **121**, 1127–31.

Costa, A., Silvestrini, R., Grignolo, E., Clemente, C., Attili, A. and Testori, A. (1987) Cell kinetics as a prognostic tool with metastatic malignant melanoma of the skin. *Cancer*, **60**, 2797–2800.

Das Gupta, T., Bowden, L. and Berg, J. W. (1963) Malignant melanoma of unknown primary origin. *Surg. Gynecol. Obstetr.*, **117**, 341–5.

Daly, J. M., Berlin, R. and Urmacher, C. (1987) Subungual melanoma: a 25-year review of cases. *J. Surg. Oncol.*, **35**, 107–12.

Day, C. L. Jr., Harrist, T. J., Gorstein F. *et al.* (1981a) Malignant melanoma. Prognostic significance of 'microscopic satellites' in the reticular dermis and subcutaneous fat. *Ann. Surg.*, **194**, 108–12.

Day, C. L. Jr., Sober, A. J., Lew, R. A. *et al.* (1981b) Malignant melanoma patients with positive nodes and relatively good prognoses: microstaging retains prognostic significance in clinical stage I melanoma patients with metastases to regional nodes. *Cancer*, **47**, 955–62.

Day, C. L., Lew, R. A., Mihm, M. C. *et al.* (1981c) The natural breakpoints for primary tumor thickness in clinical stage I melanoma. *New Engl. J. Med.*, **305**, 1155.

Day, C. L. Jr., Mihm, M. C. Jr., Sober, A. J. *et al.* (1982) Prognostic factors for melanoma patients with lesions 0.76–1.69 mm in thickness. An appraisal of 'thin' level IV lesions. *Ann. Surg.*, **195**, 30–34.

Fallowfield, M. E. and Cook, M. G. (1989) Vascular invasion in malignant melanomas. An independent prognostic variable? *Am. J. Surg. Pathol.*, **13**, 217–20.

Fallowfield, M. E. and Cook, M. G. (1990) Epidermal melanocytes adjacent to melanoma and the field change effect. *Histopathology*, **17**, 397–400.

Feun, L. G., Gutterman, J. M., Burgess, A. *et al.* (1982) The natural history of resectable metastatic melanoma (stage IVA melanoma). *Cancer*, **50**, 1656–63.

Friedman, R. J., Rigel, D. S., Kopf, A. W. *et al.* (1983) Favorable prognosis for malignant melanomas associated with acquired melanocytic nevi. *Arch. Dermatol.*, **119**, 455–62.

Gatchell, F. G. and Minor, D. (1972) Malignant melanoma of the eye, metastatic after 29 years: a case report. *O.S.M.A. J.*, **65**, 211–3.

Giuliano, A. E., Moseley, S. and Morton, D. L. (1980) Clinical aspects of unknown primary melanoma. *Ann. Surg.*, **191**, 98–104.

Gromet, M. A., Epstein, W. L. and Blois, M. S. (1978) The regressing thin malignant melanoma. A distinctive lesion with metastatic potential. *Cancer*, **42**, 2282–92.

Gussack, G. S., Reitgen, D., Cox, E., Fisher, S., Cole, T. and Seigler, H. (1983) Cutaneous melanoma of the head and neck: a review of 399 cases. *Arch. Otolaryngol.*, **109**, 803–8.

Hagen, E. C., Vennegoor, C., Schlingemann, R. O., Van der Velde, E. A. and Ruiter, D. J. (1986) Correlation of histopathological characteristics with staining patterns in human melanoma assessed by (monoclonal) antibodies reactive on paraffin sections. *Histopathology*, **10**, 689–700.

Harrist, T. J., Rigel, D. S., Day, C. L. *et al.* (1984) 'Microscopic satellites' are more highly associated with regional lymph node metastases than is primary melanoma thickness. *Cancer*, **53**, 2183–7.

Heenan, P. J., Jarvis, L. R., De Klerk, N. H. and Armstrong, B. K. (1989) Nuclear indices and survival in cutaneous melanoma. *Am. J. Dermatopathol.*, **11**, 308–12.

International Union Against Cancer (1978) *TNM Classification of Malignant Melanoma* (2nd edn.). Geneva: International Union Against Cancer.

Johnson, J. P., Lehmann, J. M., Stade, B. G., Rothbächer, U., Sers, C. and Riethmüller, G. (1989) Functional aspects of three molecules associated with metastasis development in human malignant melanoma. *Invasion Metast.*, **9**, 338–50.

Jonk, A., Kroon, B. B. R., Rümke, P., Mooi, W. J., Hart, A. A. M. and Van Dongen, J. A. (1990) Lymph node metastasis from melanoma with an unknown primary site. *Br. J. Surg.*, **77**, 665–8.

Karakousis, C. P., Emrich, L. J. and Rao, U. (1988) Prediction of survival in primary melanomas according to thickness. *Proc. Am. Assoc. Cancer Res.*, **29**, 174.

Karakousis, C. P., Emrich, L. J. and Rao, U. (1989) Tumor thickness and prognosis in clinical stage I malignant melanoma. *Cancer*, **64**, 1432–6.

Kelly, J. W., Sagebiel, R. W., Calderon, W., Murillo, L., Dakin, R. L. and Blois, M. S. (1984) The frequency of local recurrence and micro-satellites as a guide to resection margins for cutaneous malignant melanoma. *Ann. Surg.*, **200**, 759–63.

Kelly, J. W., Sagebiel, R. W., Clyman, S. and Blois, M. S. (1985a) The thin level IV malignant melanoma: a subset in which level is the major prognostic indicator. *Ann. Surg.*, **202**, 98–103.

Kelly, J. W., Sagebiel, R. W. and Blois, M. S. (1985b) Regression in malignant melanoma. A histologic feature without independent prognostic significance. *Cancer*, **56**, 2287–91.

Kernohan, N. M. and Rankin, R. (1987) S-100 protein: a prognostic indicator in cutaneous malignant melanoma? *Histopathology*, **11**, 1285–93.

Khanna, A. K., Laidler, P. and Hughes, L. E. (1986) Can late recurrence of melanoma be predicted at the time of primary treatment? *Eur. J. Surg. Oncol.*, **12**, 9–12.

Kheir, S. M., Bines, S. D., Vonroenn, J. H., Soong, S.-J., Urist, M. M. and Coon, J. S. (1988) Prognostic significance of DNA aneuploidy in stage I cutaneous melanoma. *Ann. Surg.*, **207**, 455–61.

Kirkham, N. and Cotton, D. W. K. (1984) Measuring melanomas: the Vernier method. *J. Clin. Pathol.*, **37**, 229–30.

Koh, H., Michalik, E., Sober, A. J. *et al.* (1984a) Lentigo maligna melanoma has no better prognosis than other types of melanoma. *J. Clin. Oncol.*, **2**, 994–1001.

Koh, H. K., Sober, A. J. and Fitzpatrick, T. B. (1984b) Late recurrence (beyond ten years) of cutaneous malignant melanoma. Report of two cases and a review of the literature. *J. Am. Med. Assoc.*, **251**, 1859–62.

Kopf, A. W., Gross, D. F., Rogers, G. S. *et al.* (1987) Prognostic index for malignant melanoma. *Cancer*, **59**, 1236–41.

Kuehnl-Petzoldt, C. and Fisher, S. (1987) Tumor thickness is not a prognostic factor in thin melanoma. *Arch. Dermatol. Res.*, **279**, 487–8.

Kuehnl-Petzoldt, C., Keil, H. and Schoepf, E. (1984) Prognostic significance of the patient's sex, tumor site, and mitotic rate in thin (≤1.5 mm) melanoma. *Arch. Dermatol. Res.*, **276**, 151–5.

Kuehnl-Petzoldt, C., Fisher, S. and Schoepf, E. (1987) Occurrence and prognostic significance of regression in thin malignant melanoma. *Am. J. Dermatopathol.*, **9**, 164.

Lindholm, C., Hofer, P.-A. and Jonsson, H. (1988) Karyometric findings and prognosis of stage I cutaneous malignant melanomas. *Acta Oncol.*, **27**, 227–33.

Lindholm, C., Hofer, P.-A. and Jonsson, H. (1990) Single cell DNA cytophotometry in clinical stage I malignant melanoma. Relationship to prognosis. *Acta Oncol.*, **29**, 147–50.

Manci, E. A., Balch, C. M., Murad, T. M. and Soong, S.-J. (1981) Polypoid melanoma, a virulent variant of the nodular growth pattern. *Am. J. Clin. Pathol.*, **75**, 810–5.

Mascaro, J. M., Molgo, M., Castel, T. and Castro, J. (1987) Plasma cells within the infiltrate of primary cutaneous malignant melanoma of the skin. A confirmation of its histoprognostic value. *Am. J. Dermatopathol.*, **9**, 497–9.

McGovern, V. J. (1975) Spontaneous regression of melanoma. *Pathology*, **7**, 91–99.

McGovern, V. J., Shaw, H. M., Milton, G. W. and Farago, G. A. (1979) Prognostic significance of the histological features of malignant melanoma. *Histopathology*, **3**, 385–93.

McGovern, V. J., Shaw, H. M., Milton, G. W. and Farago, G. A. (1980) Is malignant melanoma arising in Hutchinson's melanotic freckle a separate disease entity? *Histopathology*, **4**, 235–42.

McGovern, V. J., Shaw, H. M., Milton, G. W. and McCarthy, W. H. (1982) Ulceration and prognosis in cutaneous malignant melanoma. *Histopathology*, **6**, 399–407.

McGovern, V. J., Shaw, H. M. and Milton, G. W. (1983a) Prognostic significance of a polypoid configuration in malignant melanoma. *Histopathology*, **7**, 663–72.

McGovern, V. J., Shaw, H. M. and Milton, G. W. (1983b) Prognosis in patients with thin malignant melanoma: influence of regression. *Histopathology*, **7**, 673–80.

McLean, D. I., Lew, R. A., Sober, A. J., Mihm, M. C. and Fitzpatrick, T. B. (1979) On the prognostic importance of white depressed areas in the primary lesion of superficial spreading melanoma. *Cancer*, **43**, 157–61.

Mehnert, J. H. and Heard, J. L. (1965) Staging of malignant melanoma by depth of invasion. A proposed index to prognosis. *Am. J. Surg.*, **110**, 168–76.

Nambisan, R. N., Alexiou, G., Reese, P. A. and Karakousis, C. P. (1987) Early metastatic patterns and survival in malignant melanoma. *J. Surg. Oncol.*, **34**, 248–52.

Naruns, P. L., Nizze, A., Cochran, A. J., Lee, M. B. and Morton, D. L. (1986) Recurrence potential of thin primary melanomas. *Cancer*, **57**, 545–8.

Natali, P. G., Roberts, J. T., Difilippo, F. *et al.* (1987) Immunohistochemical detection of antigen in human primary and metastatic melanomas by the monoclonal antibody 140.240 and its possible prognostic significance. *Cancer*, **59**, 55–63.

Nield, D. V., Saad, M. N., Khoo, C. T. K., Lott, M. and Ali, M. H. (1988) Tumour thickness in malignant melanoma: the limitations of frozen section. *Br. J. Plast. Surg.*, **41**, 403–7.

O'Doherty, C. J., Prescot, R. J., White, H., McIntyre, M. and Hunter, J. A. A. (1986) Sex differences in presentation of cutaneous malignant melanoma and in survival from stage I disease. *Cancer*, **58**, 788–92.

Ostmeier, H. and Suter, L. (1988) Correlation of mitotic rate and Ki-67 positive cells in primary malignant melanomas. *J. Invest. Dermatol.*, **91**, 381.

Paladugu, R. R. and Yonemoto, R. H. (1983) Biologic behavior of thin malignant melanomas with regressive changes. *Arch. Surg.*, **118**, 41–44.

Pellegrini, A. E. (1980) Regressed primary malignant melanoma with regional metastases. *Arch. Dermatol.*, **116**, 585–6.

Rampen, F. H. J., Menzel, S. and Rümke, P. (1987) Satellite and in-transit metastases from melanoma are more predominant in females than in males. *Anticancer Res.*, **7**, 429–32.

Reed, K, M., Bronstein, B. R., Mihm, M. C. and Sober, A. J. (1986) Prognosis for polypoidal melanoma is determined by primary tumor thickness. *Cancer*, **57**, 1201–3.

Reintgen, D. S., Vollmer, R., Tso, C. Y. and Seigler, H. F. (1987) Prognosis for recurrent stage I malignant melanoma. *Arch. Surg.*, **122**, 1338–42.

Retsas, S., Henry, K. and MacKenzie, D. H. (1986) Missed malignant melanoma. *Br. Med. J.*, **292**, 1270–1.

Rode, J. and Dhillon, A. P. (1984) Neurone specific enolase and S-100 protein as possible prognostic indicators in melanomas. *Histopathology*, **8**, 1041–7.

Rogers, G. S., Kopf, A. W., Rigel, D. S. *et al.* (1983) Effect of anatomical location on prognosis in patients with clinical stage I melanoma. *Arch. Dermatol.*, **119**, 644–9.

Ronan, S. G., Eng, A. M., Briele, H. A., Shioura, N. N. and Das Gupta, T. K. (1987) Thin malignant melanomas with regression and metastases. *Arch. Dermatol.*, **123**, 1326–30.

Schmoeckel, C. and Braun-Falco, O. (1978) Prognostic index in malignant melanoma. *Arch. Dermatol.*, **114**, 871–3.

Schmoeckel, C., Bockelbrink, A., Bockelbrink, H. and Braun-Falco, O. (1983) Low- and high-risk malignant melanoma. II. Multivariate analysis for a prognostic classification. *Eur. J. Cancer Clin. Oncol.*, **19**, 227–35.

Shafir, R., Hiss, J., Tsur, H. and Bubis, J. J. (1983). Pitfalls in frozen section diagnosis of malignant melanoma. *Cancer*, **51**, 1168–70.

Shaw, H. M., McCarthy, W. H., McCarthy, S. W. and Milton, G. W. (1987). Thin malignant melanomas and recurrence potential. *Arch. Surg.*, **122**, 1147–50.

Shaw, H. M., McCarthy, S. W., McCarthy, W. H., Thompson, J. F. and Milton, G. W. (1989). Thin regressing malignant melanoma: significance of concurrent regional lymph node metastases. *Histopathology*, **15**, 257–65.

Slingluff, C. L., Vollmer, R. T., Reintgen, D. S. and Seigler, H. F. (1988). Lethal 'thin' malignant melanoma. Identifying patients at risk. *Ann. Surg.*, **208**, 150–61.

Smith, J. L. (1976). Histopathology and biologic behaviour of melanoma. In *Neoplasms of the Skin and Malignant Melanomas*. Chicago: Year Book Medical

Publishers, p. 293.

Smith, J. L. and Stehlin, J. S. (1965). Spontaneous regression of primary melanomas with regional metastases. *Cancer*, **18**, 1399–1415.

Sondergaard, K. and Schou, G. (1985a). Survival with primary cutaneous malignant melanoma, evaluated from 2012 cases. *Virchows Arch. A (Pathol. Anat.)*, **406**, 179–95.

Sondergaard, K. and Schou, G. (1985b). Therapeutic and clinicopathological factors in the survival of 1469 patients with primary cutaneous melanoma in clinical stage I. *Virchows Arch. A (Pathol. Anat.)*, **408**, 249–58.

Soong, S.-J. (1985). A computerized mathematical model and scoring system for predicting outcome in melanoma patients. In *Cutaneous Melanoma. Clinical Management and Treatment Results Worldwide*. Philadelphia: J. B. Lippincott, pp. 353–67.

Sørensen, F. B. (1989). Objective histopathologic grading of cutaneous malignant melanomas by stereologic estimation of nuclear volume. Prediction of survival and disease-free period. *Cancer*, **63**, 1784–98.

Sroujieh, A. S. (1988). Spontaneous regression of intestinal malignant melanoma from an occult primary site. *Cancer*, **62**, 1247–50.

Thörn, M., Adami, H.-O., Ringborg, U., Bergström, R. and Krusemo, U.-B. (1987). Long-term survival in malignant melanoma with special reference to age and sex as prognostic factors. *J. Natl Cancer Inst.*, **79**, 969–74.

Tompkins, V. N. (1953). Cutaneous melanoma: ulceration as a prognostic sign. *Cancer*, **6**, 1215–8.

Tosi, P., Luzi, P., Sforza, V. *et al.* (1989). The nuclei in cutaneous malignant melanoma, stage I, are smaller in survivors than in non-survivors. *Pathol. Res. Pract.*, **185**, 625–30.

Trent, J. M., Meyskens, F. L., Salmon, S. E. *et al.* (1990). Relation of cytogenetic abnormalities and clinical outcome in metastatic melanoma. *New Engl. J. Med.*, **322**, 1508–11.

Van der Esch, E. P., Cascinelli, N., Preda, F., Morabito, A. and Bufalino, R. (1981). Stage I melanoma of the skin: evaluation of prognosis according to histologic characteristics. *Cancer*, **48**, 1668–73.

Van Duinen, S. G., Ruiter, D. J., Broecker, E. B. *et al.* (1988). Level of HLA antigens in locoregional metastases and clinical course of the disease in patients with melanoma. *Cancer Res.*, **48**, 1019–25.

Vollmer, R. T. (1989). Malignant melanoma. A multivariate analysis of prognostic factors. *Pathol. Ann.*, **24-I**, 383–407.

Von Roenn, J. M., Kheir, S. M., Wolter, J. M. and Coon, J. S. (1986). Significance of DNA abnormalities in primary malignant melanomas and nevi, a retrospective flow cytometric study. *Cancer Res.*, **46**, 3192–5.

Walker, M. J., Beattie, C. W., Patel, M. K., Ronan, S. M. and Das Gupta, T. K. (1987). Estrogen receptor in malignant melanoma. *J. Clin. Oncol.*, **5**, 1256–61.

Wanebo, H. J., Woodruff, J. and Fortner, J. G. (1975). Malignant melanoma of the extremities: a clinicopathologic study using levels of invasion (microstage). *Cancer*, **35**, 666–76.

Wanebo, H. J., Cooper, P. H., Young, D. V., Harpole, D. H. and Kaiser, D. L. (1988). Prognostic factors in head and neck melanoma. Effect of lesion location. *Cancer*, **62**, 831–7.

Weinstock, M. A., Morris, B. T., Lederman, J. S., Bleicher, P., Fitzpatrick, T. B. and Sober, A. J. (1988). Effect of BANS location on the prognosis of clinical

stage I melanoma: new data and meta-analysis. *Br. J. Dermatol.*, **119**, 559–65.
Weissman, A., Roses, D., Harris, M. and Dibin, N. (1984). Prediction of lymph node metastasis from the histologic features of primary cutaneous malignant melanomas. *Am. J. Dermatopathol.*, **6(Suppl.)**, 35–41.

11 Extracutaneous melanocytic lesions

Melanocytic lesions outside the skin are infrequently encountered in diagnostic practice. Most occur in the eyes and juxtacutaneous mucous membranes, but they are occasionally found in a wide variety of other sites, where they may cause differential diagnostic problems with metastatic melanoma or various nonmelanocytic lesions.

The classification of *melanocytic lesions of mucous membranes* generally parallels that of cutaneous naevi and melanomas. Thus, junctional, compound, 'intramucosal' (subepithelial), blue, and combined variants of naevi, as well as a variety of melanomas are distinguished. However, there are also differences; for instance, 'junctional activity' more commonly persists into adulthood, and lesions are often larger than their cutaneous counterparts. Moreover, a histological similarity to a cutaneous lesion does not necessarily mean that the lesion has the same aetiology or pathogenesis.

'*Mucosal melanosis*' is a much used but not always strictly defined term. It is perhaps best used only in a clinical sense to indicate an area of abnormal melanotic pigmentation of a mucous membrane. Pathologically, this pigmentation can be the result of totally different situations: 1. the presence of melanocytes in mucosal sites where they are normally absent; 2. increased melanin production by mucosal melanocytes which are normal in number; 3. proliferation of mucosal melanocytes. This latter group, *mucosal melanocytic hyperplasia*, can be subdivided into forms with a lentiginous, a nested, or a combined architectural pattern of growth, with or without associated cytological atypia.

All of these pathological situations result in a patch of mucosal pigmentation, i.e. mucosal melanosis, but the forms associated with proliferation of melanocytes exhibiting nuclear atypia, are the biologically important ones because of their association with mucosal melanoma. Since 'mucosal melanosis' therefore encompasses totally innocuous lesions as well as atypical proliferations which carry a significant risk of developing into invasive melanoma, the term is not very useful in pathology and is best avoided. In the case of 'primary acquired melanosis' of the conjunctiva, use of the term is almost unavoidable, because it is so widely entrenched in the literature; nevertheless, as will be discussed below (p. 336), the same problems of nomenclature apply also to this particular site.

Nonmucosal benign melanocytic lesions can usually be likened to the cutaneous blue naevus. These lesions occur in a variety of unexpected sites, such as the prostate.

In contrast to many benign lesions, melanomas will sooner or later come to clinical attention; the question then arises, whether the tumour is a primary extracutaneous melanoma or a metastasis. *Only about 15% of all melanomas are extracutaneous and, of these, 80% are ocular neoplasms* (Scotto *et al.*, 1976). In this respect, it is important to emphasize the tendency of cutaneous melanoma to metastasize to unusual sites. The most common sites of metastasis of cutaneous melanoma were assessed in an autopsy series by Das Gupta and Brasfield (1964): in decreasing order of frequency, metastases were found in the lungs (70%), liver (68%), small bowel (58%), pancreas (53%), adrenals (50%), heart (49%), kidneys (45%), brain (39%), thyroid (39%), and spleen (36%). Other locations were found in less than 30% of cases; bone metastases were rare, but autopsy sampling of bone is often not adequate to assess the true prevalence of bone metastases. Obviously, clinical symptoms due to metastasis are less common and their relative frequencies vary from site to site; internal organ involvement as the first presentation of cutaneous melanoma is rare. Nevertheless, it will be clear that, before concluding that a particular melanoma represents an extracutaneous primary tumour, the possibility has to be considered that the tumour is in fact a metastasis from a cutaneous melanoma which was removed without histological examination, or which has regressed completely, or which is located in an extracutaneous site elsewhere.

In some instances of extracutaneous melanoma, the location, the histology and especially the presence of a pre-existent melanocytic lesion suggest a primary tumour at this site. In other instances, it remains impossible to rule out a metastasis of a cutaneous tumour with certainty. In general, the diagnosis of extracutaneous primary malignant melanoma should not be made in the presence of a clinically suspicious pigmented cutaneous lesion, or of a history suggesting regression of a pigmented skin lesion, or of a history of previous excision of a cutaneous lesion unless slides of the latter are available for re-evaluation. At clinical examination, special attention should be paid to the scalp, nail beds, interdigital folds and perianal skin, sites in which small primary melanomas easily escape clinical notice.

Relative frequencies of *sites of primary extracutaneous melanoma* were assessed on the basis of incidence figures of the Third National Cancer Survey of the United States (Scotto *et al.*, 1976). In decreasing order of frequency, these sites were: eye (78.9%), vulva (7.2%), soft tissues (2.5%), anorectum (2.3%), vagina (2.1%), upper respiratory tract (1.6%), gums and mouth (1.2%), gastrointestinal tract (0.7%), lung, lip, oesophagus, penis, bladder, remainder of urinary tract, tongue, salivary gland and nasopharynx (<0.5% each).

Mucosal melanomas, which are usually located in the upper aero-digestive tract, urogenital tract, or anus, occur most commonly in middle-aged or elderly patients; in many sites there is a male pre-dominance of cases. As compared to cutaneous melanoma, mucosal melanoma usually comes to clinical attention at a much later stage of its development, when the thickness is many millimetres, metastases are often present, and prognosis is correspondingly poor. Depending on the site and, consequently, the relationship of tumour to surgical margins, local recurrence may be a significant problem.

As indicated above, the presence of a pre-existent melanocytic lesion and the presence of tumour cells within the overlying or adjacent epithelium ('junctional activity'), are important indications that the tumour is probably a primary one (Allen and Spitz, 1953; Mills and Cooper, 1983). *'Junctional activity' is, however, not absolutely pathog-nomonic of a primary tumour*: rarely, it may be found in metastases in the skin (Kornberg *et al.*, 1978); Dail (1988) illustrated a pulmonary metastasis of melanoma where the tumour cells appear to line alveolar septa. By analogy, one can appreciate that melanoma cells metastatic to various internal organs may similarly penetrate the mucosal epi-thelium, as was indeed demonstrated in a case report of a melanoma metastatic to the gall bladder (Murphy *et al.*, 1987).

Mucosal melanomas often show a resemblance to acral lentiginous melanoma of the skin, exhibiting solitary, often dendritic, basally located tumour cells extending laterally within the surface epithelium, and inducing some reactive epithelial hyperplasia. However, pagetoid intraepithelial lateral spread and a nodular pattern of growth also occur (Kato *et al.*, 1987).

11.1   Eye and orbital cavity

Melanocytic lesions of the eye and its adnexae include a variety of benign lesions, some of which can be considered counterparts of cutaneous naevi, while others are unique to this location. There are also a number of specific melanoma subtypes which differ significantly from cutaneous melanoma. In contrast to the skin, incisional rather than excision biopsy for the diagnosis of ocular melanocytic lesions is commonly performed. Lesions of the skin covering the eyelids correspond to cutaneous melanocytic lesions at other sites.

Pigmented lesions of the conjunctiva are encountered in many pathology laboratories, but those of the uvea are submitted only in centres specializing in eye surgery: for the purposes of this book, we shall therefore concentrate on conjunctival lesions and only briefly discuss uveal ones.

11.1.1 Conjunctiva

Congenital benign melanocytic lesions of the conjunctiva include congenital melanosis and congenital naevus, oculodermal melanosis, and blue naevus (Folberg et al., 1989). Acquired benign melanocytic lesions include: ephelis, junctional, compound, and subepithelial naevi, inflamed naevus seen in adolescence, and rarely, dysplastic naevus and Spitz naevus. Primary acquired melanosis, without or with cytological atypia, is a very important conjunctival lesion lacking a cutaneous counterpart.

Hyperpigmentations without melanocytic hyperplasia occur in oriental or negroid races, and in association with previous inflammation, Peutz-Jeghers syndrome, neurofibromatosis and Addison's disease.

Congenital conjunctival melanosis occurs alone or as part of Ota's naevus ('congenital oculodermal melanocytosis'; p. 131). In contrast to primary acquired melanosis of the conjunctiva, which is an intraepithelial lesion, it consists of a subepithelial proliferation of usually heavily pigmented, spindle-shaped melanocytes, which may result clinically in a somewhat bluish discolouration (Tyndall effect).

Racial hyperpigmentation mainly involves the epibulbar conjunctiva at the interpalpebral fissure, and fades towards the fornices; it is usually bilateral but may be asymmetrical. Histologically, there is epithelial hyperpigmentation, but conjunctival melanocytes are not increased in number. The histological picture is similar in Addison's disease and *postinflammatory hyperpigmentation*, e.g. following trachoma or radiation exposure, but in the latter there is often also pigment incontinence.

Common acquired naevi of the conjunctiva appear in the first and second decade and show a predilection for the interpalpebral fissure. Acquired elevated pigmented lesions of the tarsal or forniceal conjunctiva are usually melanomas, since benign naevi are very rare at these sites (Buckman et al., 1988). Initially, conjunctival naevi are confined to the conjunctival epithelium and consist of a lentiginous and/or nested proliferation of small monomorphic melanocytes, together with epithelial hyperpigmentation; the histology of such junctional naevi, which occur practically only in childhood, may be indistinguishable from primary acquired melanosis in adulthood (see below). In such instances, some authors have used the term 'melanosis in childhood' (McDonnell *et al.*, 1989).

As with cutaneous naevi, the naevus subsequently develops a sub-epithelial component, and still later becomes completely subepithelial (Jakobiec *et al.*, 1985; Folberg *et al.*, 1989; McDonnell *et al.*, 1989). Conjunctival melanocytic naevi often consist of rather large cells and intraepithelial nests may reach almost to the surface, which may cause concern to those insufficiently familiar with these lesions. However, cellular pleomorphism is absent or minimal and cellular and nuclear size can often be seen to decrease towards the base. The absence of mitoses in the deep portion, and the presence of intralesional epithelium-lined cysts argue in favour of a benign naevus (Figure 11.1). Naevi in adolescence may exhibit a pronounced predominantly lymphocytic inflammatory response (*'inflamed naevus'*) without sinister connotation.

Rare variants of naevi of the conjunctiva and sclera include: Spitz naevus, dysplastic naevus (Jakobiec *et al.*, 1985) and common and cellular blue naevus (Smith and Brockhurst, 1976; Eller and Bernardino, 1983). Clinically, conjunctival blue naevi may be brown rather than blue, and attached to the conjunctiva rather than the sclera; histologically, the pigmented spindle-shaped melanocytes are located immediately beneath the conjunctival epithelium (Eller and Bernardino, 1983). A combined naevus ('true and blue') of the conjunctiva was reported by Kopf and Bart (1979).

Primary acquired melanosis of the conjunctiva (Reese, 1955) mainly affects middle-aged Caucasians. It appears clinically as a flat, variably pigmented conjunctival discolouration, which often involves the epibulbar conjunctiva, especially the two lower quadrants, and less commonly the forniceal and palpebral conjunctiva; it occasionally extends to the cornea and eyelid (Jakobiec *et al.*, 1989; De Wolff-Rouendaal, 1990). It may be multifocal, so that inspection of the entire conjunctiva is important. It may extend along the duct of the lacrimal gland or along the canaliculus toward the lacrimal sac. Therefore, when the lesion is seen to extend to the orifice of the lacrimal gland or to the lacrimal punctum, treatment of the visible conjunctival lesion will not guarantee eradication of the entire lesion. Completely non-pigmented examples occur: these become apparent only at histology when a conjunctival melanoma is removed (Griffith *et al.*, 1971).

Histologically, primary acquired melanosis exhibits a spectrum of

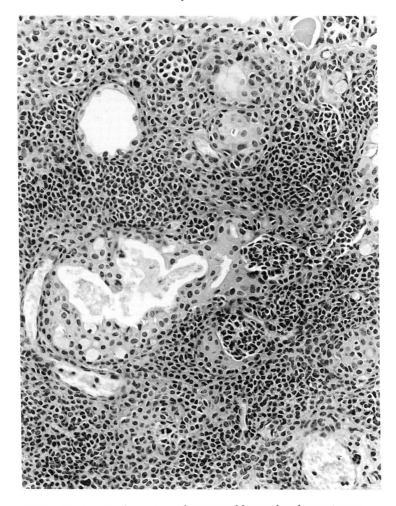

Figure 11.1   Conjunctival compound naevus. Nests of melanocytes are present within the surface epithelium and extend diffusely into the underlying tissue, in which strands and glandular structures are formed by the conjunctival epithelium (HE, × 225).

different appearances, which have hyperpigmentation and, usually, increased numbers of melanocytes as their common denominator (Figure 11.2). All melanocytes are located within the conjunctival epithelial compartment, as opposed to congenital melanosis, which is a subepithelial lesion.

There is some disagreement about the best terminology to be used in the histological classification of these lesions. Folberg and colleagues

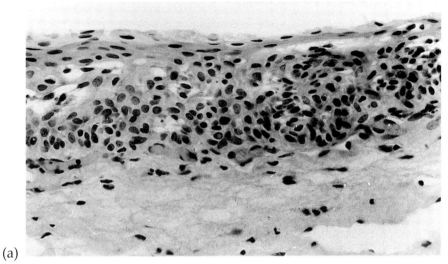

(a)

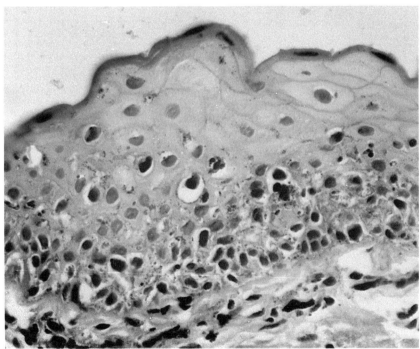

(b)

Figure 11.2 Conjunctival melanosis. (a) Proliferation of melanocytes within the epithelium; there is no significant cytological atypia (HE, × 370). (b) Melanosis with atypia of melanocytes, some of which are located above the basal cell layer (HE, × 460).

(1985a) used primary acquired melanosis as a pathological diagnosis and divided it into forms with and without atypia, the former being subdivided further according to growth pattern and cell type. Others however pointed out that primary acquired melanosis connotes a clinical appearance which may have as its pathological substrate totally different lesions, including benign melanocytic proliferations and *in situ* melanomas (Ackerman, 1985; Mihm and Guillén, 1985). We shall first summarize the former approach, since it has gained much popularity in the clinic.

As indicated above, Folberg and associates (1985a) divided acquired melanosis into forms with and without cytological atypia: this distinction is of great importance in view of the very different risks of melanoma development. Importantly, the two forms cannot be distinguished clinically, so that the distinction is based wholly on histological evaluation of biopsies. Since atypia may not be present throughout the lesion, multiple biopsies at different sites are needed.

In *primary acquired melanosis without atypia*, there may be increased pigmentation only, with normal numbers of normal-looking melanocytes, or there is a proliferation of basally located, small and monomorphic melanocytes. In these cases, the risk of development of melanoma is very small; however, it is possible that some cases later evolve into atypical melanosis if left untreated since, as already indicated, some cases show areas with and without cytological atypia adjacent to each other; also, the mean age of patients with melanosis without atypia is several years less than that of patients with atypical melanosis (Folberg *et al.*, 1985a). Clinical management of primary acquired melanosis without atypia consists of periodic clinical evaluation.

Primary acquired melanosis with atypia is associated with a definite risk of the development of invasive melanoma (Reese, 1955; Folberg *et al.*, 1985a). About three-quarters of all melanomas of the conjunctiva occur on the basis of primary acquired melanosis (Folberg *et al.*, 1985b). The melanocytes, which may be small (dendritic, polygonal or spindled) or large and epithelioid, and show varying degrees of nuclear enlargement, hyperchromasia and nucleolar prominence. The proliferation may be lentiginous, nested, pagetoid (single atypical cells scattered throughout the thickness of the epithelium) or massive.

Two subtypes of atypical primary acquired melanosis have been distinguished histologically (Folberg *et al.*, 1985a): the first is characterized by a basally located proliferation of atypical melanocytes which are not epithelioid: roughly one-fifth of such cases progress to conjunctival melanoma; the second group exhibits pagetoid spread of atypical epithelioid melanocytes: about 75–90% of this subgroup lead to invasive melanoma. There is a greater tendency for melanoma development if the lesion involves the limbus (Jakobiec *et al.*, 1989).

It may be difficult to distinguish between acquired melanosis and infiltrating melanoma, especially when there is a subepithelial inflammatory infiltrate and when sections are tangentially cut. So-called *pseudoglands of Henle*, a reactive epithelial proliferation developing in some cases of chronic conjunctivitis, may become massively involved in the process, thus mimicking invasion by tumour.

Thus, the spectrum of appearances of primary acquired melanosis of the conjunctiva ranges from a mere hyperpigmentation of the epithelium to an extensive proliferation of atypical melanocytes which in all likelihood represents *in situ* melanoma. Although some of these lesions are probably related and even constitute different phases in the development of one entity, it is equally likely that others are not. The problems associated with the use of the term 'melanosis' as a pathological diagnosis, as outlined at the start of the chapter, therefore apply also to primary acquired melanosis of the conjunctiva.

A more distinct classification of these lesions, on the basis of terminology of cutaneous pigmented lesions, is hampered by the marked variations in histology found within individual lesions, leading to sampling error on the one hand, and a blurring of seemingly distinct

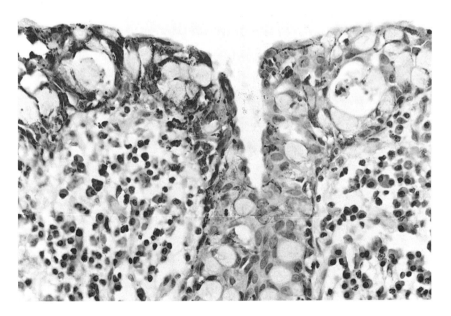

Figure 11.3   Lentigo maligna of the skin, extending in continuity to involve the conjunctival epithelium. Note pigmented dendritic processes of the tumour cells between the conjunctival epithelial cells (HE, × 370).

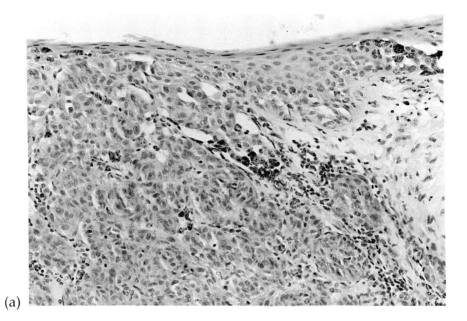

(a)

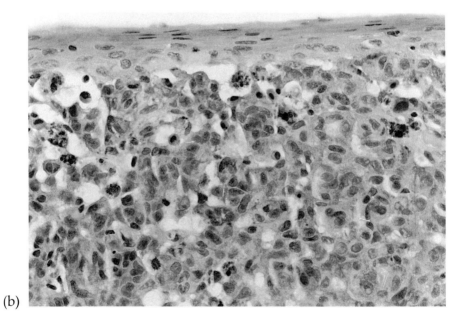

(b)

Figure 11.4 Conjunctival melanoma. (a) Atypical melanocytes arranged in nests and strands extend into the subepithelial tissue. Note irregular extension within the epithelium (right) (HE, × 185). (b) Cytological features: there is mild to moderate anisonucleosis (HE, × 370).

pathological lesions on the other. Whether this is due to insufficient data or whether it is an intrinsic property of one entity unique to this location, is not clear at this moment. Further studies correlating clinical and pathological features of these lesions, as well as further detailed follow-up studies, are needed before a wholly satisfactory clinicopathological classification becomes possible.

Ideally, primary acquired melanosis with atypia should be eradicated in its entirety, which may require several separate surgical procedures, cryosurgery and/or laser therapy. If a large portion or even the whole of the conjunctiva is affected, complete removal is impossible and cryotherapy of the clinically most affected areas is advocated, in order to slow down the course of the disease (Jakobiec et al., 1989).

The conjunctiva may become involved by extension in continuity from cutaneous lentigo maligna involving the adjacent skin (Figure 11.3).

Conjunctival melanoma (Figure 11.4; Folberg et al., 1985b) occurs mainly in adults, most commonly in the sixth decade, and affects both sexes equally. Very rarely, it occurs in childhood (McDonnell et al., 1989). About three-quarters of cases are associated with primary acquired melanosis with atypia and, in these, the chance of local recurrence is increased (De Wolff-Rouendaal, 1990). Follow-up data are difficult to interpret because of differences in treatment and, in some series, short follow-up. Increased thickness, pagetoid spread of tumour cells within the conjunctival epithelium, invasion of the cornea or episclera, and involvement of the palpebral conjunctiva, caruncle and fornix are prognostically unfavourable features (Folberg et al., 1985b; Jeffrey et al., 1986; Char, 1989; De Wolff-Rouendaal, 1990). The choice of therapy largely depends on the site and extent of the lesion. Overall tumour-related mortality is about 27% (Char, 1989).

11.1.2   Uvea

Melanocytic lesions of the *iris* exhibit a wide spectrum of histological appearances; most are benign, including spindle cell tumours lacking significant nuclear atypia (Jakobiec and Silbert, 1981).

Naevi of the ciliary body and choroid are not uncommon in the general population; the large majority occur in the posterior half of the eye. They are usually flat and relatively avascular, and consist of monomorphic cells which are either plump and polyhedral, with small and monomorphic nuclei and well-developed cytoplasm, or slender and spindled, these also being devoid of nuclear pleomorphism (Yanoff and Fine, 1982).

Melanomas of the uveal tract (Figure 11.5) are subdivided according

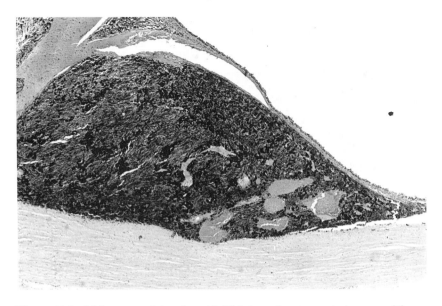

Figure 11.5 Melanoma of the choroid. This heavily pigmented tumour lifts up the retina but does not significantly invade the sclera. A few foci of necrosis are present (HE, × 35).

to the cytological features of the tumour cells rather than the architecture of the tumour. They are divided into spindle cell melanoma types A and B, epithelioid melanoma, mixed type melanoma, and a miscellaneous group of melanomas not fitting into one of these subtypes (Figure 11.6; Callender, 1931). Some tumours are totally or almost totally necrotic (McLean *et al.*, 1978).

Tumours composed wholly of type A spindle cells are traditionally designated spindle A melanomas, but follow-up studies indicated that these lesions do not metastasize and are therefore better considered naevi (McLean *et al.*, 1978). These spindle cell naevi, which are up to 10 mm in diameter and up to 3 mm in thickness, consist of elongated, slender spindle cells with monomorphic often longitudinally grooved nuclei containing finely dispersed chromatin and small, indistinct nucleoli (*'spindle A melanoma cells'*), while mitoses and necrosis are absent (McLean *et al.*, 1978).

Spindle B cells are slightly plumper than spindle A cells, and have oval, more vesicular nuclei possessing a distinct and often plump nucleolus. *Epithelioid cells* are round or polygonal and possess a generous amount of cytoplasm, while nuclei are pleomorphic and often show prominent nucleoli. Uveal melanomas commonly exhibit mixed patterns of type A and B spindle cells and epithelioid cells.

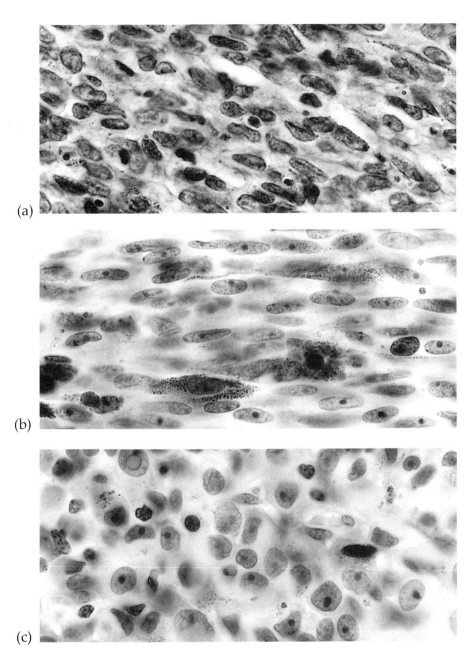

Figure 11.6 Uveal melanoma, cytological features. (a) Spindle A cells, with monomorphic oval nuclei, often longitudinally grooved or folded and devoid of conspicuous nucleoli. (b) Spindle B cells exhibiting prominent nucleoli. (c) Epithelioid cells with round or oval nuclei containing prominent nucleoli (HE, × 920).

The cell type is an important prognostic indicator: melanomas with type B cells, mixed type B/epithelioid and purely epithelioid cells have a progressively worse prognosis. However, there is significant intra- and interobserver variation when uveal melanomas are typed according to the Callender classification, so that additional, more reproducible parameters have been sought. Huntington and colleagues (1989) recently reported that the mean value of the length of the 10 largest tumour cell nucleoli present in the entire section, as measured with a micrometer eyepiece at ×1000 magnification, carries important prognostic information, which in their material was superior to the classification according to Callender. This method requires experience and regular use of a calibration slide to maintain accuracy, but does not involve specialized equipment.

Largest tumour diameter is also important prognostically: those up to 10 mm have a favourable prognosis whereas a size of 16 mm or more is an unfavourable sign (McLean et al., 1978). Furthermore, location is important: melanomas of the choroid and ciliary body have an overall mortality at least 10 times that of iris tumours; tumours of the iris are generally smaller and more often have a favourable cytological appearance. The degree of lymphocytic infiltration (Gamel et al., 1988) and the presence of necrosis, mitotic activity and orbital invasion (De la Cruz et al., 1990) are also prognostically important. It should be borne in mind that the uvea has no lymphatic drainage: metastases are therefore haematogenous and the liver is a favoured site (McLean et al., 1982).

Not all melanotic neoplasms of the uvea are melanocytic in origin: the pigment epithelium of the uvea gives rise to a variety of reactive and neoplastic melanotic lesions which are briefly mentioned in Chapter 12 (p. 394).

11.1.3   Orbital cavity

Melanoma within the orbital cavity is rare, and usually results from direct extension of an ocular tumour or metastasis of a distant melanoma. A very small number of cases however are thought to arise in the orbital cavity itself (Henderson, 1973); like the uveal melanomas, these tumours consist of spindle cells, epithelioid cells or a mixture of the two.

11.2   Nasal cavity and paranasal sinuses

Macroscopically visible pigmentation of the nasal mucosa is normally present in black Africans but is rare in Caucasians (Lewis and Martin, 1967). However, histologically, melanocytes can be found in the nasal mucosa of some Caucasians (Uehara *et al.*, 1987); they are most often located within the stroma, but may be located within the surface epithelium. *Melanocytic lentiginous hyperplasia* may lead to increased mucosal pigmentation (melanosis).

Several hundred cases of *melanoma* of the nasal cavity and paranasal sinuses have been reported. It is a disease of middle or late adult life, and most reported cases concerned Caucasians. However, when compared with the incidence of cutaneous melanoma, they are relatively more common in non-Caucasians (Uehara *et al.*, 1987). Cases present with epistaxis, nasal airway obstruction, epiphora, or facial pain and swelling (Trapp *et al.*, 1987). Adjacent mucosal pigmentation is seen in the majority of cases (Trapp *et al.*, 1987). Histologically, the tumour usually consists of a massive proliferation of atypical epithelioid and/or spindled cells; melanin may be scarce, requiring a careful search. Since undifferentiated carcinomas, olfactory neuroblastoma and a variety of other malignant tumours also occur at this site, the differential diagnosis should include these entities; thorough sampling as well as melanin stains and immunostains are very important in the differential diagnosis. There is some indication that tumour thickness is related to prognosis; however, most tumours are at least several millimetres thick, and the prognosis is poor due to local tumour recurrence as well as metastasis.

11.3   Labial mucosa, oral cavity and oropharynx

11.3.1   Labial mucosa

Congenital naevus of the labial mucosa is very rare; a recent case was described in a 7-year-old Japanese girl (Takeda, 1988). The lesion consisted of a well-circumscribed brown-black nodule, 7 mm in diameter; histologically, the lesion consisted of an intradermal naevus extending deeply into the submucosal connective tissue.

Melanotic macule and *melanoacanthoma* of the labial and oral mucosa (Horlick *et al.*, 1988) is probably not a primarily melanocytic lesion, and is discussed in the next chapter (p. 385).

Melanoma of the vermilion border of the lip is very rare (McGovern, 1976; McGinnis *et al.*, 1986; Raderman *et al.*, 1986). The invasive component may show the features of desmoplastic melanoma, i.e. fusiform tumour cells with ultrastructural features of Schwann cells, amidst increased collagen. Some show neurotropism, leading to a high rate of local recurrence, cranial neuropathies, and intracranial disease (McGinnis *et al.*, 1986; p. 255).

11.3.2   Oral cavity

Causes of mucosal hyperpigmentation in the absence of melanocytic hyperplasia include: racial pigmentations (usually located along the gums), Peutz-Jeghers syndrome and Addison's disease. In these instances, hyperpigmentation of the basal epithelial layer is seen, sometimes associated with subepithelial melanophages. '*Mucosal melanotic macule*' of the oral mucosa is dealt with in the next chapter (p. 385).

Melanocytic naevi of the oral mucosa are uncommon. They are classified in parallel with their cutaneous counterparts. The most common type is the intramucosal naevus, the mucosal counterpart of the intradermal naevus of the skin; the second most common type is the blue naevus. Junctional or compound naevi are rare; a few cases of combined naevi have been reported (Ficarra *et al.*, 1987). All these naevi can attain a size of over 1 cm (Buchner and Hansen, 1987). Recently, a congenital naevus with the histological features of Spitz naevus was reported on the palate of a 4-year-old Japanese girl (Nikai *et al.*, 1990).

Junctional naevus has been described in childhood as well as in adulthood, up to the sixth decade. It is most common on the hard palate. *Compound naevus* occurs mostly in childhood, adolescence and early adulthood, although it has also been reported up to the sixth decade; preferred sites are the hard palate and buccal mucosa. *Intramucosal (subepithelial) naevus* (Figure 11.7) occurs in a wide age range,

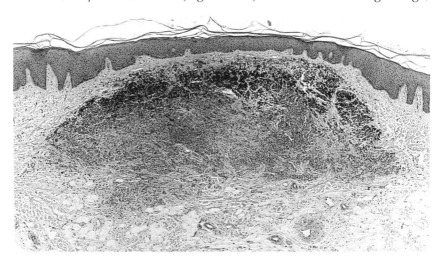

Figure 11.7   Intramucosal naevus of oral mucosa. The overlying epithelium is uninvolved. Upper parts of the naevus are pigmented. Note symmetry and regular architecture (HE, × 35).

from early childhood to late adulthood, and is most common on the hard palate, buccal mucosa, vermilion border and gingiva, but may also occur in other sites, such as the retromolar pad, labial mucosa, tip of tongue and soft palate. Compound and intramucosal naevi appear to be somewhat more common in females (Buchner and Hansen, 1987).

Blue naevus is the second commonest type of oral naevus. It is most often seen on the hard palate. There is no sex preference. Histologically, the lesion consists of a submucosal proliferation of pigmented dendritic melanocytes, similar to common blue naevus of the skin. Cellular blue naevus is very rare in the oral mucosa (Esguep *et al.*, 1983; Miller *et al.*, 1987).

A small number of *combined naevi* of the oral mucosa have been reported (Ficarra *et al.*, 1987; Barker and Sloan, 1988). The histology combines that of an intramucosal naevus and a common blue naevus.

Since it may be difficult to distinguish clinically between intraoral benign naevi and melanoma, excision of all intraoral pigmented lesions suspected to be naevi has been advised (Barker and Sloan, 1988; Buchner *et al.*, 1990).

Not all pigmented lesions of the oral mucosa are melanocytic in origin: they may be the result of haemochromatosis, various drugs (chloroquine, busulfan and other alkylating agents), tattoos (mainly of dentist's materials such as amalgam), chronic heavy metal poisoning (e.g. lead, mercury, arsenic), and haemangioma and other vascular tumours (Brocheriou *et al.*, 1985). Pigmented neuroectodermal tumour of infancy, a nonmelanocytic melanin-producing tumour, is discussed in the next chapter (p. 394).

Melanoma of the oral mucosa is a rare tumour, occurring mostly in men after the fourth decade, with a predilection for the palate and maxillary gingiva, which contrasts with the predilection sites of oral squamous carcinoma: the tongue and floor of the mouth (Snow and Van der Waal, 1986). The tumour usually presents with ulceration and bleeding; clinically, about one-third of cases are associated with pre-existing melanosis, i.e. a macular mucosal pigmentation in contiguity with the tumour (Figure 11.8; Rapini *et al.*, 1985); in Japanese patients, such melanosis has been noted in as many as two-thirds of patients (Takagi *et al.*, 1974). Histologically, such an adjacent flat pigmented lesion may represent a pre-existent mucosal melanocytic hyperplasia with atypia or an *in situ* extension of the malignancy.

Histologically, the intraepidermal component often resembles acro-lentiginous melanoma, the tumour cells being dendritic and proliferat-ing in a predominantly lentiginous pattern along the epithelial basement membrane, in association with reactive epithelial hyperplasia. The invasive component of the melanoma is epithelioid, spindled or mixed (Figure 11.9).

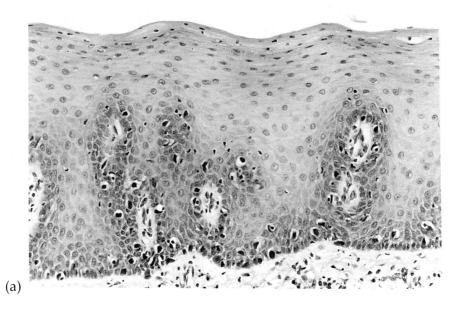

(a)

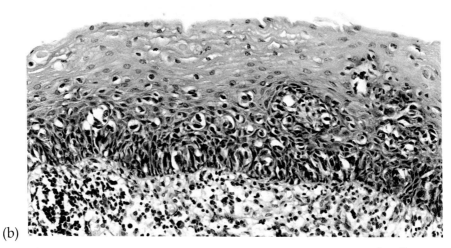

(b)

Figure 11.8 'Melanosis' of oral mucosa. (a) Atypical melanocytes, basally located as single units (HE, × 185). (b) More pronounced proliferation of partly suprabasally located melanocytes, with marked atypia. Subepithelial inflammatory infiltrate. This lesion probably represents *in situ* melanoma (HE, × 185).

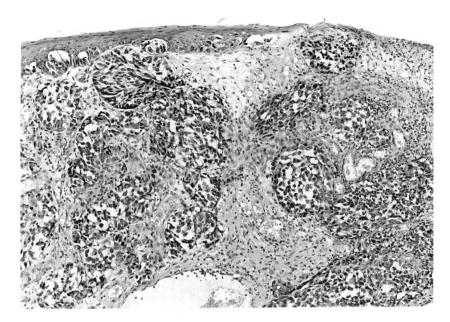

Figure 11.9   Melanoma of oral mucosa. Irregular nests and strands of atypical melanocytes infiltrate underlying tissues. Note ulceration (right) and intraepithelial spread of tumour (left) (HE, × 90).

Prognosis is generally poor, with 5-year survival rates of the order of 20–35% (Snow and Van der Waal, 1986), probably because most cases come to clinical attention relatively late, while doctor delay may also be significant, especially in cases of amelanotic tumour. Moreover, surgical margins are often narrow because of anatomical restrictions.

11.4   Larynx

Melanocytes are occasionally encountered within the basal layer of the surface epithelium of the vocal cords, or within the subjacent connective tissue and laryngeal mucosal glands (Goldman *et al.*, 1972; Busuttil, 1976). Reactive hyperactivity of these melanocytes causes the hyperpigmentation of the laryngeal mucosa sometimes seen after radiotherapy. Mucosal *melanocytic lentiginous hyperplasia* may lead to mucosal melanosis, which may attain a size of several centimetres (Goldman *et al.*, 1972).

Primary *melanoma* of the larynx is a very rare tumour, occurring mostly in middle-aged or elderly men (Goldman *et al.*, 1972). It usually presents as a large, nodular or polypoid, often ulcerating tumour, located within the epiglottis, false and true vocal cords or ventricles.

Hoarseness is the most common presenting symptom. Local recurrence is less frequent than with other mucosal melanomas of the head and neck, but the prognosis is very poor due to a high frequency of metastasic disease (Reuter and Woodruff, 1986). Histologically, laryngeal melanoma consists of atypical epithelioid or fusiform cells which may lack pigment, so that the correct diagnosis may not be immediately apparent. Melanin stains and anti-S-100 staining are then of help. In some cases, extension is present within the adjacent laryngeal epithelium; this argues in favour of a primary tumour.

11.5   Oesophagus

Melanocytes have been identified in about 4% of oesophagus specimens obtained at autopsy (De la Pava *et al.*, 1963). Oesophageal melanocytic hyperplasia may lead to the clinical picture of mucosal melanosis (DiCostanzo and Urmacher, 1987).

Oesophageal *melanoma* (Chalkiadakis *et al.*, 1985; Simpson *et al.*, 1990) is rare; reported cases usually concern Caucasians; most occur during middle or late adult life, but a case has been reported in a 7-year-old boy (Basque *et al.*, 1970). Males are affected slightly more often. There is no apparent relation to smoking, alcohol use, or family history of melanoma. Generally, clinical signs only develop when the tumour has reached a considerable size, usually of several centimetres. Presenting signs are caused by oesophageal obstruction or bleeding, as well as pain and weight loss. On barium swallow radiographs, the tumour is usually visualized as a bulky intraluminal mass. The tumour occurs more often in the middle and lower third of the oesophagus, and is characteristically polypoid and ulcerated. Focal pigmentation may be noticed endoscopically. There may be melanosis of the adjacent mucosa, which in exceptional instances involves nearly the entire oesophagus (Piccone *et al.*, 1970; Guzman *et al.*, 1989). When the tumour comes to clinical attention, metastases are detectable in about half of the cases; death often ensues within a few months (DiCostanzo and Urmacher, 1987); overall 5-year survival is about 4% (Chalkiadakis *et al.*, 1985).

In biopsy specimens, the surface may be ulcerated or intact; in the latter, an intraepithelial component of the tumour may be detected, usually consisting of rounded, epithelioid-type cells, while the invasive tumour cells are often spindled. *Melanoma should be considered in the differential diagnosis of polypoid intraoesophageal spindle cell tumours.* Usually, some melanin pigment can be detected. In resection specimens, intraepithelial lateral spread is usually demonstrable, the tumour cells extending along the basal layer in a lentiginous fashion

(Takubo *et al.*, 1983). Histologically, and especially on immunostaining with S-100, pre-existent mucosal melanocytes are often found and may have proliferated in a lentiginous pattern, even when melanosis is not apparent macroscopically (DiCostanzo and Urmacher, 1987). Hyperplasia of atypical melanocytes may be difficult or impossible to distinguish from intraepithelial spread of tumour. Both these phenomena are of help in the distinction between primary melanoma and *metastatic melanoma*, which was found in 4% of cases in an autopsy series of cutaneous melanoma, and which may also give rise to a polypoid tumour (Das Gupta and Brasfield, 1964).

11.6   Lower respiratory tract

The lungs are very commonly involved in metastatic melanoma (Das Gupta and Brasfield, 1964). Since melanocytes and benign melanocytic lesions have not been found in the bronchi and pulmonary parenchyma, a diagnosis of *primary melanoma of the lung* should be regarded with much scepticism.

There are, however, a very small number of case reports, in which the arguments provided in favour of a primary site in the bronchial mucosa are compelling, although a small element of doubt remains. These tumours occurred in middle or late adult life; some presented as polypoid, fungating intrabronchial growths leading to haemoptysis and obstructive bronchopneumonia (Salm, 1963; Gephardt, 1981; Carstens *et al.*, 1984; Alghanem *et al.*, 1987). After radical surgery, most tumours relapsed early and led to death within a few months; however, prolonged disease-free survival has also been reported (Reid and Mehta, 1966).

Macroscopically, the tumour is usually well defined, sometimes multinodular, bulging into the bronchial lumen and extending into surrounding tissues; it may or may not be pigmented. Histologically (Figure 11.10), the tumour consists of polygonal or fusiform melanocytes with atypical, mitotically active nuclei. Intraepithelial spread of tumour along the bronchial epithelial lining has been documented in some cases.

Apart from metastatic melanoma, the differential diagnosis should include several nonmelanocytic tumours: it is important to bear in mind that some bronchial carcinoids also contain melanin (p. 387). A melanotic schwannoma of the bronchus, exhibiting the characteristic architectural and ultrastructural features of schwannoma, was described by Rowlands and colleagues (1987). Furthermore, nonmelanocytic but melanin-containing malignancies at other sites, such as

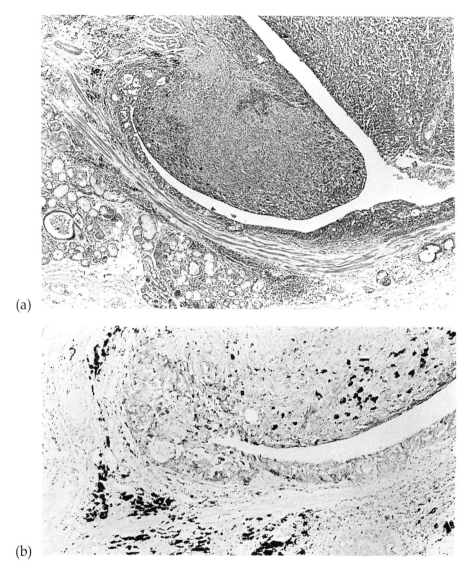

(a)

(b)

Figure 11.10 Primary melanoma of the bronchus. (a) Ulcerating, polypoid tumour mass arising from the bronchial mucosa (HE, × 35). (b) Melanin is present in tumour cells (in the polypoid mass as well as within the bronchial surface epithelial compartment) and in melanophages. Case published by Salm (1963) (Masson Fontana stain, × 90).

pigmented medullary carcinoma of the thyroid, may metastasize to the lungs.

A case of *pleural melanoma* in a 49-year-old black man was reported by Smith and Opipari (1978). There were no skin lesions and, at autopsy, no tumour was found elsewhere.

11.7 Gallbladder

Melanocytes are very rarely present within the mucosa of the gall-bladder (Breathnach, 1969). A small number of cases of primary *melanoma* of the gallbladder have been reported; these tumours occurred mainly in middle or late adult life, with a male preponderance (Mills and Cooper, 1983; Borja *et al.*, 1984; Heath and Womack, 1988). Presenting symptoms are abdominal pain related to gallbladder obstruction, jaundice, or symptoms produced by metastases.

Macroscopically, the tumour arises from the mucosa, is usually pigmented and polypoid, and usually has a diameter of several centimetres. Prognosis is generally poor; however, one patient survived for 14.5 years (Walsh, 1956). Histologically, 'junctional activity' of intra-epithelial melanocytes adjacent to the tumour has been reported by some authors; however, Murphy and colleagues (1987) demonstrated some appearances indistinguishable from 'junctional activity' in their case of uveal melanoma metastatic to the gallbladder, indicating that this phenomenon is not unique to primary tumours. Since metastases to the gallbladder are found in about 15% of cases in autopsy series (Das Gupta and Brasfield, 1964), many so-called primary melanomas of the gallbladder may in fact be metastases from undetected or regressed primaries elsewhere. Secondary melanoma of the gallbladder may also produce a polypoid pigmented tumour and clinical data are very similar.

Similar reservations are in order about a report of primary *melanoma of the common bile duct*, which also showed junctional proliferation of tumour cells (Carstens *et al.*, 1986).

11.8 Anal canal and rectum

The anal canal can be divided into three histological zones. The most proximal one, the 'colorectal zone', possesses a colon-type mucosa. Distal to it, the 'transitional zone' is covered by squamous epithelium, or mucin-producing columnar epithelium, or a stratified epithelium very similar to urothelium. This zone exhibits much histological variation, and different types of surface epithelium occur together. The most distal, 'squamous zone' is covered by nonkeratinizing squamous epithelium. The transition to perianal skin is evidenced by the emergence of skin appendages (Fenger, 1988). Melanocytes are found in the perianal skin and the squamous and transitional zones of the anal canal (Fenger and Lyon, 1982).

Melanocytic hyperplasia resulting in the clinical appearance of melanosis is usually lentiginous in architecture, but nests may also be present. There may or may not be distinct melanocytic atypia. Mucosal melanocytic hyperplasia is seen in contiguity with some anal melanomas (Fenger and Nielsen, 1986).

Primary *melanoma of the anal canal* (Morson and Volkstädt, 1963; Mason and Helwig, 1966) accounts for about 1–3% of all primary extracutaneous melanomas. There is an equal sex ratio; the large majority occur in adulthood, with a peak in the seventh decade. The tumour usually comes to clinical attention because of bleeding, pain or mass feeling (Wanebo et al., 1981). Prognosis is poor after abdominoperineal resection as well as after local excision (Kantarovsky et al., 1988): about 90% of patients succumb in the first 5 years after diagnosis (Wanebo et al., 1981).

Anal melanomas are usually at least several millimetres in thickness, and, in contrast to squamous carcinoma, may be polypoid. Most are pigmented macrosopically and ulceration is common. Histologically, the invasive component of anal melanoma is epithelioid or spindled (Figure 11.11); the latter may show the features of desmoplastic melanoma (Ackerman et al., 1985). Spindle cell melanoma at this site may mimic leiomyosarcoma and other sarcomas closely; it is therefore important that *one should seriously consider melanoma in all cases of anal (or rectal) spindle cell tumour* and perform appropriate stains to investigate this possibility. Less commonly, polygonal or round cell types predominate and a differential diagnosis of undifferentiated carcinoma or even nonHodgkin lymphoma may be considered. Generally, appropriate immunostains will readily establish the correct diagnosis.

Paget's disease of the anus may mimic *in situ* melanoma. Melanin produced by pre-existent melanocytes may be transferred preferentially to the intraepithelial carcinoma cells (p. 48). Evaluation of the cytological features of the tumour cells, mucin stains, and immunostaining for EMA, keratins and S-100 distinguish between Paget's disease and melanoma.

The large majority of anal melanomas arise in the transitional and squamous zones of the anal canal. These tumours may extend over a considerable distance at the level of the submucosa, to cause ulceration more proximally, at the level of the colorectal zone of the anus, or even within the rectum (Mills and Cooper, 1983; Kantarovsky et al., 1988). However, a case of rectal melanoma with contiguous intraepithelial

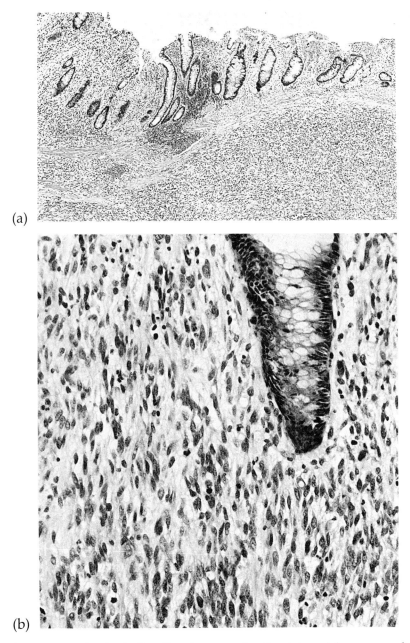

(a)

(b)

Figure 11.11 Anal spindle cell melanoma extending into rectal mucosa and submucosa. (a) The lamina propria and submucosa are diffusely infiltrated by tumour cells (HE, × 35). (b) Atypical spindle cells engulf rectal mucosal crypt (HE, × 230).

proliferation of atypical melanocytes in the adjacent rectal mucosa, which did not involve the transitional and squamous zones of the anal canal, has been published (Werdin *et al.*, 1988). In this case, pigmented dendritic melanocytes were also present in the rectal crypts. However, even though some cells were dendritic, it remains difficult to exclude beyond reasonable doubt the possibility that these cells represented metastatic tumour cells which had penetrated the epithelial basal lamina.

11.9   Genitourinary tract

11.9.1   Urinary bladder

Melanocytes are normally absent from the bladder mucosa. Mucosal melanosis of the bladder caused by the presence of melanocytes is extremely rare (Alroy *et al.*, 1986).

Primary *melanoma* of the urinary bladder is also exceedingly rare (Ainsworth *et al.*, 1976; Anichkov and Nikonov, 1982; Goldschmidt *et al.*, 1988). The tumour occurs predominantly in middle or late adult life; haematuria is generally the first symptom. At cystoscopy, the tumour usually presents as an exophytic, pigmented tumour (Ainsworth *et al.*, 1976). Squamous metaplasia of adjacent urothelium with pagetoid intraepithelial spread of tumour cells was mentioned in some reported cases. The tumour cells may be epithelioid or spindled. It remains unclear how many of these melanomas really constitute primary tumours, since metastatic melanoma of the bladder is not uncommon, although it rarely leads to clinical symptoms (Meyer, 1974). It was found in 18% of cases in one autopsy series (Das Gupta and Brasfield, 1964),

11.9.2   Urethra and penis

Primary *melanoma of the urethra* (Salm and Rutter, 1964; Kokotas *et al.*, 1981; Weiss *et al.*, 1982) occurs mostly after the age of 50, and there is probably a slight female preponderance (Barbagli *et al.*, 1988); however, a case has been reported in a 13-year-old boy (Begun *et al.*, 1984).

In males, two-thirds of cases are located distally, which may allow conservative surgery rather than amputation of the penis (Weiss *et al.*, 1982; Myskow *et al.*, 1988); about half occur in the navicular fossa (the distal widening of the urethra located within the glans penis) and some also involve the surface of the glans penis and/or prepuce. Other cases are distributed more or less evenly over the urethra. A melanocytic precursor lesion resembling a cutaneous dysplastic naevus, localized on the glans penis and in contiguity with the melanoma, was present in the case described by Weiss and co-workers (1982). Prognosis is poor: most patients succumb to metastatic disease.

Penile lentigo (Kopf and Bart, 1982), also known as 'atypical pigmented penile macule' (Leicht *et al.*, 1988) and 'melanosis' of the penis (Maize and Ackerman, 1987) consists of an irregularly shaped and variably pigmented macule, located on the glans and/or prepuce (Bhawan and Cahn, 1984), which may reach a size of several centimetres and which may exhibit 'skip areas'. It is a rare lesion, occurring in a wide age range, from childhood to late adulthood. Penile lentigo corresponds histologically to a slight increase in solitary, basally located melanocytes, usually devoid of cytological atypia, which may exhibit striking dendrites, together with an increase in pigmentation of the epithelium. Melanophages are often present in the subjacent tissue. The histological features of this lesion argue against a premalignant potential, but in a minority of cases cytological atypia is present; the significance of this has not yet been determined.

Junctional, compound and subepithelial naevi analogous to those found in the skin may also be seen on the glans and prepuce.

Melanoma of the glans penis and prepuce (Oldbring and Mikulowski, 1987; Manivel and Fraley, 1988) is rare; about two thirds of these occur on the glans (Begun *et al.*, 1984); it presents as an irregularly pigmented macule or nodule, which may later ulcerate and bleed. At the time of diagnosis, the tumour has often reached a thickness of several millimetres. Due to metastatic disease, prognosis is poor irrespective of therapy (Oldbring and Mikulowski, 1987): the tumour usually leads to death within the first 3 years after diagnosis.

11.9.3   *Prostate, spermatic cord*

Dark-greyish discolouration of prostate tissue is sometimes noted macroscopically; it is usually caused by infarcts, but sometimes by melanin produced by stromal melanocytes ('stromal melanosis', 'pigmented melanocytosis', 'prostatic blue naevus'). In other instances, a brown pigment is noticed in prostatic epithelial cells while stromal melanocytes are absent (Tannenbaum, 1974).

Prostatic blue naevus consists of a usually paucicellular proliferation of dendritic, pigment-laden melanocytes within the prostatic stroma (Figure 11.12; Gardner and Spitz, 1971; Jao *et al.*, 1971; Aguilar *et al.*, 1982; Ro *et al.*, 1988). Since the lesion generally consists of an ill-defined scatter of melanocytes rather than a focal lesion, the term *'pigmented melanocytosis'* has been proposed as an alternative to blue naevus (Botticelli *et al.*, 1989). Cases are discovered incidentally, usually in

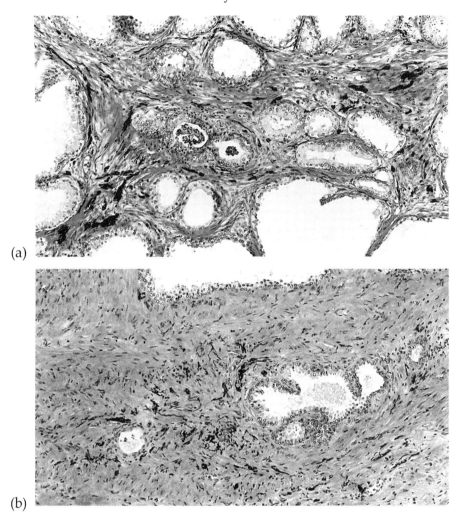

Figure 11.12 Prostatic blue naevus. (a) Scattered heavily pigmented dendritic melanocytes are present between prostatic glands (HE, × 90). (b) Melanocytes within fibromuscular stroma (HE, × 90).

transurethral resection material and, therefore, generally occur together with either prostatic hyperplasia or adenocarcinoma. Macroscopically, the tissue is evenly pigmented or shows dark brown or black streaks. Sometimes, the glandular epithelium (Gardner and Spitz, 1971), including tumour cells in cases with concomitant prostatic adenocarcinoma, also contain melanin pigment, which is located basally in the cells (Rios and Wright, 1976; Aguilar *et al.*, 1982; Furusato *et al.*, 1989). The carcinoma cells may be more heavily pigmented than the benign prostatic epithelium, which calls to mind the preferential deposition of melanin pigment in adenocarcinoma cells sometimes seen in mammary and extramammary Paget's disease (p. 48).

Occasionally, pigment is only apparent in epithelial cells, especially those lining the ducts. In these cases, it has been suggested that the epithelium is melanogenic (Goldman, 1968), since on light microscopy, intraepithelial and stromal melanocytes are not detected (Tannenbaum, 1974). It seems likely that the pigment in many such cases is not melanin but lipofuscin or a related compound, which is positive with many commonly used melanin stains. In other cases, in which isolated stromal melanocytes are present, melanin produced by melanocytes is probably transferred to the prostatic epithelium (Aguilar *et al.*, 1982; Ro *et al.*, 1988).

Melanoma may occasionally manifest itself in the prostate (Berry and Reese, 1953); secondary melanoma or extension from a urethral melanoma should then be considered.

A blue naevus occurring in the spermatic cord was mentioned by Rodriguez and Ackerman (1968).

11.9.4   *Vulva*

Benign naevi of the vulva include junctional, compound and sub-epithelial naevus, and, rarely, Spitz naevus and blue naevus.

An irregularly shaped and irregularly pigmented macule, which may reach a size of several centimetres, may be found on the vulva and sometimes extends into the introïtus. Despite its rather worrisome clinical appearance, the histology of the large majority of these lesions consists only of epithelial hyperpigmentation together with a slight increase in basally located dendritic melanocytes devoid of cytological atypia (Sison-Torre and Ackerman, 1985; Maize and Ackerman, 1987).

In a minority of cases, a more pronounced proliferation of melano-cytes is seen and such lesions may exhibit varying degrees of cellular atypia. It is unclear whether such lesions are at all related to the innocuous-appearing hyperpigmentation described above. Certainly, melanocytic hyperplasia with cellular atypia shows an association with vulvar melanoma, as witnessed by the fact that the two may be found in contiguity (Simpson *et al.*, 1988).

A small percentage of primary extracutaneous *melanomas* occur on the vulvar mucous membranes, mostly after the menopause. The tumours are generally discovered late, when they become manifest by ulceration, leading to discharge or bleeding; they are located in the anterior or posterior vulva, and may extend into the vagina. Prognosis depends on thickness, level of invasion and mitotic count (Podratz *et*

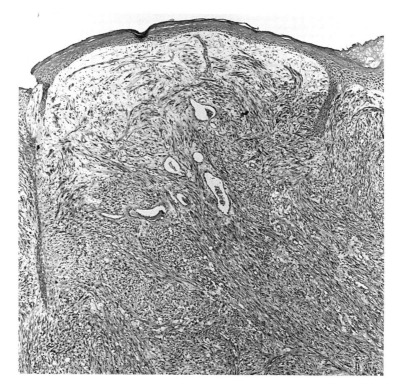

Figure 11.13 Spindle cell melanoma of vulva. An extensive proliferation of atypical spindle cells fills the greatly thickened dermis. In this field the overlying epithelium is not involved (HE, × 45).

al., 1983; Johnson *et al.*, 1986), and is generally poor when the thickness exceeds 3 mm. In a recent series (Bradgate *et al.*, 1990) age-adjusted 5- and 10-year survival rates were 35 and 22%, respectively.

Histologically, most cases show *in situ* lateral spread, with a pagetoid or lentiginous pattern. The invasive component has a remarkably variable histological appearance: spindle cell (desmoplastic and neurotropic) tumours (Figure 11.13; Warner *et al.*, 1982) may mimic spindle cell carcinoma or various histological types of sarcoma; small cell melanomas may resemble malignant lymphoma; pleomorphic tumours may be confused with liposarcoma or malignant fibrous histiocytoma.

11.9.5 Vagina

Melanocytes within the vaginal mucosa are found in 3% of vagina specimens at autopsy (Nigogosyan *et al.*, 1964) and may be the cause

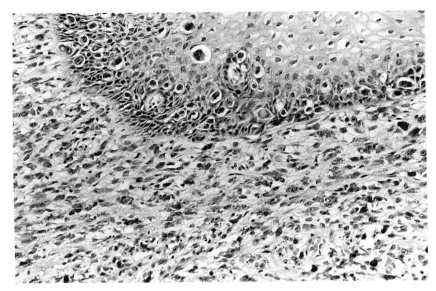

Figure 11.14   Spindle cell melanoma of vagina. Tumour cells present in the overlying vaginal squamous epithelium are epithelioid rather than spindled (HE, × 185).

of mucosal hyperpigmentation after radiotherapy. Vaginal *melanosis* consists of macroscopically visible mucosal pigmentation, corresponding histologically to the presence of pigmented melanocytes within the vaginal surface epithelium (Tsukada, 1976). Lee and co-workers (1984) reported a case of vaginal melanoma in contiguity with an intraepithelial melanocytic hyperplasia. *Blue naevus* of the vagina (Tobon and Murphy, 1977) is extremely rare.

Vaginal *melanoma* (Figure 11.14) is a rare tumour, occurring at a slightly younger age than vulvar melanoma, the mean age being around 50 years; a few cases have been described in the third decade (Musfeld and De Grandi, 1986). These tumours usually present late and may be up to several centimetres in diameter; foetid discharge and vaginal bleeding are usually the presenting symptoms. Surgery alone often fails to achieve locoregional control (Bonner *et al.*, 1988) and the prognosis is very poor indeed; only occasionally, patients survive for more than a few years.

11.9.6   Uterus

A small percentage of specimens of the uterine cervix contain melanocytes (Cid, 1959). *Melanosis of the cervix* is a macroscopically visible mucosal pigmentation due to the presence of benign pigmented melanocytes in the basal layer of the cervical squamous epithelium (Deppisch, 1983; Barter *et al.*, 1988). It is very rare; in some cases, the pigmentation also involves the vaginal mucosa.

Blue naevus is occasionally encountered in the cervix (Goldman and Friedman, 1967; Uff and Hall, 1978; Patel and Bhagavan, 1985; Casadei *et al.*, 1987), usually as a small pigmentation detected incidentally within the endocervix of hysterectomy specimens of middle-aged women. Cid (1960) found six cases in 229 consecutive hysterectomies. Rarely, the lesion is detected clinically (Patel and Bhagavan, 1985). Histologically, it consists of a proliferation of pigmented elongated or dendritic melanocytes within the stroma of the endocervix. A cellular blue naevus of the cervix and vagina was reported by Rodriguez and Ackerman (1968).

Melanoma of the cervix is very rare (Abell, 1961; Hall *et al.*, 1980); it has occasionally been diagnosed in a cervical smear (Yu and Ketabchi, 1987). The presence of an intraepithelial tumour component extending laterally, and the presence of pre-existent melanocytes in the adjacent uninvolved mucosa, argue in favour of a primary tumour. Prognosis is very poor; only few patients survive for more than 3 years.

A case of *cellular blue naevus of the myometrium* was recently reported (Martin *et al.*, 1989); there was associated hypertrophy of smooth muscle tissue, which led the authors to speculate on various histogenetic possibilities and to propose the alternative name of 'pigmented myomatous neurocristoma'.

11.10 Lymph node

Collections of small, usually nonpigmented melanocytes which strongly resemble intradermal naevus cells are occasionally seen within the capsule of lymph nodes draining the skin (Figure 11.15). These *naevus cell aggregates*, first described by Stewart and Copeland (1931), are usually small and inconspicuous, but in exceptional cases may occupy as much as one third of the node (Von Albertini, 1935; McCarthy *et al.*, 1974). Apparently, they occur only in lymph nodes draining the skin (McCarthy *et al.*, 1974), where they are encountered incidentally in lymphadenectomy specimens. They are found in a few percent of axillary lymph node dissection specimens of melanoma patients (McCarthy *et al.*, 1974; Ridolfi *et al.*, 1977); the percentage is an order of magnitude greater than their prevalence in axillary lymph nodes of breast carcinoma patients (Ridolfi *et al.*, 1977; Andreola and Clemente, 1985). The reason for this intriguing difference in prevalence has not yet been elucidated.

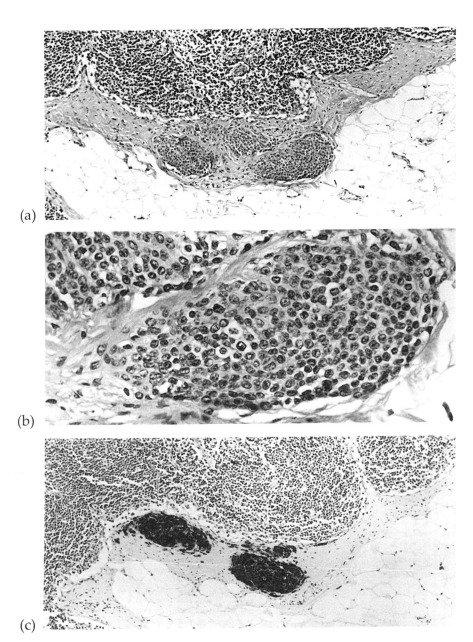

Figure 11.15 Naevus cell aggregates in lymph node capsule. (a) The location within the fibrous capsule rather than the marginal sinus helps in the distinction from micrometastases (HE, × 185). (b) The cytological features are very similar to naevus cells of intradermal melanocytic naevi (HE, × 370). (c) The naevus cells are strongly positive for S-100 (Immunoperoxidase, × 185).

Nodal naevus cell aggregates may occasionally lead to diagnostic confusion, especially in frozen sections. Obviously, almost all cases identified in lymphadenectomy and lymph node dissection specimens concern cancer patients, and they therefore must be distinguished from the patient's tumour, which can be difficult, e.g. in lobular mammary carcinoma. Importantly, the melanocytes are almost always located within the lymph node capsule and the thin fibrous trabeculae traversing the sinuses, rather than within the sinuses, afferent lymphatics or parenchyma (Johnson and Helwig, 1969). Intracytoplasmic vacuoles are absent and mucin stains are negative. Also, they are immunoreactive with S-100 and negative for epithelial markers, so that the possibility of metastatic carcinoma is usually easily ruled out, as long as the alternative diagnosis is considered. Rarely, however, these aggregates may be seen in the lymphatic tissue proper (McCarthy *et al.*, 1974), and one should bear in mind that some epithelial neoplasms are S-100 positive.

The histogenesis of these nodal melanocytic lesions has given rise to much debate. Some authors have favoured aberrant migration of melanoblasts from the neural crest during embryogenesis, pointing out that the naevus cell aggregates are usually located within the capsule rather than within the sinuses and afferent lymphatics (Epstein *et al.*, 1984). However, others favoured lymphogenous spread from a benign naevus located in the skin. Intranodal deposition of a wide variety of normal tissues, such as glandular inclusions of endometrium, endosalpinx, decidua, breast and salivary gland, is a well documented occurrence (Eckert *et al.*, 1987). Accordingly, lymphatic spread of intradermal melanocytes from cutaneous naevi has been postulated (McCarthy *et al.*, 1974). Indeed, Subramony and Lewin (1985) demonstrated naevus cell aggregates in a lymph node, together with lymphangioinvasive growth in an intradermal naevus in the area of drainage. It may be that the lymphatic tissue of the node is inimical to the survival of naevus cells reaching the node *via* afferent lymphatics, and that they penetrate and survive in the capsule.

Blue naevus of the lymph node, similar to cutaneous common blue naevus, has been described by Azzopardi and colleagues (1977). It is asymptomatic, and therefore an incidental finding. Histologically, small collections of pigmented, elongated, occasionally dendritic melanocytes are present within the lymph node capsule, where they are intermingled with melanophages (Figure 11.16); occasionally, they extend along perisinusoidal fibrous trabeculae or penetrate the surrounding fatty tissue, preferentially along blood vessels and lymphatics (Azzopardi *et al.*, 1977; Epstein *et al.*, 1984). Their presence in two separate axillary lymph nodes in the same specimen was recorded by

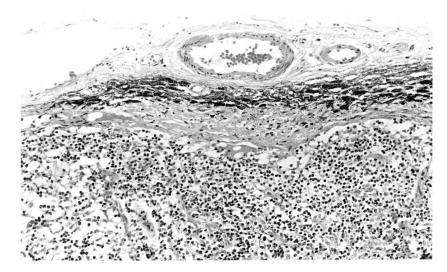

Figure 11.16   Blue naevus of lymph node. Within the fibrous capsule, an ill-defined aggregate of heavily pigmented dendritic melanocytes is present. Case published by Azzopardi *et al.*, (1977) (HE, × 185).

Goldman (1981). The intracapsular localization of these blue naevi and the dendritic, heavily pigmented nature of the constituent cells have been used as arguments in favour of a developmental anomaly (Azzopardi *et al.*, 1977; Lamovec, 1984). Since in two of seven cases reported there was a common blue naevus of the skin drained by the node (Lamovec, 1984), the alternative possibility of lymphogenous spread of a cutaneous lesion is not excluded.

Lymph nodes draining skin containing a *cellular blue naevus* occasionally exhibit collections of melanocytes closely resembling the cutaneous lesion (Rodriguez and Ackerman, 1968; Lambert and Brodkin, 1984). Clinical follow-up of such cases indicates that these nodal lesions are harmless and should not be interpreted as metastatic melanoma. This issue is discussed in Chapter 5 (p. 124).

Shenoy and colleagues (1987) reported what is probably the first documented case of a *primary melanoma* arising in a lymph node. Naevus cell aggregates were present in the nodal capsule, and the authors claimed that there was a transition from benign naevus cells to 'dysplastic naevus cells' to malignant melanoma. This case was also unique in that blue naevi were present in the capsule of three lymph nodes, including the one containing the naevus cell aggregates and the melanoma. The authors raised the intriguing possibility that a small proportion of nodal melanomas with unknown primary, which amount to at least 4% of all melanomas (p. 322), might in fact constitute primary melanomas of lymph nodes.

11.11 Melanoma of soft tissues (clear cell sarcoma)

Primary melanoma of soft tissues was originally described by Enzinger (1965) as *clear-cell sarcoma of tendons and aponeuroses*. Melanin production was noted in some tumours (Mackenzie, 1974) and the tumour was later interpreted as a soft tissue melanoma (Eckfors and Rantakokko, 1979; Raynor *et al.*, 1979; Chung and Enzinger, 1983). A benign counterpart, i.e. a melanocytic naevus of soft parts, has not been recognized. Although the term 'clear cell sarcoma' has retained considerable popularity, it is preferable to speak of melanoma of soft parts, in accordance with Chung's and Enzinger's recommendation.

Melanoma of soft parts occurs in a wide age range, with a preference for adolescence and early adulthood; females are affected slightly more often than males. Most cases in Chung and Enzinger's series of 141 cases were Caucasians, but the tumour was also seen in blacks and Mongolians. It is nearly always located in an extremity, the leg being involved three times more commonly than the arm. Here, predilection sites are: sole of foot, heel, ankle, knee, thigh. Swelling, sometimes accompanied by pain, is usually the presenting symptom. The tumour is located in the deep soft tissues and usually arises from aponeuroses, tendons and deep fascia. It may extend into the overlying structures including the dermis, but seldom causes ulceration. Erosion of underlying bone is also rare; in one extraordinary case, however, the tumour was located largely within the tibia (Morishita *et al.*, 1987); another unique case occurred at the root of the penis of a 10-year-old Chinese boy (Saw *et al.*, 1986). Not uncommonly, the tumour has been present for several years before the patient seeks medical help; there may be a history of recent more rapid increase in size.

Radical surgical excision is the treatment of choice. The tumour often recurs, sometimes after many years, and in Chung and Enzinger's series (1983), about half of the patients eventually died of recurrent tumour. Preferred sites for tumour metastasis are the regional lymph nodes and the lungs. In view of the propensity for lymphogenous spread, elective lymph node dissection may be considered. Tumour size is correlated with distant metastasis and survival (Sara *et al.*, 1990). Chemotherapy and radiotherapy are useful for palliation (Eckardt *et al.*, 1983).

Macroscopically the tumour is firm, greyish-white and often multinodular; a minority of cases show brown or black pigmentation, haemorrhage, or small cysts. Histologically the tumour is composed of

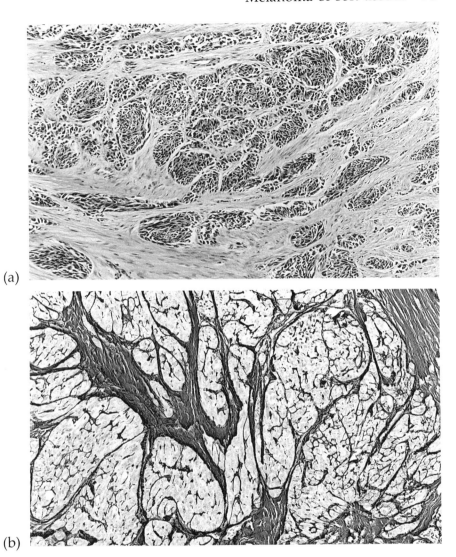

(a)

(b)

Figure 11.17   Melanoma of soft tissues (clear cell sarcoma). (a) Compact nests of pale-staining tumour cells are surrounded by dense fibrous tissue, resulting in a characteristic architecture (HE, × 185). (b) A reticulin stain highlights the pattern of well-defined nests and strands (× 185).

nests, nodules and short cords or sheets of mainly oval, elongated or occasionally polygonal cells (Figure 11.17). The tumour nests and strands are separated by fibrous septa, which are prominently outlined by a reticulin stain, highlighting the nested pattern of the tumour;

reticulin fibres do not surround individual tumour cells. Some, and rarely abundant, intercellular hyaluronic acid is occasionally present; epithelial-type mucins are absent.

The tumour cells have pale or slightly granular, poorly defined, sometimes eosinophilic cytoplasm, containing glycogen in about two-thirds of cases. The cytoplasm may have collapsed against the nucleus during fixation. Melanin is focally present in about three-quarters of cases; its demonstration often requires special stains since it is usually sparse and inconspicuous. The centrally located, vesicular nuclei have one or two prominent nucleoli (Figure 11.18). Mitoses are usually uncommon (less than 4 per 10 HPF) and in some tumours they are not found. Multinucleate tumour giant cells may be present. Some cases exhibit prominent nuclear and cellular pleomorphism. Most, but not all, tumours are at least focally positive for S-100 and HMB-45. Epithelial markers and fat stains are negative. Ultrastructural demonstration of melanosomes can be helpful in the diagnosis of difficult cases (Benson *et al.*, 1985).

Since the tumour has a characteristic clinical, architectural and cyto-logical appearance, the diagnosis usually poses no great problems.

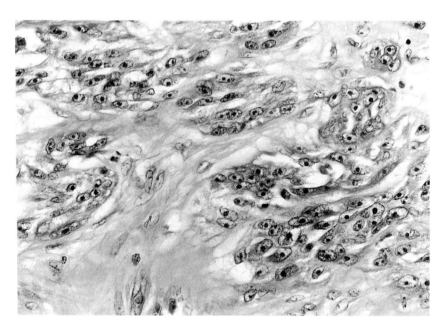

Figure 11.18   Melanoma of soft tissues (clear cell sarcoma), cellular features. Nuclei are vesicular and exhibit plump, conspicuous nucleoli. Tumour cells are arranged in nests amidst paucicellular collagenous stroma (HE, × 370).

Synovial sarcoma can usually be ruled out by appropriate stains. Cutaneous cellular blue naevus and malignant blue naevus are primarily intradermal neoplasms, and show a different distribution over body sites; also, they usually contain more melanin. Malignant blue naevus usually arises in middle or late adult life. The possibility of metastatic melanoma from a hitherto unnoticed cutaneous primary melanoma should be investigated clinically; it is hardly surprising that metastatic cutaneous melanoma may closely resemble melanoma of soft tissues (Warner *et al.*, 1983). However, in most instances, the characteristic site in a young individual, a thorough clinical examination of the patient together with the typical histology of the tumour, point to the correct diagnosis.

Clear cell sarcoma of soft tissues should not be confused with clear cell sarcoma of the kidney, a totally unrelated malignant childhood tumour of undetermined histogenesis (Sotelo-Avila *et al.*, 1986), although some favour a relation to nephroblastoma (Sandstedt *et al.*, 1987). The similarity is one of name only.

11.12   Central nervous system

11.12.1   *Meninges*

Melanocytes are normally present in the leptomeninges covering the ventrolateral surfaces of the medulla oblongata and upper spinal cord, (Gibson *et al.*, 1957); their frequency is about 325 cells per square millimetre, which is about one-third of that in the skin (Goldgeiger *et al.*, 1984). Only isolated melanocytes are found in meninges covering other parts of the brain and spinal cord. Meningeal melanocytes may give rise to macroscopic pigmentation and diffuse thickening of the meninges (*'diffuse meningeal melanosis'*; Figure 11.19) as well as a variety of tumours. Some of these lesions occur together with Ota's naevus (Hartmann *et al.*, 1989) or giant congenital naevus of the skin, which in these cases is usually located on the head and neck or midline of the trunk; this combination is known as *'neurocutaneous melanosis'*. Additional involvement of the eyes and periorbital skin is called *neurooculocutaneous melanosis*.

Meningeal melanocytoma (Limas and Tio, 1972; Winston *et al.*, 1987), also called *meningeal cellular blue naevus* because of its close resemblance to the cutaneous cellular blue naevus (Graham *et al.*, 1976; Lach *et al.*, 1988) is a very rare neoplasm. There is a wide age range, but most cases occur after the age of 40 years; the tumour is rare in childhood. There is no sex preference. It arises in close association with a nerve in its subarachnoidal course, at any level of the spine or intracranially,

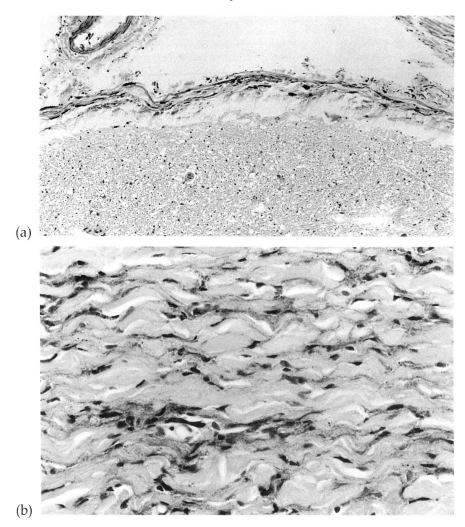

(a)

(b)

Figure 11.19 Meningeal melanosis. (a) Melanosis of leptomeninges. Heavily pigmented dendritic melanocytes are present within the leptomeninges (HE, × 90). (b) Melanosis of dura. Throughout the dural tissue, a diffuse proliferation of heavily pigmented elongated melanocytes is present (HE, × 370).

where it is most often associated with the trigeminal nerve. Symptoms are due to pressure on surrounding structures. Complete removal is curative, but may be impossible in some locations, resulting in tumour recurrence (Verma *et al.*, 1979; Winston *et al.*, 1987) and death of the patient. One case metastasized after 4 years, indicating that some of these tumours may in fact be low-grade malignancies (Cordoba *et al.*, 1989).

Macroscopically, the tumour is brown or black, and nodular. Most are intradural in location, but a few arise extradurally, in close conjunction with nerve roots. Small brown or black spots on meninges may occur in the vicinity and should not be interpreted as metastases.

Histologically a proliferation of monomorphic, oval, elongated or less commonly polygonal melanocytes is seen. The melanocytes are moderately or heavily pigmented and are arranged in fascicles, streaming patterns or sometimes whorls, reminiscent of meningioma. Sometimes, a pattern of compact nests of cells alternating with sclerotic tissue results in a striking resemblance to cutaneous cellular blue naevus (Figure 11.20). Melanophages are usually seen, especially around blood vessels. Haemorrhage and necrosis are absent.

The tumour cells have oval or elongated nuclei, which are often longitudinally grooved, and which may or may not show a distinct nucleolus (Figure 11.21). Mitoses are absent or very rare; there is little or no cellular and nuclear pleomorphism. Mutinucleate cells may be present.

Immunohistochemically, the tumour cells are positive for S-100 and NSE, and negative for EMA. Ultrastructurally, the features of melanocytes are seen; features of meningothelial cells, such as interdigitating processes and desmosomes are absent. In the earlier literature, several cases were reported as 'pigmented meningiomas'; however, the ultrastructural features clearly establish this lesion as a melanocytic tumour.

Melanotic schwannoma (p. 387) may resemble this tumour clinically and histologically. The relation of the tumour to meninges, the presence of associated meningeal melanosis and the ultrastructure of the tumour aid in the exclusion of melanotic schwannoma. The tumour cells of melanocytoma may show cellular processes and long-spacing collagen (Limas and Tio, 1972), but the absence of elaborate cellular interdigitations, well-developed basal lamina and micropinocytotic activity aid in the distinction from Schwann cells (Winston *et al.*, 1987). Meningeal melanocytoma should also be differentiated from primary and secondary melanoma of the meninges: as indicated above, necrosis is absent, while mitoses are absent or rare.

Primary melanoma of the meninges is very rare. It occurs in a wide age range, and there is a 3:2 female predominance. Most arise from the leptomeninges, but a small number of cases are confined to the dura (Narayan *et al.*, 1981; Özden *et al.*, 1984; Hartmann *et al.*, 1989; MacFarlane *et al.*, 1989). Most are located in the neurocranium, while a few arise in the spinal canal (Larson *et al.*, 1987).

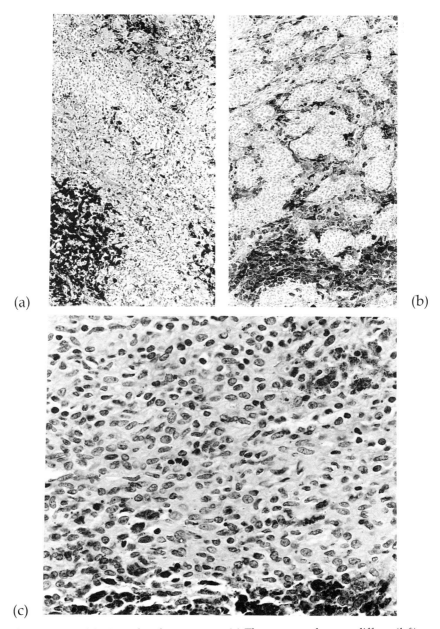

(a)

(b)

(c)

Figure 11.20   Meningeal melanocytoma. (a) The tumour shows a diffuse (*left*) or micronodular (*right*) growth pattern; pigmentation varies greatly between areas. The appearances greatly resemble cellular blue naevus of the skin (HE, × 90). (b) At higher power, a relatively monomorphic pattern of spindled melanocytes is seen, as well as groups of melanophages (HE, × 370).

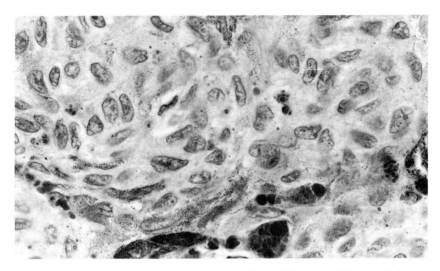

Figure 11.21   Meningeal melanocytoma, cytological features. There is little nuclear pleomorphism; nucleoli are occasionally visible. Some melanocytes contain microgranular melanin pigment. The patient also had a large, deeply pigmented congenital naevus of the scalp and neck (HE, × 920).

About two-thirds of meningeal melanomas diffusely involve the leptomeninges, leading to brown-black discolouration and thickening, with or without the formation of tumour nodules. The term *melanoblastosis* of the leptomeninges has been used for such a diffuse meningeal involvement (Bamborschke *et al.*, 1985).

Clinically, symptoms are caused by local tumour pressure or, in case of diffuse meningeal involvement, resemble those of carcinomatous meningitis or leukaemic meningeal involvement: headaches, drowsiness, psychosis, brain nerve palsy and epileptic seizures. The diagnosis is usually based on the demonstration of atypical melanocytes in the cerebrospinal fluid. Prognosis is very poor; median survival after diagnosis is about 5 months (Verma *et al.*, 1979).

Histologically, the tumour consists of highly atypical fusiform or polygonal melanocytes; in contrast to melanocytoma, mitoses are generally easily found and may be numerous; foci of necrosis are usually present.

11.12.2   Pituitary gland and pineal gland

These are rare sites of primary melanoma (Enriquez *et al.*, 1973; Scholtz and Siu, 1976; Carlson *et al.*, 1987). Probably, the tumours arise from leptomeningeal melanocytes at these sites; some cases have been associated with Ota's naevus and leptomeningeal melanosis.

11.13   Adrenal gland

Melanoma of the adrenal medulla has rarely been reported (Kinseley and Baggenstoss, 1946; Dick *et al.*, 1955; Carstens *et al.*, 1984). Since the adrenal gland is a common site of metastatic melanoma, one should be very careful indeed to exclude occult primaries elsewhere. Criteria which have been put forward for diagnosis include: no previous or simultaneous melanoma elsewhere, no previous removal of a pigmented skin or eye lesion, and preferably, exclusion by autopsy of the presence of a hidden primary lesion, and the presence of melanoma in only one adrenal gland (Carstens *et al.*, 1984). Reported cases concern large, cystic and necrotic tumours which led to widespread metastasis and death soon after clinical diagnosis of the tumour.

11.14   Miscellaneous sites

A number of purportedly primary melanomas of the *parotid gland* have been reported (Greene and Bernier, 1961): 21 cases were reviewed by Vuong and colleagues (1986), who added a case of their own. Prognosis was very poor; there were no obvious clinical or pathological differences from cases of metastatic melanoma to the parotid gland. It is not clear whether the reported cases of melanoma of the parotid really represent primary tumours; we know of no convincing examples of pre-existent melanocytes or benign melanocytic lesions in the salivary glands.

Primary melanoma of the *small bowel* was reported by Krausz and colleagues (1978). It should be emphasized that the small bowel is a favoured site for melanoma metastases (p. 332) so that a diagnosis of primary melanoma of the small bowel should be made with great reluctance. A presumably primary melanoma of Meckel's diverticulum was reported by Bloch *et al.* (1986).

A small number of primary melanomas arising within an *ovarian teratoma* have been reported (Tham *et al.*, 1981; Gregg, 1982; Parekh, 1985).

Naevus cell aggregates in placental tissue associated with giant congenital naevus are discussed in Chapter 6 (p. 154).

References

Abell, M. R. (1961) Primary melanoblastoma of the uterine cervix. *Am. J. Clin. Pathol.*, **36**, 248–55.

Ackerman, A. B. (1985) Primary acquired melanosis. *Hum. Pathol.*, **16**, 1077–8.

Ackerman, D. M., Polk, H. C. Jr. and Schrodt, G. R. (1985) Desmoplastic melanoma of the anus. *Hum. Pathol.*, **16**, 1277–9.

Aguilar, M., Gaffney, E. F. and Finnerty, D. P. (1982) Prostatic melanosis with involvement of benign and malignant epithelium. *J. Urol.*, **128**, 825–7.

Ainsworth, A. M., Clark, W. H., Mastrangelo, M. *et al.* (1976) Primary malignant melanoma of the urinary bladder. *Cancer*, **37**, 1928–36.

Alghanem, A. A., Mehan, J. and Hassan, A. A. (1987) Primary malignant melanoma of the lung. *J. Surg. Oncol.*, **34**, 109–12.

Allen, A. C. and Spitz, S. (1953) Malignant melanoma. A clinicopathological analysis of the criteria for diagnosis and prognosis. *Cancer*, **6**, 1–45.

Alroy, J., Ucci, A. A., Heaney, J. A., Mitcheson, H. D., Gavris, V. E. and Woods, W. (1986) Multifocal pigmentation of prostatic and bladder urothelium. *J. Urol.*, **136**, 96–7.

Andreola, S. and Clemente, C. (1985) Nevus cells in axillary lymph nodes from radical mastectomy specimens. *Pathol. Res. Pract.*, **179**, 616–8.

Anichkov, N. M. and Nikonov, A. A. (1982) Primary malignant melanomas of the bladder. *J. Urol.*, **128**, 813–5.

Azzopardi, J. G., Ross, C. M. D. and Frizzera, G. (1977) Blue naevi of lymph node capsule. *Histopathology*, **1**, 451–61.

Bamborschke, S., Ebhardt, G., Szelies-Stock, B., Dresbach, H. A. and Heiss, W.-D. (1985) Review and case report: primary melanoblastosis of the leptomeninges. *Clin. Neuropathol.*, **4**, 47–55.

Barbagli, G., Natali, A., Urso, C., Barbanti, G., Menchi, I. and Moroni, F. (1988) Primary malignant melanoma of the female urethra: a case report with immunohistochemical findings. *Urol. Int.*, **43**, 110–2.

Barker, G. R. and Sloan, P. (1988) An intraoral combined blue naevus. *Br. J. Oral Maxillofac. Surg.*, **26**, 165–8.

Barter, J. F., Mazur, M., Holloway, R. W. and Hatch, K. D. (1988) Melanosis of the cervix. *Gynecol. Oncol.*, **29**, 101–4.

Basque, G. J., Boline, J. E. and Holyoke, J. B. (1970) Malignant melanoma of the esophagus: first reported case in a child. *Am. J. Clin. Pathol.*, **53**, 609–11.

Begun, F. P., Grossman, H. B., Diokno, A. C. and Sogani, P. C. (1984) Malignant melanoma of the penis and male urethra. *J. Urol.*, **132**, 123–5.

Benson, J. D., Kraemer, B. B. and MacKay, B. (1985) Malignant melanoma of soft parts: an ultrastructural study of four cases. *Ultrastruct. Pathol.*, **8**, 57–70.

Berry, N. E. and Reese, L. (1953) Malignant melanoma which has its first clinical manifestations in the prostate gland. *J. Urol.*, **69**, 286–90.

Bhawan, J. and Cahn, T. M. (1984) Atypical penile lentigo. *J. Dermatol. Surg. Oncol.*, **10**, 99–100.

Bloch, T., Tejada, E. and Brodhecker, C. (1986) Malignant melanoma in Meckel's diverticulum. *Am. J. Clin. Pathol.*, **86**, 231–4.

Bonner, J. A., Perez-Tamayo, C., Reid, G. C., Roberts, J. A. and Morley, G. W. (1988) The management of vaginal melanoma. *Cancer*, **62**, 2066–72.

Borja, S. R., Meyer, W. R. and Cahill, J. P. (1984) Malignant melanoma of the gall bladder. Report of a case. *Cancer*, **54**, 929–31.

Botticelli, A. R., Di Gregorio, C., Losi, L., Fano, R. A. and Manenti, A. (1989) Melanosis (pigmented melanocytosis) of the prostate gland. *Eur. Urol.*, **16**, 229–32.

Bradgate, M. G., Rollason, T. P., McConkey, C. C. and Powell, J. (1990) Malignant melanoma of the vulva: a clinicopathological study of 50 women.

Br. J. Obstet. Gynaecol., **97**, 124–33.

Breathnach, A. S. (1969) *Pigments in Pathology*. New York: Academic Press, p. 355.

Brocheriou, C., Kuffer, R. and Verola, O. (1985) Lésions pigmentées de la cavité buccale. *Ann. Pathol. (Paris)*, **5**, 221–9.

Buchner, A. and Hansen, L. S. (1987) Pigmented nevi of the oral mucosa: a clinicopathologic study of 36 new cases and review of 155 cases from the literature. Part II: analysis of 191 cases. *Oral Surg. Oral Med. Oral Pathol.*, **63**, 676–82.

Buchner, A., Leider, A. S., Merrell, P. W. and Carpenter, W. M. (1990) Melanocytic nevi of the oral mucosa: a clinicopathologic study of 130 cases from northern California. *Oral Pathol.*, **19**, 197–201.

Buckman, G., Jakobiec, F. A., Folberg, R. and McNally, L. M. (1988) Melanocytic nevi of the palpebral conjunctiva. An extremely rare location usually signifying melanoma. *Ophthalmology*, **95**, 1053–7.

Busuttil, A. (1976) Dendritic cells within the human laryngeal mucosa. *Arch. Otolaryngol.*, **102**, 43–4.

Callender, G. R. (1931) Malignant melanotic tumors of the eye. A study of histologic types in 111 cases. *Trans-Am. Acad. Ophthalmol. Otolaryngol.*, **36**, 131–42.

Carlson, B. R., Glick, A. D. and Cushman, A. R. (1987) Primary malignant melanoma of pineal region. *J. Tennessee Med. Assoc.*, **80**, 597–9.

Carstens, P. H. B., Kuhns, J. G. and Ghazi, C. (1984) Primary melanomas of the lung and adrenal. *Hum. Pathol.*, **15**, 910–4.

Carstens, P. B., Ghazi, C., Carnighan, R. H. and Brewer, M. S. (1986) Primary malignant melanoma of the common bile duct. *Hum. Pathol.*, **17**, 1282–5.

Casadei, G. P., Grigolato, P. and Calibbo, E. (1987) Blue nevus of the endocervix. A study of five cases. *Tumori*, **73**, 75–9.

Chalkiadakis, G., Wihlm, J. M., Morand, G., Weill-Bousson, M. and Witz, J. P. (1985) Primary malignant melanoma of the esophagus. *Ann. Thorac. Surg.*, **39**, 472–5.

Char, D. H. (1989) *Clinical Ocular Oncology*. New York: Churchill Livingstone, p. 77.

Chung, E. B. and Enzinger, F. M. (1983) Malignant melanoma of soft parts. A reassessment of clear cell sarcoma. *Am. J. Surg. Pathol.*, **7**, 405–13.

Cid, J. M. (1959) La pigmentation melanique de l'endocervix. *Ann. Anat. Pathol.*, **4**, 617–28.

Cid, J. M. (1960) El nevo azul del endocervix. *An. Cir.*, **25**, 82–92.

Cordoba, A., Tunon, T. and Vazquez, J. J. (1989) Meningeal melanocytoma. Presentation of a case and review of the literature. *Arch. Neurobiol.*, **52**, 93–99.

Dail, D. H. (1988) Uncommon tumors. In *Pulmonary Pathology* (eds D. H. Dail and S. P. Hammar). New York: Springer Verlag, pp. 847–972.

Das Gupta, T. and Brasfield, R. (1964) Metastatic melanoma: a clinicopathologic study. *Cancer*, **17**, 1323–39.

De la Cruz, P. O., Specht, C. S. and McLean, I. W. (1990) Lymphocytic infiltration in uveal malignant melanoma. *Cancer*, **65**, 112–5.

De la Pava, S., Nigogosyan, G., Pickren, J. W. and Cabrera, A. (1963) Melanosis of the esophagus. *Cancer*, **16**, 48–50.

De Wolff-Rouendaal, D. (1990) *Conjunctival Melanoma in the Netherlands: a Clinicopathological and Follow-up Study*. Katwijk: All In BV., pp 151–9.

Deppisch, L. M. (1983) Cervical melanosis. *Obstet. Gynecol.*, **62**, 525–6.

Dick, J. C., Ritchie, G. M. and Thompson, H. (1955) Histological differentiation between pheochromocytoma and melanoma of the suprarenal gland. *J. Clin. Pathol.*, **8**, 89–98.

DiCostanzo, D. P. and Urmacher, C. (1987) Primary malignant melanoma of the esophagus. *Am. J. Surg. Pathol.*, **11**, 46–52.

Eckardt, J. J., Pritchard, D. J. and Soule, E. H. (1983) Clear cell sarcoma. A clinicopathologic study of 27 cases. *Cancer*, **52**, 1482–8.

Eckert, F., Schmidt, U. and Lennert, K. (1987) Immunhistologische Charakterisierung sogenannter Naevuszellnester in Lymphknoten. *Pathologe*, **8**, 81–4.

Eckfors, T. O. and Rantakokko, V. (1979) Clear cell sarcoma of tendons and aponeuroses: malignant melanoma of soft tissues? Report of four cases. *Pathol. Res. Pract.*, **165**, 422–8.

Eller, A. W. and Bernardino, V. B., Jr. (1983) Blue nevi of the conjunctiva. *Ophthalmology*, **90**, 1469–71.

Enriquez, R., Egbert, B. and Bullock, J. (1973) Primary malignant melanoma of central nervous system. Pineal involvement in a patient with nevus of Ota and multiple pigmented skin nevi. *Arch. Pathol.*, **95**, 392–5.

Enzinger, F. M. (1965) Clear-cell sarcoma of tendons and aponeuroses. An analysis of 21 cases. *Cancer*, **18**, 1163–74.

Epstein, J. I., Erlandson, R. A. and Rosen, P. P. (1984) Nodal blue nevi: a study of three cases. *Am. J. Surg. Pathol.*, **8**, 907–15.

Esguep, A., Solar, M., Encina, A. M. and Fuentes, G. (1983) Primary melanotic alterations in the oral cavity. *J. Oral Med.*, **38**, 141–6.

Fenger, C. (1988) Histology of the anal canal. *Am. J. Surg. Pathol.*, **12**, 41–55.

Fenger, C. and Lyon, H. (1982) Endocrine cells and melanin-containing cells in the anal canal epithelium. *Histochem. J.*, **14**, 631–9.

Fenger, C. and Nielsen, V. T. (1986) Precancerous changes in the anal canal epithelium in resection specimens. *Acta Pathol. Microbiol. Immunol. Scand. Sect. A.*, **94**, 63–9.

Ficarra, G., Hansen, L. S., Engebretsen, S. and Levin, L. S. (1987) Combined nevi of the oral mucosa. *Oral Surg. Oral Med. Oral Pathol.*, **63**, 196–201.

Folberg, R., McLean, I. W. and Zimmerman, L. E. (1985a) Primary acquired melanosis of the conjunctiva. *Hum. Pathol.*, **16**, 129–35.

Folberg, R., McLean, I. W. and Zimmerman, L. E. (1985b) Malignant melanoma of the conjunctiva. *Hum. Pathol.*, **16**, 136–43.

Folberg, R., Jakobiec, F. A., Bernardino, V. B. and Iwamoto, T. (1989) Benign conjunctival melanocytic lesions: clinicopathologic features. *Ophthalmology*, **96**, 436–61.

Furusato, M., Matsumoto, I., Kato, H. *et al.* (1989) Prostatic carcinoma with melanosis. *Prostate*, **15**, 65–9.

Gamel, J. W., McLean, I. W. and Greenberg, R. A. (1988) Interval-by-interval Cox model analysis of 3680 cases of intraocular melanoma shows a decline in the prognostic value of size and cell type over time after tumor excision. *Cancer*, **61**, 574–9.

Gardner, W. A. and Spitz, W. U. (1971) Melanosis of the prostate gland. *Am. J. Clin. Pathol.*, **56**, 762–4.

Gephardt, G. N. (1981) Malignant melanoma of the bronchus. *Hum. Pathol.*, **12**, 671–3.

Gibson, J. B., Burrows, D. and Weir, W. P. (1957) Primary melanoma of the meninges. *J. Pathol. Bacteriol.*, **74**, 419–38.

Goldgeiger, M. H., Klein, L. E., Klein-Angerer, S., Moellmann, G. and Nodlund, J. J. (1984) The distribution of melanocytes in the leptomeninges of the human brain. *J. Invest. Dermatol.*, **82**, 235–8.

Goldman, R. L. (1968) Melanogenic epithelium in the prostate gland. *Am. J. Clin. Pathol.*, **49**, 75–8.

Goldman, R. L. (1981) Blue naevus of lymph node capsule: report of a unique case. *Histopathology*, **5**, 445–50.

Goldman, R. L. and Friedman, N. B. (1967) Blue nevus of the uterine cervix. *Cancer*, **20**, 210–4.

Goldman, J. L., Lawson, W., Zak, F. G. and Roffman, J. D. (1972) The presence of melanocytes in the human larynx. *Laryngoscope*, **82**, 824–35.

Goldschmidt, P., Py, J. M., Kostakopoulos, A., Jacqmin, D., Grosshans, E. and Bollack, C. (1988) Primary malignant melanomas of the urinary bladder. *Br. J. Urol.*, **61**, 359–66.

Graham, D. I., Paterson, A., McQueen, A., Milne, J. A. and Urich, H. (1976) Melanotic tumours (blue naevi) of spinal nerve roots. *J. Pathol.*, **118**, 83–89.

Greene, G. W., Jr. and Bernier, J. L. (1961) Primary malignant melanomas of the parotid gland. *Oral Surg.*, **14**, 108–16.

Gregg, R. H. (1982) Primary malignant melanoma arising in an ovaian dermoid cyst. *Am. J. Obstetr. Gynecol.*, **143**, 25–8.

Griffith, W. R., Green, W. R. and Weinstein, G. W. (1971) Conjunctival malignant melanoma originating in acquired melanosis sine pigmento. *Am. J. Ophthalmol.*, **72**, 595–9.

Guzman, R. P., Wightman, R., Ravinsky, E. and Unruh, H. W. (1989) Primary melanoma of the esophagus with diffuse melanocytic atypia and melanoma *in situ*. *Am. J. Clin. Pathol.*, **92**, 802–4.

Hall, D. J., Schneider, V. and Goplerud, D. R. (1980) Primary malignant melanoma of the uterine cervix. *Obstet. Gynecol.*, **56**, 525–9.

Hartmann, L. C., Oliver, G. F., Winkelmann, R. K., Colby, T. V., Sundt, T. M. and O'Neill, B. P. (1989) Blue nevus and nevus of Ota associated with dural melanoma. *Cancer*, **64**, 182–6.

Heath, D. I. and Womack, C. (1988) Primary malignant melanoma of the gall bladder. *J. Clin. Pathol.*, **41**, 1073–7.

Henderson, J. W. (1973) *Orbital Tumors*. Philadelphia: W. B. Saunders, pp. 322–44.

Horlick, H. P., Walther, R. R., Zegarelli, D. J., Silvers, D. N. and Eliezri, Y. D. (1988) Mucosal melanotic macule, reactive type: a simulation of melanoma. *J. Am. Acad. Dermatol.*, **19**, 786–91.

Huntington, A., Haugan, P., Gamel, J. and McLean, I. (1989) A simple cytologic method for predicting the malignant potential of intraocular melanoma. *Pathol. Res. Pract.*, **185**, 631–4.

Jakobiec, F. A. and Silbert, G. (1981) Are most iris 'melanomas' really nevi? A clinicopathologic study of 189 lesions. *Arch. Ophthalmol.*, **99**, 2117–32.

Jakobiec, F. A., Zuckerman, B. D., Berlin, A. J., Odell, P., MacRae, D. W. and Tuthill, R. J. (1985) Unusual melanocytic nevi of the conjunctiva. *Am. J. Ophthalmol.*, **100**, 100–13.

Jakobiec, F. A., Folberg, R. and Iwamoto, T. (1989) Clinicopathologic characteristics of premalignant and malignant melanocytic lesions of the conjunctiva. *Ophthalmology*, **96**, 147–66.

Jao, W., Fretzin, D. F., Christ, M. L. and Prinz, L. M. (1971) Blue nevus of the prostate gland. *Arch. Pathol.*, **91**, 187–91.

Jeffrey, I. J. M., Lucas, D. R., McEwan, C. and Lee, W. R. (1986) Malignant melanoma of the conjunctiva. *Histopathology*, **10**, 363–78.

Johnson, W. T. and Helwig, E. B. (1969) Benign nevus cells in the capsule of lymph nodes. *Cancer*, **23**, 747–53.

Johnson, T. L., Kumar, N. B., White, C. D. and Morley, G. W. (1986) Prognostic features of vulvar melanoma: a clinicopathologic analysis. *Int. J. Gynecol. Pathol.*, **5**, 110–8.

Kantarovsky, A., Kaufman, Z., Zager, M., Lew, S. and Dinbar, A. (1988) Anorectal region malignant melanoma. *J. Surg. Oncol.*, **38**, 77–9.

Kato, T., Takematsu, H., Tomita, Y., Takahashi, M. and Abe, R. (1987) Malignant melanoma of mucous membranes. A clinicopathologic study of 13 cases in Japanese patients. *Arch. Dermatol.*, **123**, 216–20.

Kinseley, R. M. and Baggenstoss, A. H. (1946) Primary melanoma of the adrenal gland. *Arch. Pathol.*, **42**, 345–9.

Kokotas, N. S., Kallis, E. G. and Fokitis, P. J. (1981) Primary malignant melanoma of male urethra. *Urology*, **18**, 392–4.

Kopf, A. W. and Bart, R. S. (1979) A conjunctival pigmented lesion. *J. Dermatol. Surg. Oncol.*, **5**, 668–9.

Kopf, A. W. and Bart, R. S. (1982) Tumor conference, case 43. Penile lentigo. *J. Dermatol. Surg. Oncol.*, **8**, 637–9.

Kornberg, R., Harris, M. and Ackerman, A. B. (1978) Epidermotropically metastatic malignant melanoma. *Arch. Dermatol.*, **114**, 67–9.

Krausz, M. M., Ariel, I. and Behar, A. J. (1978) Primary malignant melanoma of the small intestine and the APUD cell concept. *J. Surg. Oncol.*, **10**, 283–8.

Lach, B., Russell, N., Benoit, B. and Atack, D. (1988) Cellular blue nevus ('melanocytoma') of the spinal meninges: electron microscopic and immunohistochemical features. *Neurosurgery*, **22**, 773–80.

Lambert, W. C. and Brodkin, R. H. (1984) Nodal and subcutaneous blue nevi: a pseudometastasizing pseudomelanoma. *Arch. Dermatol.*, **120**, 367–70.

Lamovec, J. (1984) Blue nevus of the lymph node capsule. Report of a new case with review of the literature. *Am. J. Clin. Pathol.*, **81**, 367–72.

Larson, III T. C., Houser, O. W., Onofrio, B. M. and Piepgras, D. G. (1987) Primary spinal melanoma. *J. Neurosurg.*, **66**, 47–49.

Lee, R. B., Buttoni, L., Dhru, K. and Tamini, H. (1984) Malignant melanoma of the vagina: a case report of progression from preexisting melanosis. *Gynecol. Oncol.*, **19**, 238–45.

Leicht, S., Youngberg, G. and Diaz-Miranda, C. (1988) Atypical pigmented penile macules. *Arch. Dermatol.*, **124**, 1267–70.

Lewis, M. G. and Martin, J. A. M. (1967) Malignant melanoma of the nasal cavity in Ugandan Africans: relationship to ectopic pigment. *Cancer*, **20**, 1699–1705.

Limas, C. and Tio, F. O. (1972) Meningeal melanocytoma ('melanotic meningioma'). Its melanocytic origin as revealed by electron microscopy. *Cancer*, **30**, 1286–94.

MacFarlane, R., Marks, P. V. and Waters, A. (1989) Primary melanoma of the dura mater. *Br. J. Neurosurg.*, **3**, 235–8.

Mackenzie, D. H. (1974) Clear cell sarcoma of tendon and aponeuroses with melanin production. *J. Pathol.*, **114**, 231–2.

Maize, J. C. and Ackerman, A. B. (1987) *Pigmented Lesions of the Skin*. Philadelphia: Lea & Febiger, pp. 318–20.

Manivel, J. C. and Fraley, E. E. (1988) Malignant melanoma of the penis and male urethra: 4 case reports and literature review. *J. Urol.*, **139**, 813–6.

Martin, P. C., Pulitzer, D. R. and Reed, R. J. (1989) Pigmented myomatous neurocristoma of the uterus. *Arch. Pathol. Lab. Med.*, **113**, 1291–5.

Mason, J. K. and Helwig, E. B. (1966) Ano-rectal melanoma. *Cancer*, **19**, 39–50.

McCarthy, S. W., Palmer, A. A., Bale, P. M. and Hist, E. (1974) Nevus cells in lymph nodes. *Pathology*, **6**, 351–8.

McDonnell, J. M., Carpenter, J. D., Jacobs, P., Wan, W. L. and Gilmore, J. E. (1989) Conjunctival melanocytic lesions in children. *Ophthalmology*, **96**, 986–93.

McGinnis, J. P., Greer, J. L. and Wolfe, N. L. (1986) Neurotropic melanoma of the lower lip. *J. Oral Pathol.*, **15**, 445–9.

McGovern, V. J. (1976) *Malignant Melanoma: Clinical and Histological Diagnosis.* New York: Wiley & Sons, p. 53.

McLean, I. W., Zimmerman, L. E. and Evans, R. (1978) Reappraisal of Callender's spindle A type of malignant melanoma of choroid and ciliary body. *Am. J. Ophthalmol.*, **86**, 557–64.

McLean, I. W., Foster, W. D. and Zimmerman, L. E. (1982) Uveal melanoma: location, cell type, and enucleation as risk factors in metastasis. *Hum. Pathol.*, **13**, 123–32.

Meyer, J. E. (1974) Metastatic melanoma of the urinary bladder. *Cancer*, **34**, 1822–4.

Mihm, M. C. and Guillén, F. J. (1985) Primary acquired melanosis. *Hum. Pathol.*, **16**, 1078–9.

Miller, C. S., Craig, R. M. and Mantich, N. M. (1987) Blue-black macule on the maxillary palate. *J. Am. Dent. Assoc.*, **114**, 503–4.

Mills, S. E. and Cooper, P. H. (1983) Malignant melanoma of the digestive system. *Pathol. Ann.*, **18-II**, 1–26.

Morishita, S., Onomura, T., Yamamoto, S. and Nakashima, Y. (1987) Clear cell sarcoma of tendons and aponeuroses (malignant melanoma of soft parts) with unusual roentgenologic findings. Case report. *Clin. Orthopaedics Rel. Res.*, **216**, 276–9.

Morson, B. C. and Volkstädt, H. (1963) Malignant melanoma of the anal canal. *J. Clin. Pathol.*, **16**, 126–32.

Murphy, M. N., Lorimer, S. M. and Glennon, P. E. (1987) Metastatic melanoma of the gallbladder: a case report and review of the literature. *J. Surg. Oncol.*, **34**, 68–72.

Musfeld, D. and De Grandi, P. (1986) Das Melanom in der Frauenheilkunde. *Geburtsh. Frauenheilk.*, **46**, 857–62.

Myskow, M. W., Going J. J., McLaren, K. M. and Inglis, J. A. (1988) Malignant melanoma of penis. *J. Urol.*, **139**, 817–8.

Narayan, R. K., Rosner, M. J., Povlishock, J. T., Girevendulis, A. and Becker, D. P. (1981) Primary dural melanoma: a clinical and morphological study. *Neurosurgery*, **9**, 710–7.

Nigogosyan, G., De la Pava, S. and Pickren, J. W. (1964) Melanoblasts in vaginal mucosa. Origin for primary malignant melanoma. *Cancer*, **17**, 912–3.

Nikai, H., Miyauchi, M., Ogawa, I., Takata, T., Hayashi, Y. and Okazaki, H. (1990) Spitz nevus of the palate. *Oral Surg. Oral Med. Oral Pathol.*, **69**, 603–8.

Oldbring, J. and Mikulowski, P. (1987) Malignant melanoma of the penis and male urethra. Report of nine cases and review of the literature. *Cancer*, **59**, 581–7.

Özden, B., Barlas, O. and Hacihanefioglu, U. (1984) Primary dural melanomas:

report of two cases and review of the literature. *Neurosurgery*, **15**, 104–7.

Parekh, M. A. (1985) Primary malignant melanoma in an ovarian cystic teratoma. A case report and literature review. *Mo. Med.*, **82**, 18–20.

Patel, D. S. and Bhagavan, B. S. (1985) Blue nevus of the uterine cervix. *Hum. Pathol.*, **16**, 79–86.

Piccone, V. A., Klopstock, R., LeVeen, H. H. and Sika, J. (1970) Primary malignant melanoma of the esophagus associated with melanosis of the entire esophagus. First case report. *Cardiovasc. Surg.*, **59**, 864.

Podratz, K. C., Gaffey, T. A., Symmonds, R. E., Johansen, K. L. and O'Brien, P. C. (1983) Melanoma of the vulva: an update. *Gynec. Oncol.*, **16**, 153–68.

Raderman, D., Rothem, A., Giler, S. and Ben-Bassat, M. (1986) Primary malignant melanoma of the vermilion of the lower lip. *J. Dermatol. Surg. Oncol.*, **12**, 1106–10.

Rapini, R. P., Golitz, L. E., Greer, R. O., Jr., Krekorian, E. A. and Poulson, T. (1985) Primary malignant melanoma of the oral cavity: a review of 177 cases. *Cancer*, **55**, 1543–51.

Raynor, A. C., Vargas-Cortes, F., Alexander, R. W. and Bingham, H. G. (1979) Clear-cell sarcoma with melanin pigment: a possible soft-tissue variant of malignant melanoma. Case report. *J. Bone Joint Surg.*, **61A**, 276–80.

Reese, A. B. (1955) Precancerous and cancerous melanosis of conjunctiva. *Am. J. Opthalmol.*, **39**, 96–100.

Reid, J. D. and Mehta, V. T. (1966) Melanoma of the lower respiratory tract. *Cancer*, **19**, 627–31.

Reuter, V. E. and Woodruff, J. M. (1986) Melanoma of the larynx. *Laryngoscope*, **94**, 389–93.

Ridolfi. R. L., Rosen, P. P. and Thaler, H. (1977) Nevus cell aggregates associated with lymph nodes: estimated frequency and clinical significance. *Cancer*, **39**, 164–71.

Rios, C. N. and Wright, J. R. (1976) Melanosis of the prostate gland: report of a case with neoplastic epithelium involvement. *J. Urol.*, **115**, 616–7.

Ro, J. Y., Grignon, D. J., Ayala, A. G., Hogan, S. F., Tetu, B. and Ordonez, N. G. (1988) Blue nevus and melanosis of the prostate. Electron-microscopic and immunohistochemical studies. *Am. J. Clin. Pathol.*, **90**, 530–5.

Rodriguez, H. A. and Ackerman, L. V. (1968) Cellular blue nevus. *Cancer*, **21**, 393–405.

Rowlands, D., Edwards, C. and Collins, F. (1987) Malignant melanotic schwannoma of the bronchus. *J. Clin. Pathol.*, **40**, 1449–50.

Salm, R. (1963) A primary malignant melanoma of the bronchus. *J. Pathol. Bacteriol.*, **85**, 121–6.

Salm, R. and Rutter, T. E. (1964) A double primary malignant melanoma of the fossa navicularis. *Br. J. Urol.*, **36**, 91–6.

Sandstedt, B. E., Delemarre, J. F. M., Harms, D. and Tournade, M. F. (1987) Sarcomatous Wilms' tumour with clear cells and hyalinization. A study of 38 tumours in children from the SIOP nephroblastoma file. *Histopathology*, **11**, 273–85.

Sara, A. S., Evans, H. L. and Benjamin, R. S. (1990) Malignant melanoma of soft parts (clear cell sarcoma). A study of 17 cases, with emphasis on prognostic factors. *Cancer*, **65**, 367–74.

Saw, D., Tse, C. H., Chan, J., Watt, C. Y., Ng, C. S. and Poon, Y. F. (1986) Clear cell sarcoma of the penis. *Hum. Pathol.*, **17**, 423–5.

Scholtz, C. L. and Siu, K. (1976) Melanoma of the pituitary. Case report.

J. Neurosurg., **45**, 101–3.

Scotto, J., Fraumen, J. F. and Lee, J. A. H. (1976) Melanomas of the eye and other noncutaneous sites: epidemiologic aspects. *J. Natl Cancer Inst.*, **56**, 489–91.

Shenoy, B. V., Fort, L. III and Benjamin, S. P. (1987) Malignant melanoma primary in lymph node. The case of the missing link. Case report. *Am. J. Surg. Pathol.*, **11**, 140–6.

Simpson, W. A., Burke, M., Frappell, J. and Cook, M. G. (1988) Paget's disease, melanocytic neoplasia and hidradenoma papilliferum of the vulva. *Histopathology*, **12**, 675–9.

Simpson, N. S., Spence, R. A. J., Biggart, J. D. and Cameron, C. H. S. (1990) Primary malignant melanoma of the oesophagus. *J. Clin. Pathol.*, **43**, 82–4.

Sison-Torre, E. Q. and Ackerman, A. B. (1985) Melanosis of the vulva. A clinical simulator of malignant melanoma. *Am. J. Dermatopathol.*, **7**, 51S–60S.

Smith, T. R. and Brockhurst, R. J. (1976) Cellular blue nevus of the sclera. *Arch. Ophthalmol.*, **94**, 618–20.

Smith, S. and Opipari, M. I. (1978) Primary pleural melanoma. *J. Thorac. Cardiovasc. Surg.*, **75**, 827–31.

Snow, G. B. and Van der Waal, I. (1986) Mucosal melanomas of the head and neck. *Otolaryngol. Clin. North Am.*, **19**, 537–47.

Sotelo-Avila, C., Gonzalez-Crussi, F., Sadowinski, S., Gooch III, W. M. and Pena, R. (1986) Clear cell sarcoma of the kidney. A clinicopathologic study of 21 patients with long-term follow-up evaluation. *Hum. Pathol.*, **16**, 1219–30.

Stewart, F. W. and Copeland, M. M. (1931) Neurogenic sarcoma. *Am. J. Cancer*, **15**, 1235–1320.

Subramony, C. and Lewin, J. R. (1985) Nevus cells within lymph nodes. Possible metastases from a benign intradermal nevus. *Am. J. Clin. Pathol.*, **84**, 220–3.

Takagi, M., Ishikawa, G. and Mori, W. (1974) Primary malignant melanoma of the oral cavity in Japan. *Cancer*, **34**, 358–70.

Takeda, Y. (1988) Congenital nevocellular nevus of the oral mucosa. *Ann. Dent.*, **47**, 40–42.

Takubo, K., Kanda, Y., Ishi, M. *et al.* (1983) Primary malignant melanoma of the esophagus. *Hum. Pathol.*, **14**, 727–30.

Tannenbaum, M. (1974) Differential diagnosis in uropathology. III. Melanotic lesions of the prostate: blue nevus and prostatic epithelial melanosis. *Urology*, **4**, 617–21.

Tham, K.-T., Ma, P.-H. and Kung, T. M. (1981) Malignant melanoma in an ovarian cystic teratoma. *Hum. Pathol.*, **12**, 577–9.

Tobon, H. and Murphy, A. I. (1977) Benign blue nevus of the vagina. *Cancer*, **40**, 3174–6.

Trapp, T. K., Fu, Y.-S. and Calcaterra, T. C. (1987) Melanoma of the nasal and paranasal sinus mucosa. *Arch. Otolaryngol. Head Neck Surg.*, **113**, 1086–9.

Tsukada, Y. (1976) Benign melanosis of the vagina and cervix. *Am. J. Obstet. Gynecol.*, **124**, 211–2.

Uehara, T., Matsubara, O. and Kasuga, T. (1987) Melanocytes in the nasal cavity and paranasal sinus. Incidence and distribution in Japan. *Acta Pathol. Jap.*, **37**, 1105–14.

Uff, J. S. and Hall, M. (1978) Blue naevus of the cervix: report of two cases and review of the literature. *Histopathology*, **2**, 291–9.

Verma, D. S., Spitzer, G., Legha, S. and McCredie, K. B. (1979) Chemoimmunotherapy for meningeal melanocytoma of the thoracic spinal cord. Report of a case. *J. Am. Med. Assoc.*, **242**, 2435–6.

Von Albertini, M. (1935) About a case of neuronaevus with lymph node metastasis of the same type. *Bull. Soc. Franc. Derm. Syph.*, **42**, 1273–8.

Vuong, P. N., Cassembon, F., Houissa-Vuong, S., Koubbi, G. and Balaton, A. (1986) Mélanome malin primitif de la parotide: étude anatomo-clinique. A propos d'une observation avec revue de la littérature médicale. *Ann. Oto-laryngol.* (Paris), **103**, 45–55.

Walsh, T. S. (1956) Primary melanoma of the gallbladder with cervical metastasis and fourteen and one-half years survival. *Cancer*, **9**, 518–22.

Wanebo, H. J., Woodruff, J. M., Farr, G. H. and Quan, S. H. (1981) Anorectal melanoma. *Cancer*, **47**, 1891–1900.

Warner, T. F. C. S., Hafez, G. R. and Buchler, D. A. (1982) Neurotropic melanoma of the vulva. *Cancer*, **49**, 999–1004.

Warner, T. F. C. S., Hafez, G. R., Padmalatha, C. and Lange, T. A. (1983) Acral lentiginous melanoma simulating 'clear cell sarcoma of tendons and aponeuroses'. *J. Cutan. Pathol.*, **10**, 193–200.

Weiss, J., Elder, D. and Hamilton, R. (1982) Melanoma of the male urethra: surgical approach and pathological analysis. *J. Urol.*, **128**, 382–5.

Werdin, C., Limas, C. and Knodell, R. G. (1988) Primary malignant melanoma of the rectum. Evidence for origination from rectal mucosal melanocytes. *Cancer*, **61**, 1364–70.

Winston, K. R., Sotrel, A. and Schnitt, J. (1987) Meningeal melanocytoma. Case report and review of the clinical and histological features. *J. Neurosurg.*, **66**, 50–57.

Yanoff, M. and Fine, B. S. (1982) *Ocular Pathology, a Text and Atlas*, 2nd edn. Philadelphia: Harper & Row, pp. 822–31.

Yu, H. C. and Ketabchi, M. (1987) Detection of malignant melanoma of the uterine cervix from Papanicolaou smears. A case report. *Acta Cytol.*, **31**, 73–6.

12 Other extracutaneous melanotic lesions

Melanotic pigmentation may be present in a variety of conditions unrelated to melanocytic disorders, as a result of melanocyte colonization (p. 43) and hyperactivity of melanocytes present in the vicinity. Although essentially outside the scope of this book dealing with melanocytic disorders, it may be useful to include a brief discussion of these lesions, some of which are rare and may cause diagnostic difficulties. Those occurring in the skin have been dealt with in Chapter 3; here, we shall include a discussion of the extracutaneous ones (Table 12.1).

Table 12.1 Reactive hyperpigmentation and melanocyte colonization of extracutaneous tumours

---

Squamous carcinoma
    Conjunctiva
    Upper aerodigestive tract
    Bronchus
    Genital tract

Adenocarcinomas of rectum, breast and prostate

Lesions of oral cavity:
    Melanotic macule and 'melanoacanthoma'
    Various odontogenic tumours

Carcinoid of thymus

Furthermore, some nonmelanocytic tumours are melanogenic in the sense that they produce melanosomal melanin or neuromelanin; many of these are neural crest-derived or exhibit neuroendocrine differentiation: they include a variety of primary tumours of the central and peripheral nervous system, tumours of retinal pigment epithelium, the so-called pigmented neuroectodermal tumour of infancy, medullary carcinoma of the thyroid, and certain carcinoid tumours (Table 12.2). The origin of melanin pigmentation in endocrine tumours has not been entirely resolved; in some tumours, such as thymic carcinoids, the findings are suggestive of reactive melanocytic hyperplasia; in others, such as bronchial carcinoids, melanin appears to be synthesized by the tumour cells themselves. Electron microscopical demonstration of stage II melanosomes within the cytoplasm of tumour cells has often been taken to indicate synthesis of melanin by these cells rather than transfer from adjacent melanocytes; however, Szpak and co-workers (1988) demonstrated that this is not necessarily true: therefore, the issue of melanin production *vs* melanin uptake by tumour cells is not solved conclusively by electron microscopy.

12.1   Conjunctiva

Squamous carcinoma of the conjunctiva may be pigmented due to a reactive increase in melanin production and proliferation of conjunctival melanocytes (Jauregui and Klintworth, 1976; Salisbury *et al.*, 1983).

12.2   Labial and oral melanotic lesions

Melanotic macules and 'melanoacanthomas' of the labial mucosa (Matsuoka *et al.*, 1979; Sexton and Maize, 1987; Spann *et al.*, 1987) are hyperpigmented macules, often with a slightly irregular shape and degree of pigmentation. Both occur in a wide age range with a mean of around 40 years, and are located mainly on the lower lip; females are far more commonly affected. Histologically, these lesions show acanthosis, basal keratinocyte hyperpigmentation, increased numbers of basal dendritic melanocytes, subepithelial fibrosis, teleangiectasia and pigment incontinence (Sexton and Maize, 1987); melanoacanthoma in addition exhibits colonization of the acanthotic epithelium by dendritic melanocytes in a manner similar to that seen in melanoacanthoma of the skin (p. 45). However, in view of the many clinical and

Table 12.2 Neural crest-derived and neuroendocrine tumours containing melanosomal melanin or neuromelanin

Neuroblastoma
Olfactory neuroblastoma
Ganglioglioma
Medulloblastoma
Pinealoma
Ependymoma
Choroid plexus carcinoma
Tumours of uveal pigment epithelium
Schwannoma (benign, malignant, psammomatous)
Neurofibroma
Pigmented neuroectodermal tumour of infancy ('melanotic progonoma')
Medullary carcinoma of the thyroid
Carcinoid tumours (bronchus)

histological similarities, it seems unlikely that melanotic macule and melanoacanthoma of labial and oral mucosa are really separate and unrelated entities.

Melanotic macule or melanoacanthoma of the oral mucosa (Goode *et al.*, 1983; Horlick *et al.*, 1988; Zemtsov and Bergfeld, 1989) occurs in black patients, and shows acanthosis, melanocytic proliferation, colonization of the epithelium and varying degrees of spongiosis. The clinical features (rapid growth within days or weeks, history of trauma in about half of the cases, spontaneous regression) indicate that the lesion is probably reactive in nature.

Melanocyte colonization leading to macroscopical dark pigmentation has been described in an oral *squamous carcinoma* of a black patient (Modica *et al.*, 1990).

A variety of *odontogenic tumours* may occasionally contain melanin: these include calcifying odontogenic cyst (Soames, 1982), odontogenic keratocyst (Brannon, 1977), complex odontoma (Takeda *et al.*, 1987), ameloblastic fibro-odontoma (Takeda *et al.*, 1988), odontoameloblastoma (Takeda *et al.*, 1989) and adenomatoid odontogenic tumour (Takeda, 1989).

12.3   Salivary gland

Melanocyte colonization in a salivary gland mucoepidermoid carcinoma and a poorly differentiated adenocarcinoma, in the primary tumour as well as in metastases, was reported by Thomas and colleagues (1980). Both cases occurred in Malawian patients.

12.4   Dermatopathic lymphadenopathy

Many forms of pruritic chronic dermatitis, particularly when accompanied by epidermal exfoliation, lead to enlargement of draining lymph nodes, which show marked expansion of paracortical zones, occasionally resulting in partial effacement of the architecture of the node. The paracortical zones contain numerous histiocytes, Langerhans' cells and dendritic reticulum cells (Herrera, 1987), some of which are laden with melanin, while extracellular melanin deposits may also be present. This may result in macrosocopically detectable pigmentation of the node. Especially in the presence of sheets of these S-100 positive cells, the lesion must be differentiated from metastatic melanoma, which rarely poses diagnostic difficulties, when attention is paid to the clinical context and the cytological features of the S-100 positive cells.

12.5   Endocrine organs and neuroendocrine tumours

Black discolouration of the thyroid, due to accumulation of dark-brown pigment granules in the follicular epithelium, may occur after mino-cycline treatment or, rarely, without a clear cause. The pigment shows may similarities with neuromelanin found in some parts of the brain and in some brain tumours (p. 392) and it is possibly identical (Landas *et al.*, 1986). To a lesser extent, such granules are not uncommonly found in the thyroid epithelium, especially in late adulthood.

Carcinoids of the lung and thymus occasionally contain some melanin pigment. In several cases of pulmonary carcinoid, it is very likely that the melanin is produced by the tumour cells (Cebelin, 1980; Gould *et al.*, 1981; Grazer *et al.*, 1982); however, in two thymic carcinoids (Ho and Ho, 1977; Lagrange *et al.*, 1987), melanocyte colonization was probably the underlying mechanism, since melanin-containing dendritic cells formed a second population distinct from the tumour cells. Melanocytes have been reported to occur in the murine thymus (Markert and Silvers, 1956), but they have hitherto not been noted in the human thymus. Melanin-containing carcinoids do not have sign-ificantly different clinical implications when compared to their non-pigmented counterparts.

Medullary carcinoma of the thyroid may also contain melanin, which is apparently produced by the tumour cells (Gould *et al.*, 1981; Marcus *et al.*, 1982).

12.6   Melanotic schwannoma and neurofibroma

12.6.1   *Melanotic schwannoma*

Schwann cells may occasionally contain a small amount of melanin, and since melanosomes in various stages of development can be dem-onstrated and melanocytes are absent in the vicinity, the melanin is apparently synthesized by these Schwann cells (El-Labban, 1988). It should be borne in mind that embryologically, melanocytes and Schwann cells share a common derivation from the neural crest.

Similarly, the tumour cells of schwannomas may rarely synthesize melanin. Melanin-containing Schwann cell tumours have been induced experimentally in rats by transplacental administration of ethylnitro-sourea (Spence *et al.*, 1976). The occurrence of melanin synthesis in pigmented schwannomas calls to mind the schwannian features en-countered in some cutaneous naevi and melanomas (Chapters 4 and 9).

Melanotic schwannoma occurs in a wide age range, from childhood to late adult life, the mean age of reported cases being about 38 years

(Killeen *et al.*, 1988); it affects both sexes equally. The tumour most often arises in close proximity to the neural axis, often within the sheaths of spinal nerve roots or cranial nerves, including the acoustic nerve; in one case the tumour was intramedullary in location (Solomon *et al.*, 1987). Others arise from the sympathetic chain, most often within the mediastinum, but also in cervical and lumbar locations (Fu *et al.*, 1975; Krausz *et al.*, 1984), while scattered cases have been reported at a distance from the neural axis, in a wide variety of sites including in the soft tissues of the shoulder (Font and Truong, 1984), thoracic wall (Miettinen, 1987), extremities (Ducastelle *et al.*, 1981), the oral mucosa (Janzer and Makek, 1983), mandible (Hodson, 1961), oesophagus (Assor, 1975), bronchus (Rowlands *et al.*, 1987), gastric wall (Burns *et al.*, 1983), right ventricle of the heart (Gelfland *et al.*, 1977), parotid gland (Killeen *et al.*, 1988) and skin (Webb, 1982). Symptoms may have been present for up to many years, indicating slow growth.

Macroscopically, the tumours are black and often firm and encapsulated; however, a capsule may be focally absent. The nerve from which the tumour arises may be noticed macroscopically, especially in axial sites. Recorded sizes vary between 0.8 and 26 cm.

Histologically, benign melanotic schwannoma exhibits the basic characteristics of schwannoma: an encapsulated tumour, consisting of highly cellular areas alternating with less cellular (Antoni B) areas showing mucoid and sometimes cystic change, and various other signs of degeneration. Cellular areas usually predominate and may be present exclusively. Vascular structures are usually thin-walled but occasionally show thickening and perivascular hyalinization. Whorl-like structures and psammoma bodies may be found in some instances and are a useful diagnostic feature since they are very rare in other soft tissue neoplasms (Miettinen, 1987). Nuclear palisading is often absent or inconspicuous; Verocay bodies are infrequently found. As indicated above, a fibrous capsule of varying thickness is often seen and is diagnostically important, since it is absent in melanocytic proliferations. It should be differentiated from a pseudocapsule, resulting from expansile growth pattern, seen in many tumours, albeit very rarely in melanocytic ones. A pre-existing nerve may be recognized histologically, within or adjacent to the tumour. Some lesions may show cystic degeneration, calcification, bone formation and conspicuous perivascular hyalinization, as in ancient schwannomas. The tumour cells are elongated and possess oval or elongated nuclei, which are often asymmetrical, partly rounded and partly pointed, longitudinally grooved or folded, and sometimes vacuolated; nucleoli may be prominent. There is an elongated, often buckled 'flag' of eosinophilic cytoplasm focally containing melanin pigment, and often some glycogen.

Immunohistochemically, the tumour cells are positive for vimentin and usually for S-100; positivity of a subpopulation of cells for glial fibrillary acidic protein was noted by Miettinen (1987). Ultrastructurally, the tumour cells show the characteristics of Schwann cells (interdigitating long cytoplasmic processes wrapped around one another as well as around collagen bundles and cell bodies; prominent, sometimes duplicated basal laminae; micropinocytotic vesicles; occasional microtubules, intercellular junctions; occasionally, long-spaced collagen with a periodicity of around 130 nm within the intercellular substance; (Dickersin, 1987) and contain melanosomes at various stages of maturation (Mennemeyer *et al.*, 1979).

Malignant melanotic schwannoma (Figure 12.1) shows significant mitotic activity, focal necrosis and more cytological atypia. Compact areas or diffuse sheets of more rounded or polygonal melanin-containing cells may be present and increase the resemblance to melanoma. A large proportion of these tumours metastasize and lead to the death of the patient.

The histology and biological behaviour of melanotic schwannomas show a correlation with the site of origin. Those arising in the sheaths of nerve roots are usually relatively monomorphic, with no or relatively few mitoses; these rarely metastasize, but may recur after incomplete removal. Complete surgical excision constitutes definitive treatment; however, in the case of cranial nerve involvement this may be very difficult and recurrent tumour may occasionally lead to death due to locally intractable disease. In contrast, tumours originating from the sympathetic chain (Krausz *et al.*, 1984) generally show histological evidence of malignancy, with foci of necrosis and areas of increased mitotic activity and more pronounced cellular atypia, so that the picture of malignant blue naevus or metastatic melanoma is mimicked; these tumours do metastasize. Such cases should be distinguished from metastatic melanoma with unknown primary site: in this respect, the identification of a pre-existing nerve as the site of origin is of importance. However, a benign melanotic schwannoma of the sympathetic chain has also been reported (Kayano and Katayama, 1988); the benignity was evidenced by the presence of a well-developed fibrous capsule, absence of necrosis and mitoses, and only a slight degree of cellular pleomorphism.

Tumours located at a distance from the neural axis are rare and vary in behaviour; it is therefore impossible to generalize about their clinical course. The literature on melanotic schwannoma of soft tissues before 1984 was reviewed by Font and Truong (1984). Histological assessment of tumour borders, mitotic activity, necrosis, and cellular atypia should

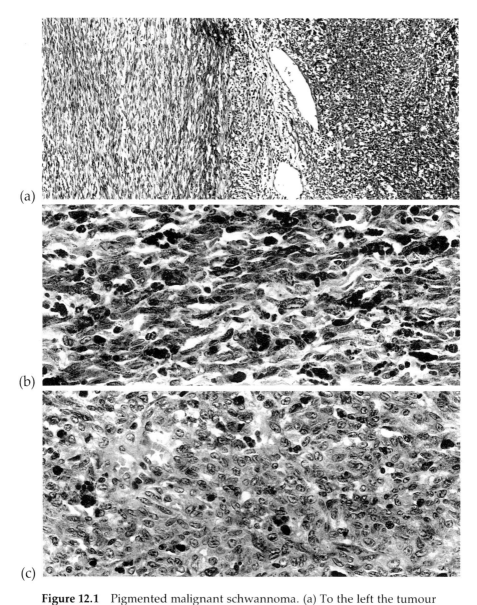

Figure 12.1 Pigmented malignant schwannoma. (a) To the left the tumour cells are spindled, whereas to the right an epithelioid cell type is seen and melanin is produced (HE, × 90). (b) Partly pigmented spindled tumour cells. The buckled and asymmetric nuclei and the undulating arrangement and shape of the tumour cells suggest a neurogenic tumour (HE, × 370). (c) In this field the cells are more plump and nucleoli become apparent. Focal melanin production. Elsewhere, the tumour was found to arise from a nerve. Case published by Krausz *et al.* (1984) (HE, × 370).

Table 12.3 Melanotic schwannoma

Clinical features
  Wide age range; no sex preference
  Most common locations: spinal and cranial nerve roots, sympathetic chain
  Prognosis varies according to histological appearance and site
  Local recurrences after incomplete excision (cranial nerves!) may lead to
    locally intractable disease

Pathological features
  Fibrous capsule, sometimes incomplete
  Spindle cells with asymmetrical nuclei and a 'flag' of eosinophilic cytoplasm
    focally containing melanin
  Melanophages
  Occasionally: variants as in other schwannomas (ancient schwannoma, bone
    formation, cytological atypia, cysts)

Remarks
  Beware misdiagnosis of melanoma on frozen sections especially
  Melanotic schwannoma with psammoma bodies: some are associated with a
    familial syndrome including myxomas of various sites, cutaneous
    pigmentations and endocrine hyperactivity syndromes

provide the basis for a guarded estimate of the malignant potential of
such lesions.

The main differential diagnoses of benign and malignant melanotic
schwannoma are cellular blue naevus and melanoma. Indeed, in some
locations such as the oral mucosa, where melanocytic tumours also
occur and may show schwannian differentiation, the distinction between a melanocytic and a Schwann cell tumour may ultimately be
impossible, unless a distinct intraepithelial component or, alternatively,
a fibrous capsule or an origin from a nerve, can be demonstrated.

The possibility of pigmented schwannoma should always be considered when a pigmented spindle cell tumour is encountered; especially on frozen section, the danger of a misdiagnosis of melanoma
is very real.

The main features of pigmented schwannoma are summarized in
Table 12.3.

12.6.2   Psammomatous melanotic schwannoma

Psammoma bodies occur in some nonmelanotic and melanotic
schwannomas. They are more variable in size than those encountered
in meningiomas, and they may coalesce to form large calcified masses,
up to several millimetres in size (Carney, 1990). When a schwannoma
contains melanin as well as psammoma bodies, there is often also a
fatty tissue component; such tumours appear to constitute a specific

entity. In about half of the pigmented schwannomas with psammoma bodies collected and reviewed by Carney (1990), there was an association with a heritable syndrome including myxomas of the heart, skin and breast, cutaneous lentigines and blue naevi, and various endocrine overactivity syndromes such as Cushing's syndrome, sexual precocity, and acromegaly, associated with pigmented adrenocortical nodules and large-cell calcifying Sertoli cell tumour. Schwannomas with melanin and psammoma bodies most commonly arise near posterior spinal nerve roots or in the alimentary canal, especially the stomach.

12.6.3   Pigmented neurofibroma

Rarely, neurofibromas contain melanin (Figure 12.2). Such cases occur with or without von Recklinghausen's disease; usually, the pigmentation is not apparent grossly. Apart from the presence of scattered melanin-containing cells, these neurofibromas do not differ significantly from their nonpigmented counterparts (Bird and Willis, 1969; Jurecka *et al.*, 1987).

12.7   Other pigmented tumours of the nervous system

A small number of melanotic meningiomas have been reported in the literature (Keegan and Mullan, 1962; Turnbull and Tom, 1963; Lesoin *et al.*, 1983); from these reports it is doubtful whether they are true meningothelial tumours or whether they in fact represent pigmented schwannomas or meningeal melanocytomas (pp. 369, 387).

A wide variety of other tumours of the nervous system may occasionally contain melanin pigment. A discussion of all individual tumour types is outside the scope of this book; a survey of pigmented tumours of the central nervous system is included in the recent report of Rosenblum and colleagues (1990). The main tumour types involved are: *neuroblastoma* (Mullins, 1980), *olfactory neuroblastoma* (Curtis and Rubinstein, 1982; Llombart-Bosch *et al.*, 1989) *medulloblastoma* (Boesel *et al.*, 1978; Jimenez *et al.*, 1987), *ganglioneuroblastoma* (Hahn *et al.*, 1976; Gonzalez-Crussi and Hsueh, 1988), *ependymoma* and *subependymoma* (McCloskey *et al.*, 1976; Rosenblum *et al.*, 1990) *choroid plexus carcinoma* (Boesel and Suhan, 1979), *pinealoma* (Herrick and Rubinstein, 1979) and *ganglioglioma* (Hunt and Johnson, 1989). No doubt, other tumours of the central nervous system could be added to this list; apparently, tumours arising from neural tissues, sharing with melanocytes an embryological derivation from the neural tube and crest, can occasionally activate the biochemical machinery required for melanin synthesis.

However, the melanin present in these tumours is not always 'mel-

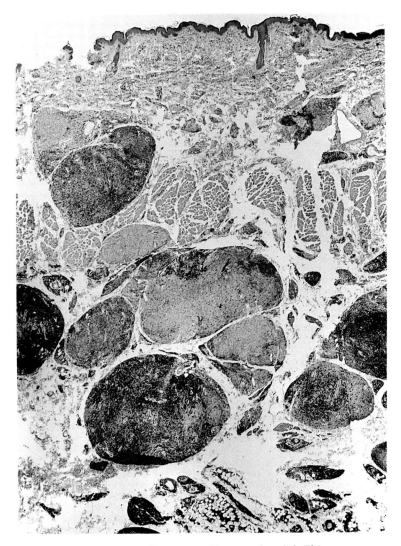

Figure 12.2   Pigmented plexiform neurofibroma of eyelid. This rare case exhibits a plexus of greatly enlarged and heavily pigmented nerves. (Case published by Bird and Willis (1969); from the collection of Dr Salm, Hammersmith Hospital, London) (HE, × 25).

anosomal' melanin: in some instances, such as neuroblastoma and one case of olfactory neuroblastoma, it is *neuromelanin* or a closely related compound. As has been discussed previously (p. 10), neuromelanin shares some of the tinctorial features of melanosomal melanin, but is in fact a different substance altogether: it is a waste product of catecholamine degradation, related to lipofuscin, and is produced in lysosomes rather than in melanosomes (Hahn *et al.*, 1976; Curtis and Rubinstein, 1982).

12.8 Tumours of uveal pigment epithelium

The pigment epithelium of iris, choroid body and retina gives rise to *hyperplasias*, either congenital or acquired; the latter are sometimes associated with previous trauma or inflammation, or with a variety of ocular or metabolic diseases, but they also occur without an apparent cause (Ts'o and Albert, 1972). *Adenomas* and *adenocarcinomas* of uveal pigment epithelium are exceedingly rare (Garner, 1970; Font *et al.*, 1972; Ramahefasolo *et al.*, 1987). All these lesions are very unlikely to be encountered in diagnostic practice outside centres specializing in ocular pathology.

12.9 Pigmented neuroectodermal tumour of infancy ('melanotic progonoma')

This rare tumor of early infancy is known under a variety of names, reflecting the many theories that have been put forward regarding its histogenesis: retinal anlage tumor, pigmented retinoblastoma, melanotic ameloblastic odontoma, pigmented adamantinoma, congenital pigmented epulis and several others. Initially the tumour was described as 'congenital melanocarcinoma' by Krompecher (1918). Later, a derivation from a misplaced remnant of the retinal anlage was hypothesized (Halpert and Patzer, 1947), or it was considered to be the result of 'fetal atavism', and was termed *melanotic progonoma* (Stowens, 1957). Others considered it a 'phylogenetic tumour related to the medial or pineal eye' (Clarke and Parsons, 1951). Indeed, there is a striking histological similarity between the tumour and the developing fetal pineal gland: both contain pigmented epithelial cells as well as small undifferentiated cells, embedded in a fibrovascular stroma (Dooling *et al.*, 1977). A neuroectodermal derivation was postulated by Borello and Gorlin (1966) on the basis of elevated urinary excretion of vanilylmandelic acid (VMA) found in their case, but this was not found in many other reported cases. Immunohistochemical and ultrastructural studies (see below) support a derivation from the neural crest.

The large majority of these tumours occur in early infancy, 95% within the first year of life (Cutler *et al.*, 1981), but a few similar lesions have been reported in adolescence and adulthood (Duckworth and Seward, 1965; Hameed and Burslem, 1970); it is not always clear whether all the latter cases represent the same entity. There is no sex predilection. About 75% occur in the maxilla, about 20% in the mandible and skull, especially around the anterior fontanelle, whereas only a few are found elsewhere (epididymis, mediastinum, scapula, shoulder, upper and lower extremities). In cases involving the skull, there may be a male preponderance and a higher incidence in blacks (De Pascalis *et al.*, 1977).

Cases located in the jaws present as a firm swelling of the jaw or gum, which may reach a size of several centimetres. Radiographically, the tumour spreads irregularly and often erodes the bone, suggesting malignancy. Since the tumour grows relatively rapidly and spreads irregularly into surrounding tissues, it is important that the diagnosis is made as soon as possible, to avoid incomplete excision and tumour recurrence. The overall recurrence rate is 10–15% (Cutler *et al.*, 1981); recurrences are often multifocal. At surgical excision, frozen-section assessment of the surgical margins approximated most closely by the tumour is advocated. Total surgical removal constitutes the definitive treatment.

Pigmented neuroectodermal tumour of infancy very seldom metastasizes; about 2–3% of cases give rise to lymph node and distant metastases and cause death due to metastatic disease (Cutler *et al.*, 1981; Navas Palacios, 1980). Recurrent tumours necessitate more extensive surgery, which in view of the location may present problems, so that locally intractable disease occasionally leads to the patient's death. On the basis of clinical data and pathological findings, it is not possible to predict malignant behaviour in advance. During the course of the disease, however, the histology of these malignant tumours may change to resemble neuroblastoma more closely (Shokry *et al.*, 1986).

Macroscopically, a firm, greyish-white or pigmented mass, well circumscribed but with irregular contours, extends into surrounding structures, and may appear multifocal in some instances. Histologically, the most characteristic feature is the presence of *two cell populations, one 'neuroblast-like'*, consisting of small immature-appearing round or oval cells with round hyperchromatic nuclei and scanty, pale cytoplasm, arranged as irregular aggregates, ribbons, small nests or pseudoalveolar patterns; rosettes and pseudorosettes are almost always absent. *The other, 'pigment epithelium-like'* cell type is larger, shows a round or oval, vesicular nucleus with a prominent nucleolus, and possesses more abundant, eosinophilic cytoplasm. Some of these cells contain small melanin granules, which may be rod-like. These larger cells are often arranged in ribbons or tubules, or line irregular cavities containing aggregates of the smaller cell type (Figure 12.3). Mitoses are usually rare. A well-developed cellular fibrovascular stroma is present. There may be a pseudocapsule formed by compressed surrounding tissues,

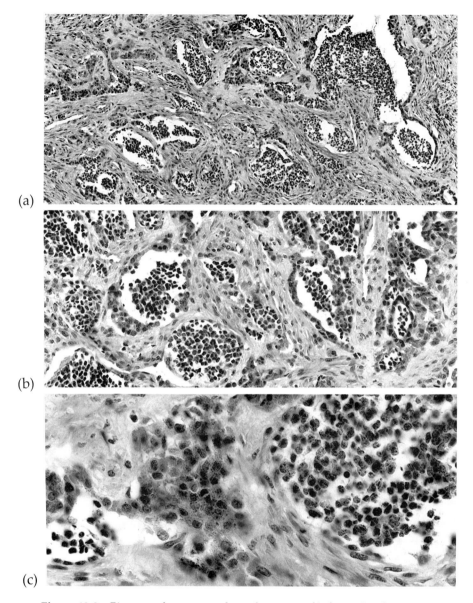

Figure 12.3 Pigmented neuroectodermal tumour of infancy ('melanotic progonoma'). (a) Irregular groups and strands of partly pigmented epithelial cells are seen within a fibrous stroma, and line irregular spaces partly filled with smaller, round cells (HE, × 90). (b) The smaller cell type is located mainly within irregular lumina lined by the larger epithelial cells (HE, × 185). (c) The larger, epithelial cells (left) contrast with the smaller round cells (right) (HE, × 370).

but more often, the borders of the tumour are irregular and indistinct.

The diagnosis is based on the identification of the two cell types, and the demonstration of melanin, which may, however, occasionally also be present in a variety of rare neurogenic (p. 387) and odontogenic (p. 385) tumours occurring at the same site. Immunohistochemically, both cell types are positive for NSE and vimentin and negative for S-100; ultrastructurally, the smaller cell type contains dense core granules and sometimes neurite-like cellular processes. The large cell type is positive with various antikeratin antibodies, and contains tonofibrils as well as melanosomes in different stages of development (Stirling *et al.*, 1988; Scheck *et al.*, 1989).

Cases occurring in sites other than the head are very rare indeed; recorded primary sites include the epididymis, subcutis of thorax, posterior mediastinum, thigh, femur and foot (Young and Gonzalez-Crussi, 1985). In these instances, misdiagnosis is a very significant danger: cases may be misinterpreted as rhabdomyosarcoma, neuroblastoma, olfactory neuroblastoma and ganglioneuroblastoma, leading to mutilating surgery or unnecessary radiotherapy and chemotherapy. Peripheral neuroepithelioma may also enter the differential diagnosis in some cases. As with cases occurring in the jaws, the diagnosis is based on the recognition of the two distinct cell types in a characteristic arrangement, perhaps with the help of immunostaining and ultrastructure as described by Stirling and associates (1988).

The main features of this tumour are summarized in Table 12.4.

Table 12.4 Pigmented neuroectodermal tumour of infancy

Clinical features
    Almost all occur in first year of life
    Over 80% occur in the jaws, usually the maxilla
    Firm swelling, sometimes with ulceration of mucosa
    Involvement of bone, irregular spread, sometimes apparently multifocal

Pathological features
    Two cell types: small, immature-appearing cells and larger, melanin-
      containing epithelial cells
    Larger cells form ribbons and alveolar structures enveloping aggregates of
      the smaller cell type
    Fibrous stroma

Remarks
    Local recurrence after incomplete removal; radical surgery constitutes
      definitive treatment
    A few metastasize: no clinical or histological features adequately distinguish
      between benign and malignant tumours

12.10   Pigmented tumours of the genital tract

Teratomas of the ovary and testis may contain melanocytes within cutaneous tissues or pigment epithelium in ocular tissues formed by the tumour (Luse and Vietti, 1968). Melanocyte colonization of an ovarian adenocarcinoma arising in an ovarian mature cystic teratoma was described by Waxman and colleagues (1986).

Three intriguing malignant tumours, two of the uterine corpus and one of the ovary, arising in adult women, have been reported which histologically somewhat resembled pigmented neuroectodermal tumour of infancy: possibly, these tumours represented variants of malignant teratoma or even of mixed müllerian tumour (Schultz, 1957; Hausman and Roitman, 1962; Hameed and Burslem, 1970).

Two partly melanotic tumours within the myometrium were described by Tavassoli (1986): they consisted of large, rounded or polyhedral S-100-negative cells, arranged in compact nests separated by fibrous septa and smooth muscle tissue. The architecture resembled that of paraganglioma; however, part of the cells synthesized melanin. Ultrastructurally, melanin synthesis was evident, and rare dense-core neuroendocrine-like secretory granules were also present.

As mentioned in the previous section, pigmented neuroectodermal tumour of infancy has been described in the epididymis (Frank and Koten, 1967; Zone, 1970). The histological features are identical to those cases located in the jaws.

References

Assor, D. (1975) A melanocytic tumor of the esophagus. *Cancer*, **35**, 1438–43.

Bird, C. C. and Willis, R. A. (1969) The histogenesis of pigmented neurofibromas. *J. Pathol.*, **97**, 631–7.

Boesel, C. P. and Suhan, J. P. (1979) A pigmented choroid plexus carcinoma: histochemical and ultrastructural studies. *J. Neuropathol. Exp. Neurol.*, **38**, 177–86.

Boesel, C. P., Suhan, J. P. and Sayers, M. P. (1978) Melanotic medulloblastoma. Report of a case with ultrastructural findings. *J. Neuropathol. Exp. Neurol.*, **37**, 531–43.

Borello, E. D. and Gorlin, R. J. (1966) Melanotic neuroectodermal tumor of infancy — a neoplasm of neural crest origin. *Cancer*, **19**, 196–206.

Brannon, R. B. (1977) The odontogenic keratocysts: a clinicopathologic study of 132 cases. Part 2. Histologic features. *Oral Surg.*, **43**, 233–55.

Burns, D. K., Silva, F. G., Forde, K. A., Mount, P. M. and Clark, H. B. (1983) Primary melanocytic Schwannoma of the stomach. Evidence of dual melanocytic and Schwannian differentiation in an extraaxial site in a patient without neurofibromatosis. *Cancer*, **52**, 1432–41.

Carney, J. A. (1990) Psammomatous melanotic schwannoma: a distinctive, heritable tumor with special associations, including cardiac myxoma and the Cushing syndrome. *Am. J. Surg. Pathol.*, **14**, 206–22.

Cebelin, M. S. (1980) Melanocytic bronchial carcinoid tumor. *Cancer*, **46**, 1843–8.

Clarke, B. E. and Parsons, H. (1951) An embryological tumor of retinal anlage involving the skull. *Cancer*, **4**, 78–85.

Curtis, J. L. and Rubinstein, L. J. (1982) Pigmented olfactory neuroblastoma. A new example of melanotic neuroepithelial neoplasm. *Cancer*, **49**, 2136–43.

Cutler, L. S., Chaudry, A. P. and Topazian, R. (1981) Melanotic neuroectodermal tumor of infancy: an ultrastructural study, literature review, and reevaluation. *Cancer*, **48**, 257–70.

De Pascalis, C., Mastroiacovo, P. and Mastrangelo, R. (1977) A melanotic neuroectodermal tumor of infancy arising from the anterior fontanel. *Tumori*, **63**, 373–80.

Dickersin, G. R. (1987) The electron microscopic spectrum of nerve sheath tumors. *Ultrastruct. Pathol.*, **11**, 103–46.

Dooling, E. C., Chi, J. G. and Gilles, F. H. (1977) Melanotic neuroectodermal tumor of infancy. Its histological similarities to fetal pineal gland. *Cancer*, **39**, 1535–41.

Ducastelle, T., Ducastelle, C., Hemet, J., Lefort, J. and Borde, J. (1981) Schwannome mélanotique (neurilemmome pigmentée) *Ann. Pathol.*, **1**, 205–12.

Duckworth, R. and Seward, G. R. (1965) A melanotic ameloblastic odontoma. *Oral Surg.*, **19**, 73–85.

El-Labban, N. G. (1988) Melanin-forming Schwann cells in some oral mucosal lesions. *Histopathology*, **12**, 301–6.

Font, R. L. and Truong, L. D. (1984) Melanotic Schwannoma of soft tissues. Electron-microscopic observations and review of literature. *Am. J. Surg. Pathol.*, **8**, 129–38.

Font, R. L., Zimmerman, L. E. and Fine, B. S. (1972) Adenoma of the retinal pigment epithelium. Histochemical and electron microscopic observations. *Am. J. Ophthalmol.*, **73**, 544–54.

Frank, G. L. and Koten, J. W. (1967) Melanotic hamartoma ('retinal anlage tumor') of the epididymis. *J. Pathol. Bacteriol.*, **93**, 549–54.

Fu, Y.-S., Kaye, G. I. and Lattes, R. (1975) Primary malignant melanocytic tumors of the sympathetic ganglia, with an ultrastructural study of one. *Cancer*, **36**, 2029–41.

Garner, A. (1970) Tumors of the retinal pigment epithelium. *Br. J. Ophthalmol.*, **73**, 715–23.

Gelfland, E. T., Taylor, R. F., Roa, S., Hendin, D., Akabutu, J. and Callaghan, J. C. (1977) Melanotic Schwannoma of the right atrium. *J. Thorac. Cardiovasc. Surg.*, **74**, 808–12.

Gonzalez-Crussi, F. and Hsueh, W. (1988) Bilateral adrenal ganglioneuroblastoma with neuromelanin. Clinical and pathologic observations. *Cancer*, **61**, 1159–66.

Goode, R. K., Crawford, B. E., Callihan, M. D. and Neville, B. W. (1983) Oral melanoacanthoma. Review of the literature and report of ten cases. *Oral Surg. Oral Med. Oral Pathol.*, **56**, 622–8.

Gould, V. E., Memoli, V. A., Dardi, L. E., Sobel., H. J., Somers, S. C. and Johannessen, J. V. (1981) Neuroendocrine carcinomas with multiple immunoreactive peptides and melanin production. *Ultrastruct. Pathol.*, **2**, 199–217.

Grazer, R., Cohen, S. M., Jacobs, J. B. and Lucas, P. (1982) Melanin-containing peripheral carcinoid of the lung. *Am. J. Surg. Pathol.*, **6**, 73–8.

Hahn, J. F., Netsky, M. G., Butler, A. B. and Sperber, E. E. (1976) Pigmented ganglioneuroblastoma: relation of melanin and lipofuscin to schwannomas and other tumors of neural crest origin. *J. Neuropathol. Exp. Neurol.*, **35**, 393–403.

Halpert, B. and Patzer, R. (1947) Maxillary tumor of the retinal anlage. *Surgery*, **22**, 837–41.

Hameed, K. and Burslem, M. R. (1970) A melanotic ovarian neoplasm resembling the 'retinal anlage' tumor. *Cancer*, **25**, 564–7.

Hausman, D. H. and Roitman, H. B. (1962) A malignant melanotic tumor of the uterus. *Bull. Ayer Clin. Lab.*, **4**, 79–87.

Herrera, G. A. (1987) Light microscopic, S-100 immunostaining and ultra-structural analysis of dermatopathic lymphadenopathy, with and without associated mycosis fungoides. *Am. J. Clin. Pathol.*, **87**, 187–95.

Herrick, M. K. and Rubinstein, L. J. (1979) The cytological differentiating potential of pineal parenchymal neoplasms (true pinealomas). A clinico-pathological study of 28 tumours. *Brain*, **102**, 289–320.

Ho, F. C. S. and Ho, J. C. I. (1977) Pigmented carcinoid tumour of the thymus. *Histopathology*, **1**, 363–9.

Hodson, J. J. (1961) An intra-osseous tumor combination of biological importance — invasion of melanotic Schwannoma by an adamantinoma. *J. Pathol. Bacteriol.*, **82**, 257–66.

Horlick, H. P., Walther, R. R., Zegarelli, D. J., Silvers, D. N. and Eliezri, Y. D. (1988) Mucosal melanotic macule, reactive type: a simulation of melanoma. *J. Am. Acad. Dermatol.*, **19**, 786–91.

Hunt, S. J. and Johnson, P. C. (1989) Melanotic ganglioglioma of the pineal region. *Acta Neuropathol.*, **79**, 222–5.

Janzer, R. C. and Makek, M. (1983) Intraoral malignant melanotic Schwannoma. Ultrastructural evidence for melanogenesis by Schwann's cells. *Arch. Pathol. Lab. Med.*, **107**, 298–301.

Jauregui, H. O. and Klintworth, G. K. (1976) Pigmented squamous cell carcinoma of cornea and conjunctiva. A light microscopic, histochemical, and ultrastructural study. *Cancer*, **38**, 778–88.

Jimenez, C. L., Carpenter, B. F. and Robb, I. A. (1987) Melanotic cerebellar tumor. *Ultrastruct. Pathol.*, **11**, 751–9.

Jurecka, W., Mainitz, M., Metze, D., Gebhart, W., Bruck, H. G. and Kofler, K. (1987) Pigmented neurofibroma. *Am. J. Dermatopathol.*, **9**, 175–6.

Kayano, H. and Katayama, I. (1988) Melanotic schwannoma arising in the sympathetic ganglion. *Hum. Pathol.*, **19**, 1355–8.

Keegan, H. R. and Mullan, S. (1962) Pigmented meningiomas: an unusual variant. Report of a case with review of the literature. *J. Neurosurg.*, **19**, 696–8.

Killeen, R. A., Davy, C. L. and Bauserman, S. C. (1988) Melanocytic schwannoma. *Cancer*, **62**, 174–83.

Krausz, T., Azzopardi, J. G. and Pearse, E. (1984) Malignant melanoma of the sympathetic chain: with a consideration of pigmented nerve sheath tumours. *Histopathology*, **8**, 881–94.

Krompecher, E. (1918) Zur Histogenese und Morphologie der Adamantinome und sonstiger Kiefergeschwülste. *Beitr. Pathol.*, **64**, 165–97.

Lagrange, W., Dahm, H.-H., Karstens, J., Feichtinger, J. and Mittermayer, C. (1987) Melanocytic neuroendocrine carcinoma of the thymus. *Cancer*, **59**, 484–8.

Landas, S. K., Schelper, R. L., Fermin, O. T., Turner, J. W., Moore, K. C. and Bennett-Gray, J. (1986) Black thyroid syndrome: exaggeration of a normal process? *Am. J. Clin. Pathol.*, **85**, 411–8.

Lesoin, F., Leys, D., Verier, A., Krivosic, I., Vaneecloo, F. M. and Jomin, M. (1983) Les tumeurs mélanotiques primitives du système nerveux central. A propos d'une observation de méningiome mélanocytique de l'angle ponto-cérébelleux. *Rev. Otoneuro-ophthalmol.*, **55**, 443–8.

Llombart-Bosch, A., Carda, C., Peydro-Olaya, A., Noguera, R., Boix, J. and Pellin, A. (1989) Pigmented esthesioneuroblastoma showing dual differentiation following transplantation in nude mice. An immunohistochemical, electron microscopical, and cytogenetic analysis. *Virchows Arch. A. (Pathol. Anat.)*, **414**, 199–208.

Luse, S. A. and Vietti, T. (1968) Ovarian teratoma. Ultrastructure and neural component. *Cancer*, **21**, 38–52.

Marcus, J. N., Dise, C. A. and LiVolsi, V. A. (1982) Melanin production in a medullary thyroid carcinoma. *Cancer,* **49**, 2518–26.

Markert, C. L. and Silvers, W. K. (1956) The effects of genotype and cell environment on melanoblast differentiation in the house mouse. *Genetics*, **41**, 429–50.

Matsuoka, L. Y., Glasser, S. and Barsky, S. (1979) Melanoacanthoma of the lip. *Arch. Dermatol.*, **115**, 1116–7.

McCloskey, J. J., Parker, J. C., Brooks, W. H. and Blacker, H. M. (1976) Melanin as a component of cerebral gliomas. The melanotic cerebral ependymoma. *Cancer*, **37**, 2373–9.

Mennemeyer, R. P., Hammar, S. P., Tytus, J. S., Hallman, K. O., Raisis, J. E. and Bockus, D. (1979) Melanotic schwannoma. Clinical and ultrastructural studies of three cases with evidence of intracellular melanin synthesis. *Am. J. Surg. Pathol.*, **3**, 3–10.

Miettinen, M. (1987) Melanotic Schwannoma: coexpression of vimentin and glial fibrillary acidic protein. *Ultrastruct. Pathol.*, **11**, 39–46.

Modica, L. A., Youngberg, G. A. and Avila, F. O. (1990) Melanocyte colonization of an oral carcinoma. *Histopathology*, **17**, 477–8.

Mullins, J. D. (1980) A pigmented differentiating neuroblastoma. A light and ultrastructural study. *Cancer*, **46**, 522–8.

Navas Palacios, J. J. (1980) Malignant melanotic neuroectodermal tumor. Light and electron microscopic study. *Cancer*, **46**, 529–36.

Ramahefasolo, S., Coscas, G., Regenbogen, L. and Godel, V. (1987) Adenocarcinoma of retinal pigment epithelium. *Br. J. Ophthalmol.*, **71**, 516–20.

Rosenblum,, M. K., Erlandson, R. A., Aleksic, S. N. and Budzilovich, G. N. (1990) Melanotic ependymoma and subependymoma. *Am. J. Surg. Pathol.*, **14**, 729–36.

Rowlands, D., Edwards, C. and Collins, F. (1987) Malignant melanotic schwannoma of the bronchus. *J. Clin. Pathol.*, **40**, 1449–55.

Salisbury, J. A., Szpak, C. A. and Klintworth, G. K. (1983) Pigmented squamous cell carcinoma of the conjunctiva. A clinicopathologic ultrastructural study. *Ophthalmology*, **90**, 1477–81.

Scheck, O., Ruck, P., Harms, D. and Kaiserling, E. (1989) Melanotic neuroectodermal tumor of infancy occurring in the left thigh of a 6-month-old female infant. *Ultrastruct. Pathol.*, **13**, 23–33.

Schultz, D. (1957) A malignant melanotic neoplasm of the uterus resembling the retinal anlage tumor. *Am. J. Clin. Pathol.*, **28**, 524–32.

Sexton, F. M. and Maize, J. C. (1987) Melanotic macules and melanoacanthomas of the lip. A comparative study with census of the basal melanocyte
population. *Am. J. Dermatopathol.*, **9**, 438–44.

Shokry, A., Briner, J. and Marek, M. (1986) Malignant melanotic neuroectodermal tumor of infancy: a case report. *Pediatr. Pathol.*, **5**, 217–23.

Soames, J. V. (1982) A pigmented calcifying odontogenic cyst. *Oral Surg.*, **52**,
395–400.

Solomon, R. A., Handler, M. S., Sedelli, R. V. and Stein, B. M. (1987)
Intramedullary melanotic Schwannoma of the cervicomedullary junction.
Neurosurgery, **20**, 36–8.

Spann, C. R., Owen, L. G. and Hodge, S. J. (1987) The labial melanotic
macule. *Arch. Dermatol.*, **123**, 1029–31.

Spence, A. M., Rubinstein L. J., Conley F. K. and Herman, M. M. (1976)
Studies on experimental malignant nerve sheath tumors maintained in tissue
and organ culture systems. III. Melanin pigment and melanogenesis in
experimental neurogenic tumors: a reappraisal of the histogenesis of
pigmented nerve sheath tumors. *Acta Neuropathol.*, **35**, 27–45.

Stirling, R. W., Powell, G. and Fletcher, C. D. M. (1988) Pigmented neuroectodermal tumour of infancy: an immunohistochemical study. *Histopathology*,
12, 425–35.

Stowens, D. (1957) A pigmented tumor of infancy: the melanotic progonoma. *J.
Pathol. Bacteriol.*, **73**, 43–51.

Szpak, C. A., Shelburne, J., Linder, J. and Klintworth, G. K. (1988) The
presence of stage II melanosomes (premelanosomes) in neoplasms other
than melanomas. *Modern Pathol.*, **1**, 35–43.

Takeda, Y. (1989) Pigmented adenomatoid odontogenic tumour. Report of an
undescribed case and review of the literature of pigmented intraosseous
odontogenic tumours. *Virchows Arch. A (Pathol. Anat.)*, **415**, 571–5.

Takeda, Y., Suzuki, M., Kuroda, M. and Yamazaki, Y. (1987) Melanin-pigment
in complex odontoma. *Int. J. Oral Maxillofac. Surg.*, **16**, 222–6.

Takeda, Y., Suzuki, A., Kuroda, M., Itagaki, M. and Shimono, M. (1988)
Pigmented ameloblastic fibro-odontoma: detection of melanin pigment in
enamel. *Bull. Tokyo Dent. Coll.*, **29**, 119–23.

Takeda, Y., Kudora, M. and Suzuki, A. (1989) Melanocytes in odontoameloblastoma. A case report. *Acta Pathol. Jap.*, **39**, 465–8.

Tavassoli, F. A. (1986) Melanotic paraganglioma of the uterus. *Cancer*, **58**,
942–8.

Thomas, K. M., Hutt, M. S. R. and Borgstein, J. (1980) Salivary gland tumors
in Malawi. *Cancer*, **46**, 2328–34.

Ts'o, M. O. M. and Albert, D. M. (1972) Pathological condition of the retinal
pigment epithelium. Neoplasms and nodular non-neoplastic lesions. *Arch.
Ophthalmol.*, **88**, 27–38.

Turnbull, H. R. and Tom, M. I. (1963) Pigmented meningioma. *J. Neurosurg.*,
20, 76–80.

Waxman, M., Vuletin, J. C., Rosenblatt, P. and Herzberg, F. P. (1986)
Melanocyte colonization of adenocarcinoma arising in an ovarian dermoid.
Histopathology, **10**, 207–15.

Webb, J. N. (1982) The ultrastructure of a melanotic Schwannoma of the skin.
J. Pathol., **137**, 25–36.

Young, S. and Gonzalez-Crussi, F. (1985) Melanocytic neuroectodermal tumor
of the foot. Report of a case with multicentric origin. *Am. J. Clin. Pathol.*, **84**,
371–8.

Zemtsov, A. and Bergfeld, W. F. (1989) Oral melanoacanthoma with prominent spongiotic intraepithelial vesicles. *J. Cutan. Pathol.*, **16**, 365–9.

Zone, R. M. (1970) Retinal anlage tumor of the epididymis. A case report. *J. Urol.*, **103**, 106–7.

13 Cytological diagnosis of melanoma

In the past two decades it has been clearly established that melanoma can be identified confidently in cytological specimens and that *especially for the recognition of metastatic disease, fine needle aspirates (FNA) are of great practical value.* In the past, FNA diagnosis of primary cutaneous melanocytic lesions has been advocated, for example by Woyke and co-workers (1980), who used FNA for preoperative diagnosis of cutaneous melanoma, enabling the surgeon to excise the tumour with a wide margin in the first instance. However, as we have discussed in the previous chapters, architectural features are of paramount importance in the microscopic diagnosis of primary cutaneous melanocytic lesions. Therefore, the definitive diagnosis of primary lesions should be based on histology.

The accuracy of FNA in the detection of melanoma metastases of various sites (skin, subcutis, lymph node, lung, liver, kidney, vagina, cervix, endometrium, bone, brain and eye) is impressive, as witnessed, for instance, by the large series of Perry and colleagues (1986b) in which FNA findings were correlated with either subsequent histology or with clinical follow up. Prior to the advent of FNA, a surgical biopsy for histology was necessary to detect metastases. FNA may be applied to sites not easily accessible for excisional biopsy, such as the eye (Czerniak *et al.*, 1983; Folberg *et al.*, 1985; Char *et al.*, 1989; Scroggs *et al.*, 1990). Malignant melanoma of soft parts (clear cell sarcoma) diagnosed on FNA was reported recently by Schwartz and Zollars (1990).

Shafir and colleagues (1983) advocated the use of imprint cytology as an adjunct to frozen sections in the intraoperative diagnosis of primary melanoma. However, we do not favour operative frozen section diagnosis of primary melanoma, for reasons discussed elsewhere (p. 21).

There are several reports of the cytological findings on melanoma in genital smears (Ehrmann *et al.*, 1962; Linthicum, 1971; Lewis and Chapman, 1975; Masubuchi *et al.*, 1975; Sagebiel *et al.*, 1978; Takeda *et al.*, 1978; Yu and Ketabchi, 1987; Nagy *et al.*, 1990), oral cavity scrapings (Medak *et al.*, 1969), oesophageal washings and brushings (Johnson *et al.*, 1955; Broderick *et al.*, 1972; Aldovini *et al.*, 1983), sputum (Yamada *et al.*, 1972; Hajdu and Savino, 1973), serous fluids (Yamada *et al.*, 1972; Hajdu and Savino, 1973; Angeli *et al.*, 1988; Keller *et al.*, 1990) and urinary sediment (Piva and Koss, 1964; Woodard *et al.*, 1978; Valente *et al.*, 1985).

While cytology clearly has a role in the diagnosis of metastatic melanoma, it should be pointed out that, since primary melanocytic lesions are not suitable for FNA diagnosis, very little is known about the cytology of benign melanocytic lesions. In this chapter, the cyto-logical features of melanoma are discussed.

13.1 Methods

13.1.1 Conventional staining techniques

The cytological diagnosis of melanoma can be achieved on either *Papanicolaou-* or *Romanowsky*-stained specimens, independently of whether direct smears, imprints or cytocentrifuge preparations are used. Other stains such as haematoxylin and eosin (HE) are also applicable. Pathologists differ in their preference; the distribution and the details of the nuclear chromatin are crisper in Papanicolaou-stained specimens, while intra- and extracellular pigments and metachromatically staining substances such as mucin are much more obvious when the Romanowsky method is used. A Papanicolaou stain of high quality requires prompt fixation of the specimen before any air-drying occurs. Conversely, to achieve optimal results on smears stained by a Romanowsky technique such as May-Grünwald-Giemsa, rapid drying is crucial.

13.1.2 Cytochemical methods for identification of melanin

In the diagnosis of melanoma, the correct identification of the intra- or extracellular melanin is important.

Since other pigments, most commonly haemosiderin, lipofuscin, ceroid, neuromelanin and rarely argentaffin pigment, can be mistaken for melanin, confirmatory stains are commonly used (Pearse, 1985). The *Masson-Fontana* and *Schmorl stains* can be used on both air-dried and alcohol-fixed cytological specimens (Plate 1). Wilander *et al.* (1985) showed that in cytological specimens melanin displays a positive Masson's argentaffin reaction, irrespective of the fixation used (air drying, formalin, Bouin's fluid, acetone-alcohol). Interestingly, formalin fixation of the cytological specimen was a prerequisite for the demonstration of argentaffinity of serotonin-containing small intestinal carcinoids. Therefore, Masson's argentaffin stain can be used in conjunction with different fixatives to discriminate melanin from serotonin-containing granules. Masson-Fontana and Schmorl stains are not entirely specific for melanin as they stain chromolipids and neuromelanin as well (Wolman, 1980; Pearse, 1985). The latter two pigments can be differentiated from melanin by their positivity with Sudan black and oil-red-O stain, and their yellow or orange auto-fluorescence on UV illumination. Sudan black staining and auto-fluorescence can be best demonstrated after bleaching the melanin moiety (Wolman, 1980). It is prudent to use Perls' prussian blue reaction for haemosiderin, in parallel with melanin stains.

Melanin can be removed by *bleaching techniques*, in contrast to lipofuscin and haemosiderin, which are resistant to bleaching. It is especially useful in heavily pigmented specimens, to confirm that the pigment is melanin, and to reveal the cytological details of the heavily melanized cells (Lefer and Johnston, 1972).

The *DOPA oxidase technique* is useful for the detection of traces of melanin synthesis in hypo- or amelanotic melanomas. Curiously, granules of mast cells also stain by this technique; however, their metachromatic characteristics differentiate them from melanin.

The pigment in ochronosis is similar to melanin and gives the same histochemical reactions, but it emits yellow autofluorescence (Pearse, 1985).

13.1.3 *Use of immunocytochemistry in the cytological diagnosis of malignant melanoma*

Immunocytochemistry can be a valuable adjunct in difficult cases, but its use must be selective. A panel of antibodies to give complementary data should be applied in order to minimize the chance of error, and the results should be evaluated together with the cytological features and the clinical data (Shoup *et al.*, 1990). Positive and negative controls should be used in all instances.

The number of spare slides required for immunocytochemistry depends on the differential diagnostic problem and the cellularity of the sample. In case of a malignant effusion, the preparation of additional slides is usually not a problem, but the number of spare smears of an FNA is usually small. This limitation can be partially circumvented by using cytocentrifuge preparations from needle washings or by partitioning smears on to separate glass slides by applying Diatex compound (American Scientific Products, Edison, New Jersey; Chess and Hajdu, 1986; Lozowski and Hajdu, 1987). Immunocytochemical staining can also be performed on smears previously stained by the Papanicolaou method (Travis and Wold, 1987). Decolourization of the stained smear is inadvisable as this is brought about also by the immunocytochemical procedure, and it may have a deleterious effect on antigen preservation. Recently, Domagala *et al.* (1990) and Kung *et al.* (1990) reviewed the application of immunocytochemical techniques to cell block preparations from fine needle aspirates.

The use of poly-L-lysine coated slides is recommended for immuno-staining in order to ensure good adherence of the cells to the slide.

For the demonstration of most antigens, the indirect immuno-peroxidase, the alkaline phosphatase antialkaline phosphatase and the avidin-biotin complex techniques are most commonly used.

In smears containing a mixed population of cells, it is vital to differentiate between positive staining of the 'target' cells and the background population. Degenerate cells may produce aberrant staining patterns, a problem encountered by the histologist also. Furthermore, inadequate blocking of endogenous peroxidase can lead to false-positive staining. Rarely, phagocytosis by malignant cells can lead to aberrant staining.

The differential diagnosis of anaplastic malignant tumours usually includes amelanotic melanoma, undifferentiated carcinoma and malignant lymphoma. In such instances, the primary panel should include antibodies to *S-100 protein, vimentin, cytokeratins, and common leukocyte antigen.*

Melanoma is usually positive for *S-100 protein,* which is localized in the cytoplasm as well as in the nucleus. It is important to note that S-100 protein may be present in a large variety of epithelial and mesenchymal neoplasms (p. 291). *Melanoma specific antibody (HMB-45)* is considerably more specific but less sensitive than S-100 (Gown *et al.,* 1986; Hachisuka *et al.,* 1986; Drier *et al.,* 1987; Duray *et al.,* 1988; Ordonez *et al.,* 1988; Walts *et al.,* 1988). However, sweat glands, breast lobules and ducts, a few breast carcinomas, peripheral nerve sheath tumours, and neuroectodermal tumours of infancy, have been reported positive with HMB-45 (Bonetti *et al.,* 1989; Pelosi *et al.,* 1990). Further assessment of this antibody is desirable. Antibodies against *neuron specific enolase (NSE),* and *protein gene product 9.5 (PGP 9.5)* can also be used.

Melanoma is vimentin positive and generally cytokeratin negative, but low molecular weight cytokeratins can be detected in a minority of cases (Gatter *et al.,* 1985; Zarbo *et al.,* 1990). It is important to bear in mind that some 'noncarcinomas' may express cytokeratin (epithelioid sarcoma, synovial sarcoma, mesothelioma, leiomyosarcoma and rarely rhabdomyosarcoma, especially the alveolar variant, and chondrosarcoma). It is therefore advisable to include an antibody to *epithelial membrane antigen (EMA)* in the panel; EMA is almost always negative in melanomas, but it is positive in a large majority of epithelial tumours and mesotheliomas, as well as in some mesenchymal tumours, plasmacytomas, T-cell lymphomas and Ki-1 lymphomas (Pinkus and Kurtin, 1985).

Common leucocyte antigen (CD 45) is negative in melanoma. It is present on the cell surface in the majority of non-Hodgkin's lymphomas, and is a rather specific marker for lymphoid cells; however, some large cell lymphomas are negative. Some of these CD 45-negative lymphomas are positive for Ki-1 antigen recognized by Ber-H2 antibody.

The final result, the successful cytological diagnosis of melanoma, depends not only on the technical preparation and staining, but on the cellularity and quality of the sample and on the skill of the pathologist, who should always take the clinical and morphological data into consideration.

13.2   Microscopic features: general remarks

Most of the following morphological discussion of melanoma is based on FNA material; however, the cytological features described are also applicable to imprints, scrapings, brush specimens, or spontaneously exfoliated cells in fluids, sputum, vaginal smears or other cytological preparations. The wide morphological spectrum displayed by melanoma overlaps with several other neoplasms, which may make the diagnosis difficult or impossible in the absence of appropriate clinical information. However, despite the high variability of the cytological findings, the diagnosis of melanoma can usually be achieved on the basis of features commonly associated with this neoplasm (Hajdu and Savino, 1973; Friedman *et al.*, 1980; Woyke *et al.*, 1980, Kline and Kannan, 1982; Gupta *et al.*, 1985; Perry *et al.*, 1986a,b; Layfield and Ostrzega, 1989).

Generally FNA of melanoma are highly cellular. As in histological specimens, *epithelioid* and *spindle cell* types can be recognized and frequently occur in combination, resulting in the so-called *mixed-cell* type. Woyke *et al.* (1980) recognized two further types: smears with predominance of giant cells and smears with predominance of small, round cells. Since both giant cells and small round melanoma cells occur rather frequently in epithelioid malignant melanoma, these two additional types can be regarded as variants of the latter group (Table 13.1).

When considering a diagnosis of melanoma, pathologists usually look for *melanin pigment* as the most convincing morphological

Table 13.1 Cell types in malignant melanoma

Epithelioid cells
    Round, oval or polygonal cells with moderate to abundant cytoplasm and
        eccentric, round nuclei
    Small, round cells
        May be confused with plasmacytoma and lymphoma
        Usually intermixed with large epithelioid cells
    Binucleate cells
        Various sizes, intermixed with other cell types
    Giant cells
        Mononuclear, multilobated or multinucleated forms with abundant
        cytoplasm, polygonal or bizarre shapes
        Usually intermixed with other cell types

Spindle cells
    Bipolar or dendritic cells with long, thin cytoplasmic processes and
        centrally placed elongated or ovoid nucleus
    Occur in isolation or together with other cell types

evidence of melanocytic differentiation. However, in most cases, only a small number of cells contain pigment and as many as 25–60% of cytological specimens of melanoma are amelanotic (Friedman *et al.*, 1980; Woyke *et al.*, 1980; Perry *et al.*, 1986a; Layfield and Ostrzega, 1989). In contrast, in some cases there is a very marked degree of pigmentation, to an extent where the cytological morphology is obscured by the pigment (Plate 2). In such cases, bleaching is necessary in order to see whether the heavily pigmented cells are melanophages or tumour cells. Aspirates from large, necrotic metastases often contain cell debris and free background pigment without recognizable tumour cells. In such a situation one can make a presumptive diagnosis of a melanocytic tumour. As haemorrhage and necrosis may result in the deposition of haemosiderin, it is strongly advisable to carry out stains for iron as well as melanin.

    Melanin in melanocytes often appears finely granular or dusty, contrasting with the irregular and clumped melanin granules seen in melanophages (Plate 3). However, the different appearance of intracytoplasmic melanin is not always discriminatory between melanocytes and melanophages, as coarse and irregular melanin granules may also be observed in melanocytes. The colour of melanin differs according to the stain: it is light to dark brown or brownish-yellow in Papanicolaou and HE stains, but varying shades of blue and/or green in May-Grünwald-Giemsa stains (Plates 2 and 3).

Table 13.2 Cytological features of FNA of epithelioid-cell melanoma

General features
  Highly cellular smear
  Noncohesive, dispersed cell pattern
  Anisocytosis of round or polygonal cells
  'Triphasic-sized' cell population frequent

Cytoplasmic features
  Moderate to abundant cytoplasm
  Dusty or finely granular melanin; rarely coarsely granular or clumped
    melanin
  Amelanotic in 25–60%
  Homogeneous, granular or vacuolated cytoplasm
  Microvacuolization common; extreme degree: balloon cell melanoma
  Large solitary cytoplasmic vacuole; usually seen in few cells; many cells
    affected: signet-ring cell melanoma

Nuclear features
  Eccentric nucleus
  Round nucleus with smooth, regular outline
  Evenly distributed chromatin; finely granular on Papanicolaou,
    homogeneous or reticulated on Giemsa
  Intranuclear cytoplasmic inclusions
  Prominent nucleoli; macronucleoli in 56%
  Binucleate cells frequently present
  Cells with multilobed nuclei and/or multinucleated cells variably present

13.3   Epithelioid-cell melanoma

This commonest type of melanoma is characterized cytologically by a *predominant population of round, oval or polygonal epithelioid tumour cells with eccentric nuclei* (Table 13.2).

A *dispersed cell pattern* due to lack of cohesion between melanoma cells is a constant and diagnostically important feature (Plate 4). In FNA a minority of cells may form loose sheets or clusters, but these lack the mosaic pattern or intercellular bridges seen in some carcinomas.

Anisocytosis, due to striking variability of cell size combined with a variable number of mono-, bi- or multinucleated giant cells, is a characteristic feature (Plate 5). Kline and Kannan (1982) recognized a so-called 'triphasic-sized' cell population in 50% of epithelioid melanomas: on Papanicolaou-stained specimens (alcohol-fixed) the majority of cells measured between 10 and 20 μm, but, smaller cells between 4 and 9 μm and giant cells between 20 and 50 μm were also present. On air-dried smears, the range of tumour cells varies between 10 and 300 μm (Hajdu and Savino, 1973).

In some specimens, anisocytosis is less conspicuous and the cells

Plate 1 Masson-Fontana stain in the identification of melanin. Black silver granules corresponding to melanin are present in the cytoplasm of several cells (Masson-Fontana, x 480).

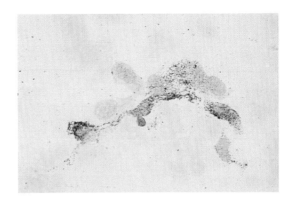

Plate 2 Heavily pigmented melanoma. Cytological details are obscured by brownish-yellow melanin. (Papanicolaou, x 300).

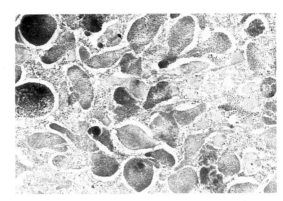

Plate 3 Fine dusty melanin in the cytoplasm of epithelioid melanoma cells, contrasting with coarsely granular pigment in macrophages. The colour of the melanin varies from light to dark blue or greenish (Giemsa, x 300).

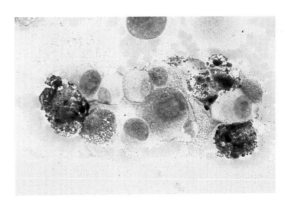

Plate 4 Typical noncohesive pattern of melanoma. Round or polygonal cells with eccentric nuclei are typical of epithelioid cell melanoma (Papanicolaou, x 200).

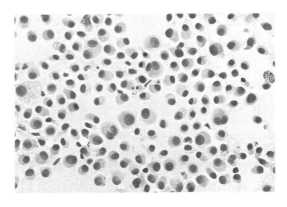

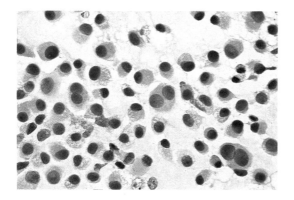

Plate 5 Amelanotic epithelioid melanoma. Anisocytosis and binucleation without significant nuclear pleomorphism are common features. Nuclei are round, eccentrically positioned, with evenly dispersed, finely granular chromatin. The cytoplasm is homogenous or finely vacuolated (Papanicolaou, x 300).

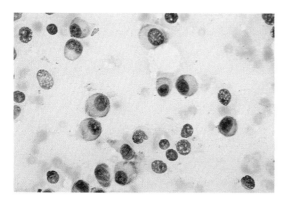

Plate 6 Amelanotic epithelioid melanoma of small round cell type. The cytological features of this melanoma type can be confused with those of plasmacytoma (Giemsa, x 300).

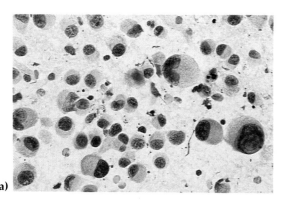

(a)

Plate 7 Epithelioid malignant melanoma. Giant cells mixed with smaller melanoma cells result in a pleomorphic picture.
(a) Papanicolaou, (x 300);
(b) Giemsa, (x 200).

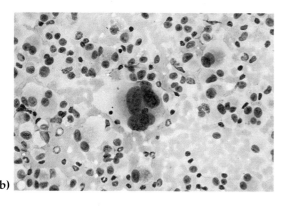

(b)

are smaller. Such *small round cell melanomas* can be confused with myeloma, mainly on the basis of cell size and eccentrically positioned nucleus (Plate 6). However, the evenly dispersed nuclear chromatin in melanoma cells clearly differs from that seen in plasmacytoma.

The other extreme, the so-called *pleomorphic variant*, contains a high proportion of giant tumour cells (Plate 7). This tumour type can be mistaken for anaplastic carcinoma or some kind of pleomorphic sarcoma (osteosarcoma, MFH, etc.). However, the non-giant cell population exhibits a surprisingly bland appearance of nuclei (see below), which is an important feature in this differential diagnostic problem. When melanin is present in such cases, the diagnosis is clear.

Giant melanoma cells may be up to 300 μm in May-Grünwald-Giemsa stained smears. Their nuclei are most commonly multilobated or the cells are multinucleated, containing up to 15 nuclei of various sizes. However, mononuclear variants also occur (Plate 14); intact nuclei and mitotic figures may occur together in the same cell. The frequent occurrence of giant cells in some smears results in a pleomorphic appearance.

Cannibalism, i.e. tumour cells enveloping other tumour cells, is occasionally observed (Plate 15) and was present in three cases out of 50 studied by Woyke and colleagues (1980).

Metastatic melanoma with prominent myxoid stroma (Bhuta et al., 1986) containing abundant, hyaluronidase-sensitive, myxoid matrix may cause considerable diagnostic confusion. The cytological features of such cases were described by Rocamora et al. (1988) and Lindholm and De la Torre (1988).

13.3.1 Cytoplasmic features

Epithelioid cell melanoma consists mainly of round, oval or polygonal cells with a well-defined cytoplasmic margin. There is a moderate to abundant amount of cytoplasm; in air-dried specimens, the ratio of cellular to nuclear diameter is 2:1 or greater (Layfield and Ostrzega, 1989). This ratio is smaller on alcohol-fixed, Papanicolaou-stained specimens. Pigmentation of the cytoplasm has already been discussed. The appearance of the cytoplasm is often variable, even in the same smear: it may be homogeneous or granular, micro- or macrovacuolated.

In Romanowsky-stained specimens, the cytoplasmic staining varies from deep blue to very pale (Plate 8); very faint cytoplasmic staining is often but not always due to microvacuolation of the cytoplasm. In smears stained by the Papanicolaou method, there is no obvious variability of the staining intensity between individual tumour cells.

Gupta and colleagues (1985) described the presence of multiple, well-defined, clear *microvacuoles* in the cytoplasm of many melanoma cells and similar nuclear vacuolation in some cells, which occurred in about 40% of melanoma aspirates. These vacuoles, of equal size, are prominent in May-Grünwald-Giemsa stained smears (Plate 9), but only faintly visible in Papanicolaou stained specimens. The vacuolization is probably related to abnormal melanogenesis (p. 92; Hashimoto and Bale, 1972); the cells with microvacuolization probably represent intermediate forms between the nonvacuolated cells and the hyper-vacuolated cells of balloon cell melanoma. We agree with Gupta and colleagues (1985) that cytoplasmic microvacuolation is a rather frequent finding in melanoma and share their surprise that this striking mor-phological feature has not received more attention in the literature. The presence of multiple small vacuoles in the nuclei of a few tumour cells could be the result of intranuclear cytoplasmic invagination (Sobel *et al.*, 1969). This type of intranuclear vacuolization is different mor-phologically from the much larger, single cytoplasmic intranuclear inclusion discussed below.

Hypervacuolated cells of *balloon cell melanoma* have been described in fine needle aspirates by Friedman and colleagues (1982). Balloon cells are larger than the microvacuolated intermediate cells described above, measuring from 50 to 100 μm in diameter. Their nuclei are often com-pressed against the cell membrane and have a scalloped appearance.

Occasionally, melanomas contain cells with a single, large, cyto-plasmic vacuole, which replaces a large part of the cytoplasm, resulting in a *signet-ring appearance*. Sometimes, several such large vacuoles can be observed in the cytoplasm (Plate 10). In our experience, a few isolated signet-ring cells are commonly present in melanoma. They were present in 51% of the 71 cases studied by Layfield and Ostrzega (1989). 'Signet-ring cell melanoma', a rare morphological variant of melanoma containing large numbers of such cells, has been described histologically (p. 282; Sheibani and Battifora, 1988). The content of these vacuoles needs elucidation.

In the cells of some melanomas, most of the cytoplasm, with the exception of a narrow peripheral rim, has a dense, homogeneous, ground-glass appearance, staining pale on Papanicolaou and deep blue on May-Grünwald-Giemsa. A *spherical inclusion-like cytoplasmic mass* may be formed, which consists of bundles of vimentin filaments, which may impinge on and distort the nucleus, giving it a crescentic shape.

13.3.2   Nuclear features

In the majority of epithelioid melanoma cells, independent of their size, the nuclei are eccentrically located, and are often in direct contact

Plate 8 Epithelioid amelanotic melanoma. Dispersed round to polygonal cells with a moderate amount of pale blue cytoplasm (Giemsa, x 300).

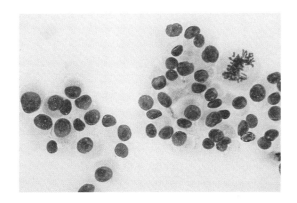

Plate 9 Epithelioid amelanotic melanoma.
(a) Microvesicular cytoplasmic vacuolization; when this change is pronounced and involves the whole of the cytoplasm, the term 'balloon cell' applies (Giemsa, x 480).
(b) Microvesicular vacuolization affecting the nucleus as well (Giemsa, x 770).

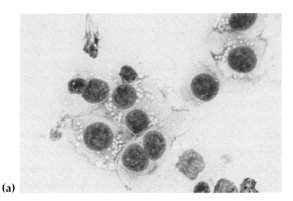

(a)

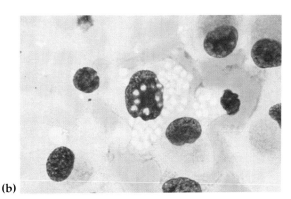

(b)

Plate 10 Epithelioid melanoma, macrovesicular cytoplasmic vacuolization (Giemsa, x 770).

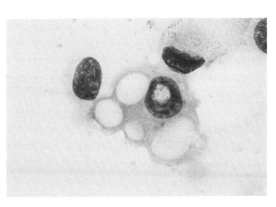

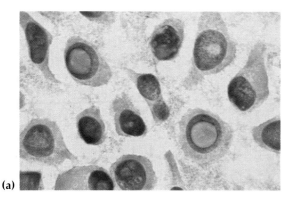

(a)

Plate 11 Epithelioid melanoma, intranuclear cytoplasmic inclusions are frequent.
(a) Papnicolaou, (x 770);
(b) Giemsa, (x 480).

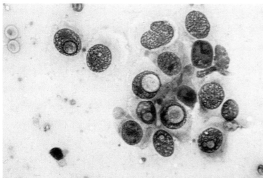

(b)

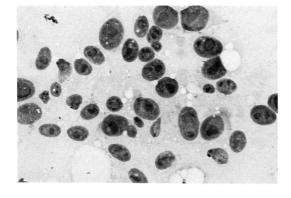

Plate 12 Epithelioid melanoma. Prominent, irregular, single or multiple nucleoli are present (Giemsa, x 300).

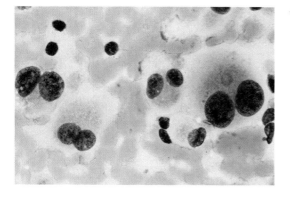

Plate 13 Epithelioid melanoma. Four binucleate melanoma cells of different sizes are seen. Binucleate cells occur frequently in melanomas (Giemsa, x 480).

with the cell membrane. The nuclei are generally round with a smooth, regular contour, but some are convoluted or lobated. An evenly dispersed, fine chromatin pattern is rather characteristic (Plate 5) and was observed in 97% of the cases studied by Layfield and Ostrzega (1989). A finely granular chromatin pattern is apparent in Papanicolaou-stained smears, while with the May-Grünwald-Giemsa stain, a homogeneous or a finely reticular pattern is seen.

Intranuclear cytoplasmic inclusions (p. 230) are helpful in the cytological diagnosis of melanoma (Yamada *et al.*, 1972), though they are not completely specific, since they are also observed in other neoplasms such as papillary carcinoma of thyroid, hepatocellular carcinoma, adenocarcinoma of lung and meningioma (Apitz, 1937; Sobel and Schwarz, 1969). The intranuclear cytoplasmic inclusion appears as a large, single, sharply defined, round or ovoid intranuclear body with a regular outline in air-dried as well as in alcohol-fixed specimens (Plate 11). They were present in 60% of the cases reported by Layfield and Ostrzega (1989) and 84% in the series studied by Woyke *et al.* (1980). Rarely, melanin granules are present within the inclusion. The number of cells containing such intranuclear cytoplasmic inclusions varies greatly.

Prominent nucleoli are present in the majority but by no means all epithelioid-cell melanomas. Their number varies from one to three and they show marked pleomorphism (Plate 12). Perry *et al.* (1986a) reported macronucleoli in 56% of epithelioid melanomas; however, importantly, in about 3% of cases nucleoli were inconspicuous.

Mitotic figures, including atypical ones, can usually be demonstrated but they may be sparse (Layfield and Ostrzega, 1989).

Binucleated cells (Plate 13) are present in practically all epithelioid-cell melanomas, though they may be rare. The nuclei of the binucleated cells are also located at the periphery of the cell, often in contact with each other or even partially overlapping. When they are arranged in a mirror-image fashion, and especially when prominent nucleoli are present, they can be mistaken for Reed-Sternberg cells. The shape, the nuclear outline and chromatin distribution are similar to those seen in the mononuclear tumour cells.

13.4 Spindle cell melanoma

This is the rarest form of melanoma; its incidence in published series of FNA of melanoma is around 13% (Perry *et al.*, 1986a; Layfield and Ostrzega, 1989).

The neoplasm consists of spindle-shaped cells with long *bipolar cytoplasmic processes* (Plate 16; Table 13.3). Less frequently, the

Table 13.3 Cytological features of FNA of spindle cell melanoma

---

General features
  Highly cellular smear
  Noncohesive cell pattern with loose groupings
  Elongated, fusiform cells
  Bipolar and dendritic cells
  Frequently combined with epithelioid cells, resulting in mixed cell type

Cytoplasmic features
  Thin, long cytoplasmic processes; highlighted by melanin granules in
    pigmented cases
  Homogeneous or granular cytoplasm, often pale staining

Nuclear features
  Centrally placed nucleus
  Oval or elongated nuclei with round ends
  Smooth, regular nuclear outline
  Evenly distributed, finely granular chromatin
  Intranuclear cytoplasmic inclusions are less frequent than in epithelioid cell
    melanoma
  Inconspicuous nucleoli in about one-third of cases
  Macronucleoli in about one-third of cases
  Binucleate and giant cells are less frequent than in epithelioid-cell melanoma

---

tumour cells exhibit *arborizing dendritic cytoplasmic extensions*. In air-dried smears, the spindle-shaped cells may reach a length of 100–400 µm (Friedman *et al.*, 1980). The cytoplasmic processes are thin and often stain only faintly. The different types of cytoplasmic vacuolation commonly seen in epithelioid melanoma cells are usually absent. When the tumour is pigmented, then the bipolar and dendritic cytoplasmic processes are highlighted by the melanin granules (Plate 17).

The characteristic lack of cohesion, resulting in a dissociated cell pattern in this type of melanoma as well; however, cell groups with loosely attached cells are more common than in epithelioid melanoma (Plate 18).

The *nuclei* of spindle cell melanoma are oval or elongated with rounded ends. The nucleus is centrally placed, oriented along the long axis, and usually fills the entire width of the cell. This is in sharp contrast to the round, eccentrically placed nucleus of epithelioid melanoma. However, the chromatin is also evenly distributed and finely granular in distribution, and the nuclear outline is smooth (Plate 19). Intranuclear cytoplasmic inclusions are less frequent than in epithelioid melanoma.

Not uncommonly, nucleoli are inconspicuous in spindle cell melanoma. In the series of Perry and colleagues (1986a), this was

Plate 14 Melanoma. Giant cells with single, multilobated or multiple nuclei are frequently observed in melanomas.
(a) Papanicolaou, (x 480);
(b) Giemsa, (x 480);
(c) Papanicolaou, (x 480).

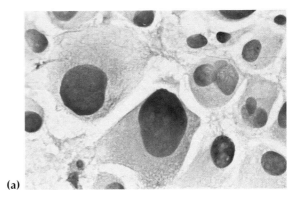

(a)

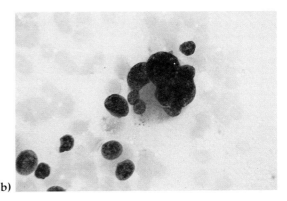

(b)

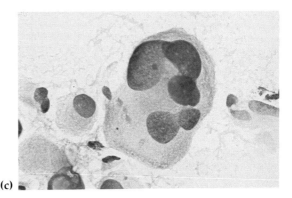

(c)

Plate 15 Melanoma; tumour cell cannibalism. In the centre of the field the phagocytosed cell has undergone degeneration, resulting in a false signet-ring appearance of the host cell (Giemsa, x 770).

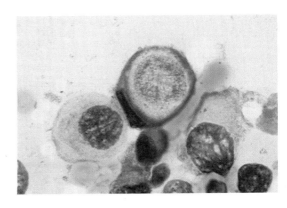

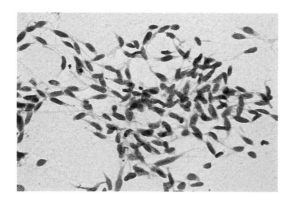

Plate 16 Amelanotic spindle cell melanoma. Loose aggregate of rather uniform spindle-shaped cells with long cytoplasmic processes. This appearance may lead to confusion with that of a mesenchymal neoplasm (Papanicolaou, x 200).

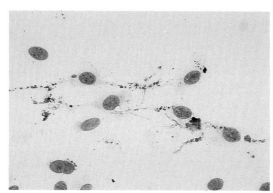

Plate 17 Spindle cell melanoma. The presence of melanin granules highlights the long cytoplasmic processes (Giemsa, x 300).

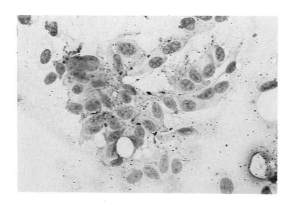

Plate 18 Spindle cell melanoma. Cohesive groups of melanoma cells are more frequent in spindle cell than in epithelioid melanomas. Intra- and extracytoplasmic melanin is also seen (Giemsa, x 300).

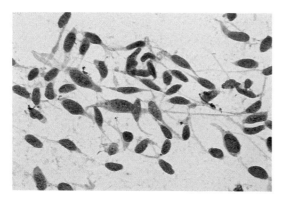

Plate 19 Amelanotic spindle cell melanoma. Bipolar, spindle-shaped melanocytes having slender to plump ovoid nuclei with evenly dispersed, finely granular chromatin (Papanicolaou, x 300).

Plate 20 Spindle cell melanoma. Prominent nucleoli (in contrast to Plate 19) are present in this case, which also shows myxoid degeneration (Giemsa, x 200).

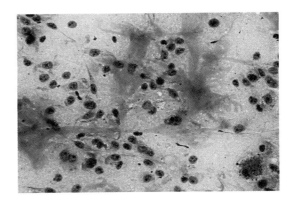

Plate 21 Malignant melanoma of mixed-cell type. Both spindle and epithelioid cells with and without intracytoplasmic melanin (Papanicolaou, x 300).

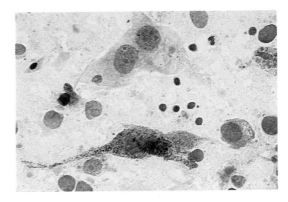

Plate 22 Pleural fluid, metastatic malignant melanoma.
(a) dispersed malignant cells with eccentric nuclei and prominent nucleoli intermixed with inflammatory cells and occasional mesothelial cells. The cytological features of the malignant cells show similarities to those of epithelioid melanoma, illustrated previously (Papanicolaou, x 300).

(a)

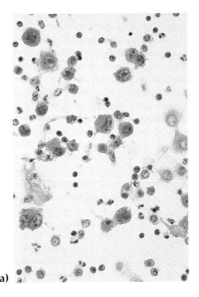

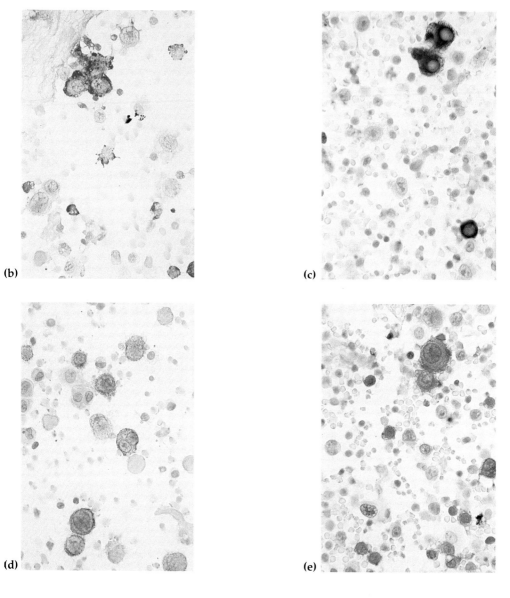

(b) PAS reveals glycogen in mesothelial cells and inflammatory cells but not in the malignant cells; however rarely melanoma cells also contain glycogen (PAS, x 300).
(c) Immunostaining for cytokeratin discriminates between positive mesothelial cells and negative melanoma cells (Immunoperoxidase, x 200).
(d) Melanoma-specific antibody HMB-45 gives a positive reaction with some of the malignant cells. This antibody is often useful in the diagnosis of melanoma (Immunoperoxidase, x 300).
(e) S-100 antibody reacts with the majority of the tumour cells. However, two mesothelial cells (top) are also positive, which can lead to diagnostic confusion (Immunoperoxidase, x 300).

the case in 29% of spindle cell melanomas, contrasting to 3.4% of epithelioid melanomas. In the same series, 29% of spindle cell melanomas had macronucleoli (Plate 20).

Binucleated cells, which are such a distinctive feature of epithelioid melanoma, also occur but they are less frequent. In such cases the nuclei in the spindle cells are usually placed in tandem along the long axis of the cell, and only rarely are they found side by side (Woyke *et al.*, 1980).

Giant cells and multinucleated cells are generally sparse in spindle cell melanomas.

Amelanotic spindle cell melanomas can be mistaken cytologically for benign and malignant soft tissue tumours (schwannomas, fibro-sarcomas, etc.). An admixture of epithelioid cells, the presence of intranuclear pseudoinclusions and the presence of very small traces of melanin are of help in the differential diagnosis. Often, additional cytochemical and immunocytochemical studies are required.

13.5 Melanomas of mixed cell type

This second most common type of melanoma consists of a mixture of epithelioid and spindle cells in varying proportions, but with each cell type present in a significant number (Plate 21). The cytological features of epithelioid and spindle cells have been described in the previous sections.

The mixture of spindle and epithelioid cells intermixed with bi-nucleated and multinucleated giant cells imparts a pleomorphic appearance to the tumour.

13.6 Uveal melanomas

The clinical diagnosis of uveal melanoma is difficult and, on the basis of the few reported series, FNA appears adequate to establish a cytological diagnosis (Jakobiec *et al.*, 1979; Czerniak *et al.*, 1983; Char *et al.*, 1989; Scroggs *et al.*, 1990). Other methods, such as aspiration of fluid from the anterior chamber or from the subretinal space, are less successful.

As discussed in Chapter 11 (p. 342), four types of intraocular melanoma are distinguished on cytological grounds: epithelioid cell and spindle cell type A and B and melanomas of mixed-cell type. These tumours share many cytological features of melanomas of extraocular sites; therefore only a few relevant microscopical features will be discussed.

Epithelioid-cell melanoma is the rarest type of intraocular melanoma.

FNA of this melanoma type exhibits dissociated round or polygonal cells with abundant cytoplasm and eccentric round nuclei. Cytoplasmic processes can be seen in some cases, but a regular cytoplasmic outline is more common. Large, irregular nucleoli are frequent in this type of melanoma. Anisocytosis and binucleation are also prominent.

Spindle cell melanoma type A, the second rarest form of intraocular melanoma, is characterized by the presence of uniform, spindle cells with long, thin, bipolar cytoplasmic processes. The centrally positioned elongated or oval nuclei have a regular outline and uniformly distributed chromatin. The nuclei often have longitudinal folds. Most importantly, no prominent nucleoli can be found, in contrast to type B melanoma. Mitotic figures are rare.

Spindle cell melanoma type B is a common form of intraocular melanoma and also consists of fusiform cells; however, these cells are larger and have more abundant cytoplasm than type A cells. The cytoplasmic processes are also thicker. The nuclei are oval rather than elongated and contain a single large nucleolus.

Apart from tumours with a predominance of one of the above cell types, melanomas with *mixed-cell type* are recognized. This is the commonest type of intraocular melanoma. It consists of epithelioid and type B spindle cells.

The subdivision of intraocular melanomas into the above four cytological categories is important in view of their very different biological behaviour (p. 342).

13.7   Cytological features of melanoma in specimens other than FNA

The site of the tumour and the method by which the cells are obtained may have an effect on the smear pattern, although the microscopical features of melanoma cells are essentially identical.

Samples obtained by brushing and scraping often contain large clumps of melanoma cells, contrasting with the more dispersed pattern commonly seen in FNA (Woyke *et al.*, 1980). In *vaginal smears* or in *sputum*, the number of melanoma cells is often scanty, which can make a specific diagnosis in cases of hypo- or amelanotic melanoma very difficult indeed. Moreover, in sputum, the haemosiderin and/or carbon-containing macrophages may obscure the presence of pigmented melanoma cells.

Melanuria in association with generalized melanosis can result in accumulation of benign pigmented cells and pigment casts in the urine (p. 294). It is necessary to identify malignant nuclear features in pigment-filled cells before making the diagnosis of melanoma involving the urinary tract (Valente *et al.*, 1985).

In *serous effusions* it is often problematic to distinguish between activated mesothelial cells and malignant cells. Since metastatic carcinomas in pleural or ascitic fluid are more frequent, the recognition of metastatic melanoma without a history of a previous primary tumour is a considerable diagnostic challenge. This is one of the situations where immunocytochemistry can be very helpful (Plate 22). As ever, there are pitfalls; for example, S-100 stains not only melanomas but some metastatic carcinomas as well. Moreover, S-100 positivity has also been documented in some mesotheliomas (Rasmussen and Larsen, 1985). However, as discussed before, a panel of carefully selected antibodies is often very useful, in conjunction with conventional morphology and taking into account the clinical data.

References

Aldovini, D., Detassis, C. and Piscioli, F. (1983) Primary malignant melanoma of the oesophagus. Brush cytology and histogenesis. *Acta Cytol.*, **27**, 65–8.

Angeli, S., Koelma, I. A., Fleuren, G. J. and Van Steenis, G. J. (1988) Malignant melanoma in fine needle aspirates and effusions. *Acta Cytol.*, **32**, 707–12.

Apitz, K. (1937) Ueber die Pigmentbildung in dem Zellkernen melanotischer Geschwülste: I. Beitrag zur Pathologie des Zell Kernes. *Virchows Archiv A (Pathol. Anat.)*, **300**, 89–112.

Bhuta, S., Mirra, J. M. and Cochran, A. J. (1986) Myxoid malignant melanoma. A previously undescribed histologic pattern noted in metastatic lesions and a report of four cases. *Am. J. Surg. Pathol.* **10**, 203–11.

Bonetti, F., Colombari, E., Zamboni, G., Martignoni, G., Mombello, A. and Chilosi, M. (1989) Breast carcinoma positive for melanoma marker (HMB-45). *Am. J. Clin. Pathol.*, **22**, 491–5.

Broderick, P. A., Allegra, S. R. and Corvese, N. (1972) Primary malignant melanoma of the esophagus: A case report. *Acta Cytol.*, **16**, 159–64.

Char, D. H., Miller, T. R., Ljung, B.-M., Howes, E. L. and Stoloff, A. (1989) Fine needle aspiration biopsy in uveal melanoma. *Acta Cytol.*, **33**, 599–605.

Chess, Q. and Hajdu, S. I. (1986) The role of immunoperoxidase staining in diagnostic cytology. *Acta Cytol.*, **30**, 1–7.

Czerniak, B., Woyke, S., Domagala, W. and Krzysztolik, Z. (1983) Fine needle aspiration cytology of intraocular malignant melanoma. *Acta Cytol.*, **27**, 157–65.

Domagala, W. M., Markiewski, M., Tuziak, T., Kram, A., Weber, K. and Osborn, M. (1990) Immunocytochemistry on fine needle aspirates. *Acta Cytol.*, **34**, 291–6.

Drier, J. K., Swanson, P. E., Cherwitz, D. L. and Wick, M. R. (1987) S-100 protein immunoreactivity in poorly differentiated carcinomas. Immunohistochemical comparision with malignant melanoma. *Arch. Pathol. Lab. Med.*, **111**, 447–52.

Duray, P. H., Palazzo J., Gown, A. M. and Ohuchi, N. (1988) Melanoma cell heterogeneity. A study of two monoclonal antibodies compared with S-100 protein in paraffin sections. *Cancer*, **61**, 2460–8.

Ehrmann, R. L., Younge, P. A. and Lerch, V. L. (1962) The exfoliative cytology and histogenesis of an early primary malignant melanoma of the vagina. *Acta Cytol.*, **6**, 245–54.

Folberg, R., Augsburger, J. J., Gamel, J. W., Shields, J. A. and Lang, W. R. (1985) Fine-needle aspirates of uveal melanomas and prognosis. *Am. J. Ophthalmol.*, **100**, 654–7.

Friedman, M., Forgione, H. and Shanbhag, V. (1980) Needle aspiration of metastatic melanoma. *Acta Cytol.*, **24**, 7–15.

Friedman, M., Rao, U. and Fox, S. (1982) The cytology of metastatic balloon cell melanoma. *Acta Cytol.*, **26**, 39–43.

Gatter, K. C., Ralfkiaer, E., Skinner, J. *et al.* (1985) An immunocytological study of malignant melanoma and its differential diagnosis from other malignant tumours. *J. Clin. Pathol.*, **38**, 1353–7.

Gown, A. M., Vogel, A. M., Hoak, D., Gough, F. and McNutt, M. A. (1986) Monoclonal antibodies specific for melanocytic tumors distinguish subpopulations of melanocytes. *Am. J. Pathol.*, **123**, 195–203.

Gupta, S. K., Rajwanshi, A. K. and Das, D. K. (1985) Fine needle aspiration cytology smear patterns of malignant melanoma. *Acta Cytol.*, **29**, 983–8.

Hachisuka, H., Sakamoto, F., Nomura, H., Mori, O. and Sasai, Y. (1986) Immunohistochemical study of S-100 protein and neuron specific enolase (NSE) in melanocytes and related tumors. *Acta Histochem.*, **80**, 215–23.

Hajdu, S. I. and Savino, A. (1973) Cytologic diagnosis of malignant melanoma. *Acta Cytol.*, **17**, 320–7.

Hashimoto, K. and Bale, G. (1972) An electron microscopic study of balloon cell nevus. *Cancer*, **30**, 530–40.

Jakobiec, F. A., Coleman, D. J. and Chattick, A. (1979) Ultrasonographically guided needle biopsy and cytologic diagnosis of solid intraocular tumors. *Ophthalmology*, **86**, 1662–78.

Johnson, W. D., Koss, L. G., Papanicolaou, G. N. and Seybolt, J. F. (1955) Cytology of esophageal washings: evaluation of 364 cases. *Cancer*, **8**, 951–7.

Keller, J. M., Listrom, M. B., Hart, J. B., Olson, N. J. and Jordan, S. W. (1990) Cytologic detection of penile malignant melanoma of soft parts in pleural effusion using monoclonal antibody HMB-45. *Acta Cytol.*, **34**, 393–6.

Kline, T. S. and Kannan, V. (1982) Aspiration biopsy cytology and melanoma. *Am. J. Clin. Pathol.*, **77**, 597–601.

Kung, I. T. M., Chan, S. K. and Lo, E. S. F. (1990) Application of the immuno-peroxidase technique to cell block preparation from fine needle aspirates. *Acta Cytol.*, **34**, 297–303.

Layfield, L. J. and Ostrzega, N. (1989) Fine needle aspirate smear morphology in metastatic melanoma. *Acta Cytol.*, **33**, 606–12.

Lefer, L. G. and Johnston, W. W. (1972) Hydrogen peroxide bleach technique in the diagnosis of malignant melanoma. *Acta Cytol.*, **16**, 505–6.

Lewis, B. V. and Chapman, P. A. (1975) Cytological diagnosis of primary malignant melanoma of the vagina. *Br. J. Obstet. Gynaecol.*, **82**, 74–6.

Lindholm, K. and De la Torre, M. (1988) Fine needle aspiration cytology of myxoid metastatic malignant melanoma. *Acta Cytol.*, **32**, 719–21.

Linthicum, C. M. (1971) Primary malignant melanoma of the vagina: a case report. *Acta Cytol.*, **15**, 179–81.

Lozowski, W. and Hajdu, S. I. (1987) Cytology and immunocytochemistry of bronchioloalveolar carcinoma. *Acta Cytol.*, **31**, 717–25.

Masubuchi, S., Nagai, I., Hirata, M., Kubo, H. and Masubuchi, K. (1975) Cytologic studies of malignant melanoma of the vagina. *Acta Cytol.*, **19**, 527–32.

Medak, H., McGrew, E. A., Burkalow, P. and Jans, R. B. (1969) Definitive cytopathologic characteristics of primary oral melanoma. *Oral Surg. Oral Med. Oral Pathol.*, **27**, 237–46.

Nagy, P., Csaba, I. and Kadas, I. (1990) Malignant melanoma mestastatic to the endometrium. Cytologic findings in an endometrial sample. *Acta Cytol.*, **34**, 382–4.

Ordonez, N. G., Sneige, N., Hickey, R. C. and Brooks, T. E. (1988) Use of monoclonal antibody HMB-45 in the cytologic diagnosis of melanoma. *Acta Cytol.* **32**, 684–8.

Pearse, A. G. E. (1985) *Histochemistry, Theoretical and Applied*, 4th edn. Edinburgh: Churchill Livingstone.

Pelosi, G., Bonetti, F., Colombari, R., Bonzanini, M. and Iannucci, A. (1990) Use of monoclonal antibody HMB-45 for detecting malignant melanoma cells in fine needle aspiration biopsy samples. *Acta Cytol.*, **34**, 460–2.

Perry, M. D., Gore, M., Seigler, H. F. and Johnston, W. W. (1986a) Fine needle aspiration biopsy of metastatic melanoma. A morphologic analysis of 174 cases. *Acta Cytol.*, **30**, 385–96.

Perry, M. D., Seigler, H. F. and Johnston, W. W. (1986b) Diagnosis of metastatic malignant melanoma by fine needle aspiration biopsy: a clinical and pathologic correlation of 298 cases. *J. Natl. Cancer Inst.*, **77**, 1013–9

Pinkus, G. S. and Kurtin, P. J. (1985) Epithelial membrane antigen — a diagnostic discriminant in surgical pathology: immunohistochemical profile in epithelial, mesenchymal, and hematopoietic neoplasms using paraffin sections and monoclonal antibodies. *Hum. Pathol.*, **16**, 929–40.

Piva, A. E. and Koss, L. G. (1964) Cytologic diagnosis of malignant melanoma in urinary sediment. *Acta Cytol.*, **8**, 398–402.

Rasmussen, O. O. and Larsen, K. E. (1985) S-100 protein in malignant mesotheliomas. *Acta Pathol. Microbiol. Scand. (A)*, **93**, 199–201.

Rocamora, A., Carrillo, R., Vives, R. and Solera, J. C. (1988) Fine needle aspiration biopsy of myxoid metastasis of malignant melanoma. *Acta Cytol.*, **32**, 94–100.

Sagebiel, R., Gates, E. and Hill, L. C. (1978) Cytologic detection of recurrent vaginal melanoma. *Acta Cytol.*, **22**, 353–7.

Schwartz, J. G. and Zollars, P. R. (1990) Malignant melanoma of soft parts: report of two cases. *Acta Cytol.*, **34**, 397–400.

Scroggs, M. W., Johnston W. W. and Klintworth, G. K. (1990) Intraocular tumors. A cytopathologic study. *Acta Cytol.*, **34**, 401–8.

Shafir, R., Hiss, J., Tsur, H. and Bubis, J. J. (1983) Imprint cytology in the intraoperative diagnosis of malignant melanoma. *Acta Cytol.*, **27**, 255–7.

Sheibani, K. and Battifora, H. (1988) Signet-ring cell melanoma. A rare morphologic variant of malignant melanoma. *Am. J. Surg. Pathol.*, **12**, 28–34.

Shoup, S. A., Johnston, W. W., Siegler, H. F. *et al.* (1990) A panel of antibodies useful in the cytologic diagnosis of metastatic melanoma. *Acta Cytol.*, **34**, 385–92.

Sobel, H. J., Schwarz, R. and Marquet, E. (1969) Nonviral nuclear inclusions. *Arch. Pathol.*, **87**, 179–92.

Takeda, M., Diamond, S. M., DeMarco, M. and Quinn, D. M. (1978) Cytologic diagnosis of malignant melanoma metastatic to the endometrium. *Acta Cytol.*, **22**, 503–6.

Travis, W. D. and Wold, L. E. (1987) Immunoperoxidase staining of fine needle aspiration specimens previously stained by the Papanicolaou technique. *Acta Cytol.*, **31**, 517–20.

Valente, P. T., Atkinson, B. F. and Guerry, D. (1985) Melanuria. *Acta Cytol.*, **29**, 1026–8.

Walts, A. E., Said, J. W. and Shintaku, P. (1988) Cytodiagnosis of malignant melanoma. Immunoperoxidase staining with HMB-45 antibody as an aid to diagnosis. *Am. J. Clin. Pathol.*, **90**, 77–80.

Wilander, E., Norheim, I. and Oberg, K. (1985) Application of silver stains to cytologic specimens of neuroendocrine tumors metastatic to the liver. *Acta Cytol.*, **29**, 1053–7.

Wolman, M. (1980) Lipid pigments (chromolipids): their origin, nature and significance. *Pathobiol. Ann.*, **10**, 253–67.

Woodard, B. H., Ideker, R. E. and Johnston, W. W. (1978) Cytologic detection of malignant melanoma in urine. A case report. *Acta Cytol.*, **22**, 350–2.

Woyke, S., Domagala, W., Czerniak, B. and Strokowska, M. (1980) Fine needle aspiration cytology of malignant melanoma of the skin. *Acta Cytol.*, **24**, 529–38.

Yamada, T., Itou, U., Watanabe, Y. and Ohashi, S. (1972) Cytologic diagnosis of malignant melanoma. *Acta Cytol.*, **16**, 70–76.

Yu, H. C. and Ketabchi, M. (1987) Detection of malignant melanoma of the uterine cervix from Papanicolaou smears. A case report. *Acta Cytol.*, **31**, 73–76.

Zarbo, R. J., Gown, A. M., Visscher, D. W. and Crissman, J. D. (1990) Anomalous cytokeratin expression in malignant melanoma: one- and two-dimensional Western blot analysis and immunohistochemical survey of 100 melanomas. *Modern Pathol.*, **3**, 494–501.

Index